Diane de Anda, PhD
Editor

Social Work with Multicultural Youth

Social Work with Multicultural Youth has been co-published simultaneously as *Journal of Ethnic & Cultural Diversity in Social Work*, Volume 11, Numbers (1/2) and (3/4) 2002.

Pre-publication REVIEWS, COMMENTARIES, EVALUATIONS . . .

"INSIGHTFUL–really captures the anguishing dilemmas and challenges of working with ethnic youth . . . . Makes a significant contribution to the evidence-based practice literature. . . . Practitioners, educators, and researchers will benefit immensely from these findings and recommendations. . . . This distinguished group of authors offers important information on 'culturally syntonic interventions' that take into account strengths and resiliency as well as risk and protective factors, aiming toward health and well-being for this population. The research on Latinas particularly highlights the importance of gender differences indelivering culturally competent practices."

Rowena Fong, MSW, EdD
Professor of Social Work
The University of Texas at Austin

Social Work with Multicultural Youth

Social Work with Multicultural Youth has been co-published simultaneously as *Journal of Ethnic & Cultural Diversity in Social Work*, Volume 11, Numbers (1/2) and (3/4) 2002.

The *Journal of Ethnic & Cultural Diversity in Social Work* Monographic "Separates"

(formerly the *Journal of Multicultural Social Work* series)*

Below is a list of "separates," which in serials librarianship means a special issue simultaneously published as a special journal issue or double-issue *and* as a "separate" hardbound monograph. (This is a format which we also call a "DocuSerial.")

"Separates" are published because specialized libraries or professionals may wish to purchase a specific thematic issue by itself in a format which can be separately cataloged and shelved, as opposed to purchasing the journal on an on-going basis. Faculty members may also more easily consider a "separate" for classroom adoption.

"Separates" are carefully classified separately with the major book jobbers so that the journal tie-in can be noted on new book order slips to avoid duplicate purchasing.

You may wish to visit Haworth's Website at . . .

http://www.HaworthPress.com

. . . to search our online catalog for complete tables of contents of these separates and related publications.

You may also call 1-800-HAWORTH (outside US/Canada: 607-722-5857), or Fax 1-800-895-0582 (outside US/Canada: 607-771-0012), or e-mail at:

docdelivery@haworthpress.com

Social Work with Multicultural Youth, edited by Diane de Anda, PhD (Vol. 11, No. 1/2, 3/4, 2002). *Illustrates the diversity within the U.S. adolescent popluation, examines the factors that serve as barriers or facilitators to development, and identifies strengths and protective factors contributing to resilience as well as needs and risk factors.*

Violence: Diverse Populations and Communities, edited by Diane de Anda, PhD, and Rosina M. Becerra, PhD* (Vol. 8, No. 1/2, 3/4, 2000). *Provides new empirical research and theoretical models to help you understand the impact of violence in various ethnic and cultural communities and populations. The book covers violence in the community, adolescents and violence, plus dating violence and sexual assault and domestic violence/child abuse, spouse/partner abuse, and elder abuse.*

The Challenge of Permanency Planning in a Multicultural Society, edited by Gary R. Anderson, PhD, Angela Shen Ryan, DSW, and Bogart R. Leashore, PhD* (Vol. 5, No. 1/2/3, 1997). *"Hits home the importance of cultural knowledge, sensitivity, and skill for putting permanency and stability into the lives of at-risk children." (Juvenile & Family Court Journal)*

Innovations in Delivering Culturally Sensitive Social Work Services: Challenges for Practice and Education, edited by Yvonne W. Asamoah, PhD* (Vol. 4, No. 4, 1997). *"A unique look at different approaches, programs, and studies that include cultural diversity and sensitivity from a management perspective." (American Public Welfare Association)*

School Social Workers in the Multicultural Environment: New Roles, Responsibilities, and Educational Enrichment, edited by Paul R. Keys, PhD, MSW* (Vol. 3, No. 1, 1994). *"Provides concrete, practical help for those designing curricula on multicultural social work or teaching courses in that field." (Leon Ginsberg, PhD, Carolina Research Professor, College of Social Work, University of South Carolina)*

Multicultural Human Services for AIDS Treatment and Prevention: Policy, Perspectives, and Planning, edited by Julio Morales, PhD, and Marcia Bok, PhD* (Vol. 2, No. 3, 1993). *"Can help increase social workers' often limited knowledge and experience with various social and ethnic groups. It provides specific suggestions and recommendations for program development." (Lambda Book Report)*

Social Work with Immigrants and Refugees, edited by Angela Shen Ryan, DSW* (Vol. 2, No. 1, 1993). *"Provides guidance for those assisting in the settlement and adjustment of people newly arrived in an unfamiliar country." (Public Welfare)*

Social Work with Multicultural Youth

Diane de Anda, PhD
Editor

Social Work with Multicultural Youth has been co-published simultaneously as *Journal of Ethnic & Cultural Diversity in Social Work*, Volume 11, Numbers (1/2) and (3/4) 2002.

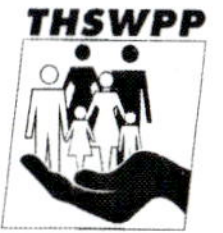

The Haworth Social Work Practice Press
An Imprint of
The Haworth Press, Inc.
New York • London • Oxford

Published by

The Haworth Social Work Practice Press, 10 Alice Street, Binghamton, NY 13904-1580 USA

The Haworth Social Work Practice Press is an imprint of The Haworth Press, Inc., 10 Alice Street, Binghamton, NY 13904-1580 USA.

Social Work with Multicultural Youth has been co-published simultaneously as *Journal of Ethnic & Cultural Diversity in Social Work*, Volume 11, Numbers (1/2) and (3/4) 2002.

Cover design by Lora Wiggins

Library of Congress Cataloging-in-Publication Data

Social Work with Multicultural Youth / Diane de Anda, editor.
p. cm.
Includes bibliographical references and index.
ISBN 0-7890-2189-7 (hbk. : alk. paper) – ISBN 0-7890-2190-0 (pbk: alk. paper)
1. Social work with youth–United States. 2. Social work with minorities–United States. 3. Minority youth–Services for–United States. I. De Anda, Diane.
HV1431.S63 2003
362.7′089–dc21 2003006683

Indexing, Abstracting & Website/Internet Coverage

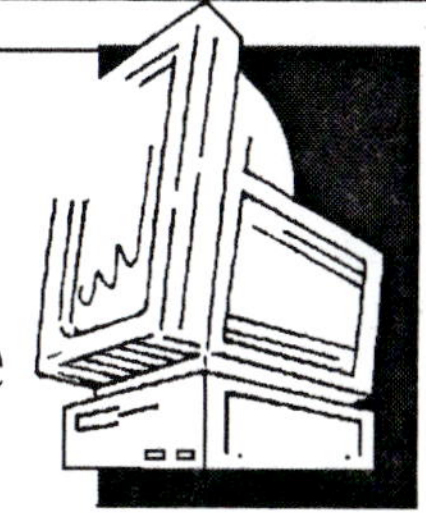

This section provides you with a list of major indexing & abstracting services. That is to say, each service began covering this periodical during the year noted in the right column. Most Websites which are listed below have indicated that they will either post, disseminate, compile, archive, cite or alert their own Website users with research-based content from this work. (This list is as current as the copyright date of this publication.)

Abstracting, Website/Indexing Coverage . . . . Year When Coverage Began

- *Academic Abstracts/CD-ROM* **1994**
- *Academic Search: data base of 2,000 selected academic serials, updated monthly: EBSCO Publishing* **1996**
- *Academic Search Elite (EBSCO)* **2001**
- *Book Review Index* **1994**
- *caredata CD: the social & community care database <www.nisw.org.uk>* **1994**
- *Chicano Studies Collections* **1991**
- *CINAHL (Cumulative Index to Nursing & Allied Health Literature), in print, EBSCO, and SilverPlatter, Data-Star, and PaperChase. (Support materials include Subject Heading List, Database Search Guide, and Instructional video)* **2001**
- *CNPIEC Reference Guide: Chinese National Directory of Foreign Periodicals* **1996**
- *Criminal Justice Abstracts* **1997**
- *ERIC Clearinghouse on Rural Education & Small Schools* **1991**

(continued)

- *Expanded Academic ASAP <www.galegroup.com>* 2001
- *Family & Society Studies Worldwide <www.nisc.com>* 1996
- *Family Violence & Sexual Assault Bulletin* 1999
- *IBZ International Bibliography of Periodical Literature* 1996
- *Index Guide to College Journals (core list compiled by integrating 48 indexes frequently used to support undergraduate programs in small to medium sized libraries* 1999
- *Index to Periodical Articles Related to Law* 1991
- *International Bulletin of Bibliography on Education* 1992
- *MasterFILE: updated database from EBSCO Publishing* 1996
- *Multicultural Education Abstracts* 1994
- *Psychological Abstracts (PsycINFO) <www.apa.org>* 2001
- *Public Library FULLTEXT: EBSCO Publishing* 1996
- *Referativnyi Zhurnal (Abstracts Journal of the All-Russian Institute of Scientific and Technical Information–in Russian)* . . . 1991
- *Sage Public Administration Abstracts (SPAA)* 1991
- *School Organisation & Management Abstracts* 1994
- *Social Science Source: coverage of 400 journals in the social sciences area; updated monthly; EBSCO Publishing* 1996
- *Social Sciences Index (from Volume 1 & continuing) <www.hwwilson.com>* 1999
- *Social Services Abstracts <www.csa.com>* 1991
- *Social Work Abstracts* 1991
- *Sociological Abstracts (SA) <www.csa.com>* 1991
- *Special Educational Needs Abstracts* 1991
- *Studies on Women Abstracts* 1994
- *Violence and Abuse Abstracts: A Review of Current Literature on Interpersonal Violence (VAA)* 1994
- *Vocational Search: keyword access covering 400 trade related periodicals; monthly updates; EBSCO Publishing* 1996

(continued)

Special Bibliographic Notes related to special journal issues (separates) and indexing/abstracting:

- indexing/abstracting services in this list will also cover material in any "separate" that is co-published simultaneously with Haworth's special thematic journal issue or DocuSerial. Indexing/abstracting usually covers material at the article/chapter level.
- monographic co-editions are intended for either non-subscribers or libraries which intend to purchase a second copy for their circulating collections.
- monographic co-editions are reported to all jobbers/wholesalers/approval plans. The source journal is listed as the "series" to assist the prevention of duplicate purchasing in the same manner utilized for books-in-series.
- to facilitate user/access services all indexing/abstracting services are encouraged to utilize the co-indexing entry note indicated at the bottom of the first page of each article/chapter/contribution.
- this is intended to assist a library user of any reference tool (whether print, electronic, online, or CD-ROM) to locate the monographic version if the library has purchased this version but not a subscription to the source journal.
- individual articles/chapters in any Haworth publication are also available through the Haworth Document Delivery Service (HDDS).

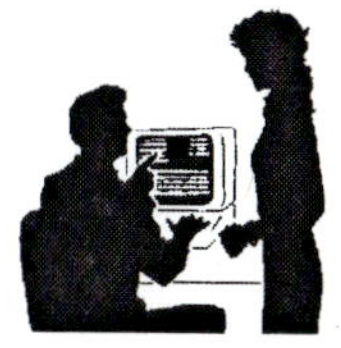

ABOUT THE EDITOR

Diane de Anda, PhD, is Associate Professor in the Department of Social Welfare at the UCLA School of Public Policy and Social Research, where she teaches cognitive behavioral theory and methods and advanced crosscultural awareness research methods. The Editor of *Controversial Issues in Multicultualism* and a reviewer for *Children and Youth Services Review*, *Journal of Teaching in Social Work*, and *The Journal of Early Adolescence*, Dr. de Anda's articles have appeared in numerous scholarly journals, including *Social Work in Education, Journal of Youth and Adolescence. Journal of Social Service Research, Journal of Adolescent Research*, *Children & Youth Services Review*, and *Hispanic Journal of Behavioral Sciences*.

Dr. de Anda's research interests include adolescent pregnancy and motherhood, stress and coping in adolescence, violence prevention among youth, ethnic identity among adolescents, and bicultural socialization. Her most recent book is entitled *Violence: Diverse Populations and Communities* (Haworth).

Social Work with Multicultural Youth

Social Work with Multicultural Youth has been co-published simultaneously as *Journal of Ethnic & Cultural Diversity in Social Work*, Volume 11, Numbers (1/2) and (3/4) 2002.

ALL HAWORTH SOCIAL WORK PRACTICE PRESS BOOKS AND JOURNALS ARE PRINTED ON CERTIFIED ACID-FREE PAPER

Social Work with Multicultural Youth

CONTENTS

Preface

MULTICULTURAL YOUTH

The face of American youth is changing. American adolescents are a more ethnically diverse population than they have ever been, and this diversity is projected to increase over the next half century. The Asian/Pacific Islander youth population alone is comprised of 43 different ethnic groups. Latino youth are also a heterogeneous population, which includes those with family origins in Mexico, Central and South America, Puerto Rico, Cuba, the Dominican Republic, etc. In the year 2000, ethnic minority youth constituted one-third of the adolescent population; by mid-century, the combined ethnic minority youth population will exceed the White adolescent population (U.S. Census, Census 2000).

Multicultural youth constitute a continuum in terms of level of acculturation, from those with several generations in the United States to recent immigrants. Those "in between" include the U.S. born sons and daughters of recent immigrants and refugees and the 1.5 generation, who entered the U.S. in childhood so that by adolescence their socialization experiences have often been quite divergent. For African American and American Indian youth, their cultural distinctiveness exists generally without ties to specific cultures outside of the country. As a result, most ethnic youth live in multiple cultures, their family's culture of origin with its level of acculturation and cultural adaptation, the broader mainstream culture, and the youth culture they share with their peers.

The developmental changes and tasks of adolescence place additional adaptation pressures on youth in multiple areas of their lives

---

[Haworth co-indexing entry note]: "Preface." de Anda, Diane. Co-published simultaneously in *Journal of Ethnic & Cultural Diversity in Social Work* (The Haworth Social Work Practice Press, an imprint of The Haworth Press, Inc.) Vol. 11, No. 1/2, 2002, pp. xv-xx; and: *Social Work with Multicultural Youth* (ed: Diane de Anda) The Haworth Social Work Practice Press, an imprint of The Haworth Press, Inc., 2002, pp. xiii-xviii. Single or multiple copies of this article are available for a fee from The Haworth Document Delivery Service [1-800-HAWORTH, 9:00 a.m. - 5:00 p.m. (EST). E-mail address: docdelivery@haworthpress.com].

http://www.haworthpress.com/store/product.asp?sku=J051

(cognitive, psychological, social, physical, and sexual). Coping skills needed to deal with the attendant stressors are also in a process of development, and, therefore, vary in their effectiveness in dealing with these demands and adaptations. Identity development is the primary task of adolescence, but for multicultural youth with multiple points of reference, this may be an even more complex task. Finally, the developmental processes of adolescence are future oriented. However, with the sense of unease and instability created by the world-changing events of September 11 and domestic economic uncertainties, the development of a youthful vision of a positive future that motivates the present may not be as likely as it was for prior generations of youth.

These are also new challenges for social workers and other helping professionals, as well as educators, who serve youth populations. It is not enough to be aware of the general developmental issues of adolescence. To meet the needs of the youth of today, it is necessary to recognize that their needs, issues, and strengths may be as diverse as the youth population itself, and that effective action is dependent upon understanding the cultural contexts of each youth cohort and the structural factors that determine their unique relationship with the society at large. The purpose of this volume is to begin such a task: to recognize the diversity within the adolescent population; to examine the factors which serve as barriers and as facilitators of their development; to identify strengths and protective factors contributing to resilience as well as needs and risk factors; to develop accurate conceptual frameworks for understanding their experiences; and to create culturally syntonic interventions to promote their well-being.

The first article in this volume ("A Profile of Adolescent Health: The Role of Race, Ethnicity and Gender"), provides the overall context for addressing today's youth by offering a comprehensive epidemiological profile of adolescent populations with current data on multiple areas which contribute to adolescents' health and well-being. Differentiations by ethnicity and gender allow the reader to recognize population-specific risk factors and trends in morbidity and mortality that can assist practitioners and policymakers in devising intervention agendas. The authors (Brindis, Park, Paul and Burg) emphasize the importance of recognizing assets and strengths as well as needs and risks, the cultural context, and structural factors in the broader society that contribute significantly to risk and the health status of ethnic minority youth populations.

The next two articles move from a problem-focused perspective to employ cultural strengths and resilience models to meet the developmental needs and provide enhanced opportunities for Latino and African American youth. Authors of both articles address the structural barriers that impinge upon minority youth and cultural assets which can be used to counter these forces.

Zambrana and Zoppi ("Latina Students: Translating Cultural Wealth into Social Capital to Improve Academic Success") provide an overview of academic disparities between Latina adolescents and their cohorts in other ethnic groups. Contributory factors are identified at the individual, familial, community, and societal/structural levels. The authors then present an innovative conceptualization, defining "cultural wealth" within this population and identifying it as an untapped source of strength and resilience. They argue for the need to translate this resource (cultural wealth) into social capital that will promote academic opportunities and success among Latina adolescents.

Hopps, Tourse and Christian ("From Problems to Personal Resilience: Challenges and Opportunities in Practice with African American Youth") employ Conflict Theory to place the disadvantaged status and position of African American youth in a proper context. Balancing concern for risk factors within the population with a recognition of strengths and potential protective factors within the culture and community, they advocate for a group intervention approach based on a resilience framework that integrates race and ethnicity as well as values and ethics into the group process. They further suggest that interventions are enhanced by the inclusion of a justice based model, which encourages personal mastery and self-efficacy through advocacy efforts aimed at structural barriers and inequities.

Iglehart and Becerra ("Hispanic and African American Youth: Life After Foster Care Emancipation") provide a bridge between broad conceptualizations of issues and phenomenological understandings of the impact of these issues upon individuals within the identified population. After an overview of the literature with regard to issues and problems affecting foster care youth, personal, and often poignant, testimony with regard to their circumstances is provided by Latino and African American emancipated foster care youth. The qualitative analysis identifies major themes that emerged from ethnographic interviews. Descriptions of barriers, hopes, and hardships move the reader beyond abstract terms to specific events, feelings, and relationships that shaped the lives and future expectations of these youth. The authors distill these individual and thematic experiences into specific, culturally sensitive recommendations for modifying the process of preparing foster care youth for emancipation in order to enhance the welfare and future trajectory of these youth.

Longitudinal data analyzed by Seyfried and Chung ("Parent Involvement as Parental Monitoring of Student Motivation and Parent Expectations Predicting Later Achievement Among African American and European American Middle School Age Students") offer information regarding factors differentially impacting academic achievement between African American youth and their European American cohorts. The data indicate that while high parental expectations positively affect later academic achievement for European American youth, the high expectations of African American parents do not have the same effect on the academic achievement of their children. For African American children, structural factors are again implicated, as it is the African American child's early academic achievement that is the best predictor of later (middle school) academic achievement. In other words, the ability of the educational institution to prepare African American children at the early elementary school level determines their ability to succeed academically as adolescents. The authors identify a need to shift interventions with parents to a focus on empowerment to bring about institutional changes that will enhance the opportunities for earlier academic achievement and promote a more positive academic trajectory.

The last half of the volume examines specific issues related to adolescent populations and interventions proposed to address specific problem areas.

The article by Franke, Huynh-Hohnbaum, and Chung ("Adolescent Violence: With Whom They Fight and Where") moves the examination of adolescent violence beyond the consideration of incidence rates to an attempt to uncover the context in which violence occurs. Differences in the person with whom the adolescent fights (e.g., family member, friend, stranger) and the place the fights occur most frequently (e.g., school, home, neighborhood) are examined by race/ethnicity, gender, and age. Complex relationships among variables are analyzed to identify risk and protective factors, with attachment to family and school found to be particularly salient protective factors.

The next two articles deal with the area of substance use in specific adolescent populations.

Lee, Law, Eo, and Oliver ("Perception of Substance Use Problems in Asian American Communities by Chinese, Indian, and Vietnamese American Youth") contribute to the limited literature on substance use in Asian/Pacific Islander (API) populations. To obtain an "insider's" perspective, a sample of Chinese, Indian, and Vietnamese American youth were surveyed regarding their knowledge and perceptions of alcohol and drug use within the API population as well as attitudes towards help seeking for substance abuse problems. Important implications for substance abuse interventions are offered inasmuch as discrepancies between the stated value of treatment and the preference for self-help rather than familial support and professional treatment were indicated. The authors caution against assumptions of cultural homogeneity within the API populations and acknowledge the importance of recognizing that the cultural context is population-specific. Differences in treatment preferences among the three groups of youth provide an example of intervention strategies that will need to be adapted to the differing cultural perspectives of the targeted population.

Resilience and protective factors emerge from the qualitative data collected by Marsiglia, Miles, Dustman and Sills ("Ties That Protect: An Ecological Perspective on Latino/a Urban Pre-Adolescent Drug Use") from seventh grade Latino/a adolescents. Although risk factors were identified in the young respondents' neighborhoods, attachment to and support primarily from family members and secondarily from school personnel served as protective factors against drug use. The establishment of a collaborative relationship between these two positive sources is encouraged to strengthen the resilience of Latino/a youth in high risk neighborhoods.

The final two articles focus on issues related to adolescent sexual behavior.

Diversity within the population of Latina adolescents, based on level of acculturation, is explored in the article by Jimenez, Potts, and Jimenez ("Reproductive Attitudes and Behavior Among Latina Adolescents"). A number of differences in behavior and attitudes were found between Latina adolescents born outside the U.S. and U.S. born adolescents, irrespective of whether English or Spanish was the primary language in the home. Foreign born Latina adolescents maintained a more conservative stance, having a lower incidence of sexual activity and professing a desire to wait until marriage. These findings might have been expected given their more traditional cultural background in contrast to the U.S. born groups, however other findings were not so clearly predictable. For example, in contrast to the other two groups, U.S. born adolescents who spoke Spanish in the home (presumably second generation offspring of immigrants) demonstrated the greatest concern for their parents wishes; those who refrained from sexual activity did so primarily because it would "upset" their parents. Moreover, this group also had the highest percentage with college aspirations, possibly another instance of attempting to fulfill parental expectations. The article discerns within-group differences that need to be taken into account in planning interventions aimed at prevention; for example, acculturation differences need to be accommodated particularly with regard to risk factors. Finally, the authors suggest that the desire to attend college be perceived not only as a desirable end in itself, but as a protective factor against adolescent pregnancy.

In the last article, de Anda ("The GIG: An Innovative Intervention to Prevent Adolescent Pregnancy and Sexually Transmitted Infection in a Latino Community") presents an evaluation of a unique intervention aimed at changing the knowledge and attitudes of Latino youth with regard to pregnancy and STIs. The manner in which the intervention and evaluation were designed to be congruent with the participants' cultural and social context is described. The intensive intervention takes place over a five hour period, providing educational activities in an entertainment format. The effectiveness of this approach is demonstrated by significant improvement in knowledge and attitudes fostering risk reduction and pregnancy and STI prevention. Implications for designing of interventions aimed at youth populations are presented with a recognition that contexts may vary and feedback from the youth in the community is critical to the development of a successful intervention.

Despite the varying foci of the different articles, each shared common perspectives and admonitions, the importance of: recognizing diversity both across and within youth populations; considering the context specific to the youth population in order to understand needs, strengths, and circumstances and to plan service delivery and interventions congruent with this understanding; recognizing structural factors that contribute to problems faced by youth; noting cultural, familial, and community resilience and protective factors available to different youth populations, and finally, employing a strengths based approach in meeting the needs and fostering the development of multicultural youth.

Diane de Anda, PhD

A Profile of Adolescent Health: The Role of Race, Ethnicity and Gender

Claire Brindis
M. Jane Park
Tina Paul
Scott Burg

SUMMARY. As the adolescent population living in this country undergoes dramatic demographic changes in the 21st Century, increasing both in numbers and ethnic/racial diversity, practitioners and policy makers need to understand the prevalence of and trends in adolescent risk-taking behaviors, morbidity and mortality. Significant disparities in health status exist by ethnicity/race and gender in areas including: unintentional injury, violence, mental health, substance use, sexual behavior, and disease preven-

Claire Brindis, DrPH, is Professor of Pediatrics and Health Policy and Executive Director, National Adolescent Health Information Center (NAHIC) and the Public Policy Analysis and Education Center for Middle Childhood and Adolescent Health (Center), University of California, San Francisco. M. Jane Park, MPH, is Coordinator of NAHIC and the Center. Tina Paul, MPH, CHES, is Project Associate at NAHIC and the Center. Scott Burg, BA, formerly served as a Research Assistant at NAHIC and the Center.

Address correspondence to: Claire Brindis, DrPH, University of California, San Francisco, 3333 California Street Suite, San Francisco 265, CA 94143-0936.

The development of this article was supported by grants from the Maternal and Child Health Bureau, Health Resources and Services Administration, U.S. Department of Health and Human Services, 4H06MC00002, 6U93MC0023, and 2T71MC00003).

[Haworth co-indexing entry note]: "A Profile of Adolescent Health: The Role of Race, Ethnicity and Gender." Brindis et al. Co-published simultaneously in *Journal of Ethnic & Cultural Diversity in Social Work* (The Haworth Social Work Practice Press, an imprint of The Haworth Press, Inc.) Vol. 11, No. 1/2, 2002, pp. 1-32; and: *Social Work with Multicultural Youth* (ed: Diane de Anda) The Haworth Social Work Practice Press, an imprint of The Haworth Press, Inc., 2002, pp. 1-32. Single or multiple copies of this article are available for a fee from The Haworth Document Delivery Service [1-800-HAWORTH, 9:00 a.m. - 5:00 p.m. (EST). E-mail address: docdelivery@haworthpress.com].

http://www.haworthpress.com/store/product.asp?sku=J051

10.1300/J051v11n01_01

tion. The epidemiological profile can help mobilize communities to address adolescent health issues. Developing effective interventions will require an ecological approach that builds on adolescents' assets and takes into account the contexts in which they live.

KEYWORDS. Adolescent health, morbidity and mortality, risk-taking behavior, resiliency

INTRODUCTION

The health and well-being of adolescents has a major impact on the overall social and economic health of the country. Today's adolescents are tomorrow's workforce, parents, and leaders, and their future is shaped by the opportunities made available to them today. Adolescence is a unique developmental stage and represents a time of accelerated growth during which a number of physiological, cognitive, social and emotional changes occur simultaneously. During adolescence (ages 10-19) young people confront new issues that affect their physical and mental health–issues that face young adults (ages 20-24) as well (Clayton, Brindis, Hamor, Raiden-Wright, & Fong, 2000). Adolescents are particularly prone to risk-taking and experimentation as they learn to manage new capabilities and greater freedom. These behaviors are often a normal part of establishing independence, but they can also lead to negative and potentially serious health consequences.

The health issues of adolescents and young adults are easy to overlook because they are not, for the most part, acute illnesses or chronic diseases. The majority of adolescents are healthy when assessed by traditional medical markers, such as disease patterns and health care utilization. A recent analysis of the 1997 National Health Interview Survey indicated that more than 80% of children and adolescents report good or excellent health (Bloom & Tonthat, 2002). Adolescents have relatively low rates of cancer, hypertension, and other physical disorders (Ozer, Brindis, Milllstein, Knopf, & Irwin, 1998). Relatively few adolescents and young adults are hospitalized, with most depending on ambulatory care for medical treatment (Bloom & Tonthat, 2002).

Adolescent health problems are largely behavioral and social in nature, with the most serious adolescent health problems having their origins in health-damaging behaviors. These behaviors affect not only adolescent health, but also contribute to the leading causes of adult morbidity and mortality. The following categories of risk-taking behavior–which often begin in adolescence–are related to the leading causes of adolescent and adult mortality and morbidity: drug and alcohol use, unsafe sexual activity, violence, injury-related behavior, tobacco use, inadequate physical activity, and poor dietary habits (Kann et al., 2000). Thus, investment in adolescent health has the potential to reduce the burden of morbidity and mortality among adults. The importance of risk-taking behaviors in adolescent health is underscored by the adolescent focus of the Healthy People 2010 Initiative. The Initiative has identified 21 critical objectives among the 108 that address adolescents and young adults. Of these 21 objectives, 10 address specific risk-taking behaviors, and many of the remaining 11 are outcomes directly linked to behaviors.

There are significant disparities in adolescent health status, including the initiation of risk-taking behaviors, with some populations facing much greater risks to their health. Disparities in health status are found throughout the lifespan, and, indeed, the Healthy People 2010 Initiative has as one of its two over-arching goals, the elimination of disparities in health status for all Americans. Among adolescents, poorer health status is correlated with lower income, less education, racial or ethnic minority status, and other social variables (Montgomery, Kiely, & Papas, 1996). As reflected in this article, there exists a relative wealth of data demonstrating adolescent health disparities by race/ethnicity and gender. However, data demonstrating how income moderates the effect of ethnic and racial status is rarely available for this age group (Ozer et al., 1998). In addition, special populations of adolescents also face greater health problems. These include adolescents who (1) have chronic physical or mental health conditions; (2) live in foster or group homes; (3) are homeless or who have run away from home; (4) are incarcerated or involved in the juvenile justice system; and (5) are pregnant and parenting. Other groups, such as adolescents who are undocumented, migrant, or new immigrants and/or whose English skills are limited, face special challenges in accessing care (Brindis, VanLandeghem, Kirkpatrick, Lee, & Macdonald, 1999). Adolescents in more than one of the aforementioned categories are even more likely to face multiple risks. For example, adolescents who experience mental health problems are more likely to be living away from home and involved in the juvenile justice system. These adolescents are more likely to have complex health care needs (Irwin, Brindis, Holt, & Langlykke, 1994).

The nation's capacity to monitor individual adolescent risk-taking behaviors has increased tremendously since the early 1990s. Ongoing national and state surveys monitor prevalence of behaviors and related outcomes including substance use, unintended injuries, violent behaviors, unintended pregnancy, and STIs. The major national sources of data provide information on the prevalence of risk-taking behavior by gender and race/ethnicity. However, specific income data on these populations is absent in these data sets, thus limiting the ability to further disentangle the relationship between income and racial and ethnic status. In spite of this important limitation, available information allows program managers and policy makers to identify populations at greater risk of adverse outcomes, allowing more strategic use of limited resources.

While it is important to measure the disparities in risk-taking behaviors among youth, it is also necessary to understand the factors behind these disparities. This information is key to undertaking effective action to reduce or eliminate health disparities. In the last decade, the adolescent health field has broadened its approach from a relatively narrow focus on reducing risk among individuals to a more comprehensive approach–one that both looks at the context in which young people make health-related decisions and promotes healthy adolescent development (Brindis, Ozer, Handly, Knopf, Millstein, & Irwin, 1998). This broader approach is essential for better understanding and addressing disparities in adolescent health. It also points to the limitations of relying solely on racial and ethnic labels as providing a comprehensive picture of the health of adolescents.

Focusing on individual behavior de-emphasizes the importance of the context in which young people live and make health-related decisions. In response to this, researchers have increasingly turned to holistic or ecological models over the last decade to better understand the many contexts that influence adolescents' lives and health-related decision-making. The holistic model recognizes that the behavior of adolescents has environmental influences, such as families, peers, school, community, media, and policy. Rather than looking to correct deficiencies in the adolescents themselves, this approach turns the attention to creating healthy and supportive environments (National Research Council, 1993). Other researchers call for the importance of developing a new paradigm encompassing a more inclusive perspective on interethnic and interracial relations in order to account for the increasingly cultural and linguistic diversity that is reflected in American society (Taylor-Gibbs, 1999).

The traditional focus on risk-taking behaviors has also engendered a primary emphasis on measuring and preventing "problem" behaviors, rather than on developing and strengthening young people's assets. It has also led to the development of distinct fields and categorical thinking about behaviors that often are inter-related and have common root causes (e.g., substance abuse and violence). It has also contributed to a focus on attempting to change individual behavior, without adequate consideration of antecedent factors (e.g., familial patterns of engaging in similar behaviors such as tobacco use), social, environmental, economic, and other contextual factors influencing individual behavior (e.g., prevalence of tobacco sales as a result of tobacco farmer subsidies, level of social stress contributing to tobacco dependence, lack of opportunities to access prevention programs). This long established perspective demonstrates the limited adoption of an Ecological Risk and Resiliency Approach (Bogenschneider, 1996) in collecting national data that considers individual and social context factors and their interactions. The lack of contextual data, specifically basic social conditions, limits the ability to develop the most effective targeted interventions. Furthermore, although membership in particular ethnic communities is not in itself a risk factor, it does influence access to both prevention resources and effective service delivery systems (see Marsiglia, Miles, Dustman and Sills, 2002) and has often been used as a short-hand to summarize far more complex interactions. Furthermore, by reliance on racial and ethnic labels, stereotyped images have contributed to further balkanization of ethnic and racial sub-groups of adolescents.

A small, but significant change in the overall approach for addressing adolescent health, called "youth development," has emerged over the past decade. Although research incorporating youth development and holistic perspectives is relatively new, studies have yielded findings about individual and contextual factors influencing young people's risk-taking behavior–findings with important implications for promoting adolescent health. For example, data from the National Longitudinal Survey of Adolescent Health (or "Add Health") point to the significant role played by home, school and after-school environments on adolescents' health-related decisions. Adolescents are less likely to engage in risk behaviors if they have a sense of physical, emotional, and economic security, are able to make a contribution to the community, have input into decision-making, and have opportunities to participate in engaging and challenging activities that build skills and competencies (Resnick et al., 1997).

Add Health found that young people who feel a strong sense of connectedness, or feelings of love and caring, to their parents and/or other family members typically demonstrate resiliency and a lower frequency of engaging in risk-taking behavior. Conversely, adolescents who report a lower sense of connectedness to their families tend to engage in much higher levels of risk-taking behaviors, including tobacco, alcohol, and other substance use. Add Health findings also indicated that perceived parental expectations regarding their adolescent's school attainment is associated with healthy behavior. In addition, adolescents who have problems with schoolwork and who have substantial unstructured leisure time are more likely to engage in high-risk behaviors. The study also found that adolescents are at an increased risk of suicide, involvement in interpersonal violence, and substance use in homes with easy access to guns, alcohol, tobacco, or drugs (Resnick et al., 1997).

These findings demonstrate the importance of context in shaping adolescents' risk-taking behavior. It also substantiates the need for a youth development approach that promotes assets in young people–for example, psychosocial strengths such as negotiating skills and resiliency or pro-social behaviors, such as community service or participation in sports (Clayton et al., 2000). Unfortunately, while extensive data exist on the risk-taking behaviors, morbidity and mortality of adolescence, there is little ongoing national data collection providing information on both the positive and negative antecedent factors (individual, familial and community), as well as political, social and economic contextual factors influencing health. National efforts to collect these data are needed to help communities reframe their approach to improving adolescent health, from an approach that perceives adolescents to have deficits and problems to one that recognizes adolescents as important community assets and emphasizes the creation of safe and supportive environments.

In this article, the authors review adolescent health status beginning with a demographic profile of the adolescent population, followed by health status data with a specific focus on comparing markers of adolescent health (including risk behaviors, morbidity, and mortality) by ethnicity/race and gender. In interpreting these data, it is important to bear in mind the aforementioned lack of contextual data to explain why disparities exist. In the Discussion section, the implications of these data are addressed along with the need for national data on assets and contextual influences to complement existing adolescent health data sets.

A DEMOGRAPHIC PROFILE OF ADOLESCENTS

Background

More people were added to the U.S. population during the 1990s than at any other time, except the 1950s. This focus on adolescents comes at a critical time, with the population of adolescents in the U.S. ages 10-19 expected to grow by almost 2 million by the year 2010, from 39.9 million to 41.7 million. Though large in absolute numbers, this represents a much smaller percentage increase than that of the overall population (4.6% vs. an expected 8.6% increase for the total U.S. population). Because the adolescent population is projected to grow more slowly than the overall U.S. population, the proportion of adolescents is projected to decrease from 14.5% of the U.S. population in 2000 to 13% in 2020. Nonetheless, by 2020, the adolescent population is projected to reach 42.4 million, and a record 50 million adolescents are projected by the year 2040 (Census Bureau, 2000).

The growth of the adolescent population will not be distributed evenly across the United States. The Western states are expected to experience the greatest growth among adolescents ages 10-19, with a projected 23.5% increase from 1998 to 2010. This compares to a 10.6% increase in the South, an 8.8% increase in the Midwest, and a 2.3% increase in the Northeast. In addition to the increasing concentration of adolescents in the Western and Southern regions of the country, the adolescent population is increasingly located within metropolitan areas (Census Bureau, 2001).

The size, mean age, and ethnic/racial composition of the adolescent population experienced significant changes during the 1990s, and the demographic profile of this population is projected to continue changing in the coming decades. Key trends include: the decrease of White youth as a proportion of the adolescent population; a shift from Black to Hispanic/Latino youth as the second most populous ethnic/racial group; and a greater ethnic/racial diversity among the adolescent population than the U.S. population as a whole (see Figure 1) (Census Bureau, 2000).

Non-Hispanic White youth comprised 66% of the adolescent population in the year 2000, a decrease from 76% in 1980. It is projected that this percentage will continue to decrease, reaching 56% in the year 2020, and that, by 2040, non-Hispanic White youth will no longer represent a majority of adolescents. As of 2000, Black youth comprised 15% of the adolescent population. For Hispanic/Latino, Asian/Pacific

FIGURE 1. Actual and Projected Adolescent Population Growth by Ethnicity/Race, Ages 10-19, 1998-2010

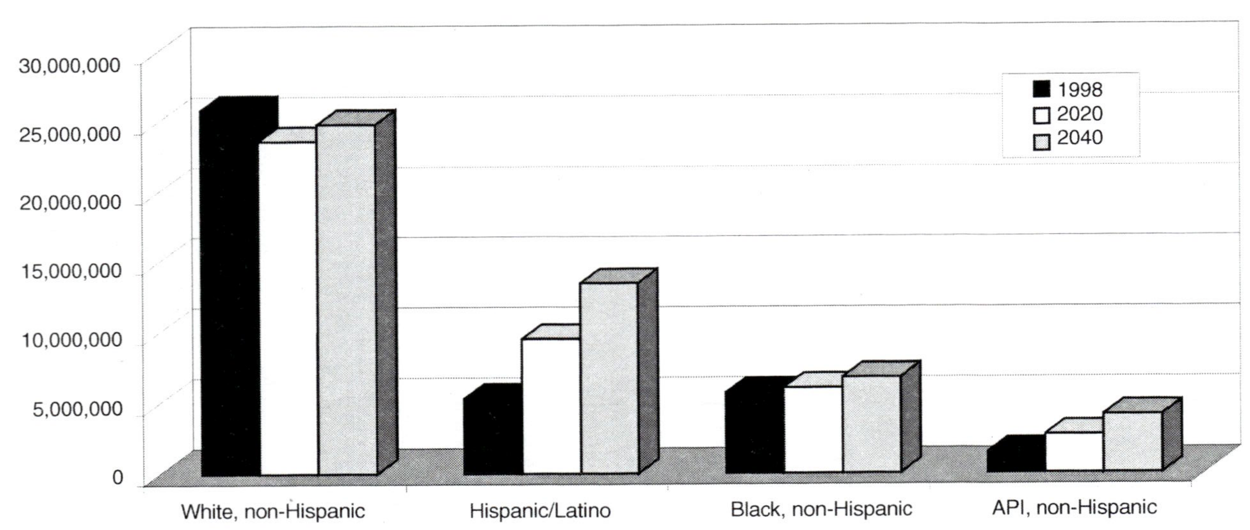

Source: Census Bureau, 2000

Islander and American Indian/Alaska Native youth, this figure was 14%, 4%, and 1%, respectively. However, the Hispanic/Latino adolescent population is expected to nearly double by the year 2020, when it will comprise a projected 23% of all adolescents. In comparison, the proportion of Black adolescents will decrease to 14%, and the American Indian/Alaska Native youth population will remain at 1%. The Asian/Pacific Islander population will also experience rapid growth, rising to 6% of the adolescent population by 2020 (Census Bureau, 2000).

The shift in the ethnic/racial makeup of the nation's youth stems from the higher immigration of Hispanic/Latino and Asian/Pacific Islander populations. In addition, as birth and fertility rates among non-Hispanic White and Black populations have decreased over the past two decades, there has been an increase in birth and fertility rates among Hispanic/Latino populations (Mackay, Fingerhut, & Duran, 2000). As the adolescent population grows in diversity and size, it will compete for limited resources with an aging population that is increasing rapidly both in absolute numbers and as a proportion of the overall population. This will pose challenges for advocates for adolescents who seek educational, social, and community resources needed to maintain and improve the health of young people.

Socioeconomic Profile

Family structure has an important influence on adolescent health, with children from single-parent households faring worse on many indicators of health. This is due to both the higher average income of two-parent households and the additional support and supervision often afforded when two adults are present in the home. Nearly half of all marriages end in divorce, and more than half of all children will spend some time in a single-parent family (Zill & Nord, 1994). Roughly 69% of adolescents currently live with two parents; of these, one in five do not live with both biological parents. Thirty-one percent of all adolescents live with only one parent, typically the mother. Roughly half a million adolescents live in foster care (Dryfoos, 1998).

Income is also associated with many measures of adolescent health status, with poorer children faring worse than their higher-income counterparts. Almost one in five adolescents in this country live in families with incomes below the federal poverty line. More than one-third of African American and Hispanic/Latino adolescents live in financially disadvantaged families, as do 13% of White adolescents (see Figure 2) (Dryfoos, 1998). The National Research Council Panel on High Risk Youth (1993) noted that a combination of social factors makes it difficult for families to rise out of poverty, including inner-city deterioration, discrimination, deteriorating public schools, single-parent households, and low-paying jobs. Such adverse social factors have a negative impact on adolescent health (Rickel & Becker, 1997).

A PROFILE OF ADOLESCENT HEALTH

This section presents a profile of adolescent health, organized around five major categories:

- Injury (Intentional and Unintentional),
- Reproductive health,
- Substance use,
- Disease Prevention and Health Promotion, and
- Chronic Health Conditions

In part, this organization reflects the preponderance of data on risk-taking behaviors and their consequences–itself a reflection of the current approach to adolescent health. As mentioned in the introduction, a more comprehensive approach would also present data on healthy development as well as the contexts in which adolescents make health-related decisions. The authors present topics separately as reflected in national data, which generally offer profiles of individual behaviors. It is worth noting, however, that studies have demonstrated that risk-taking behaviors are often clustered among specific groups of adolescents. We describe ethnic/racial and gender differences among adolescents wherever national data are available. For ethnic/racial data, the category names presented (e.g., African American or Black, Hispanic or Latino) are those used by the data collection agency or survey sponsor. When used in the following sections, these identifiers reflect standard census and other national data set categories of race and ethnicity used by the sponsoring agency. Risk-taking behavior is also reviewed as it is linked to morbidity and mortality, for example, poor nutrition as it is linked to obesity or other types of eating disorders.

FIGURE 2. Percent of Adolescents Under Age 18 Living in Poverty, 1980-1999

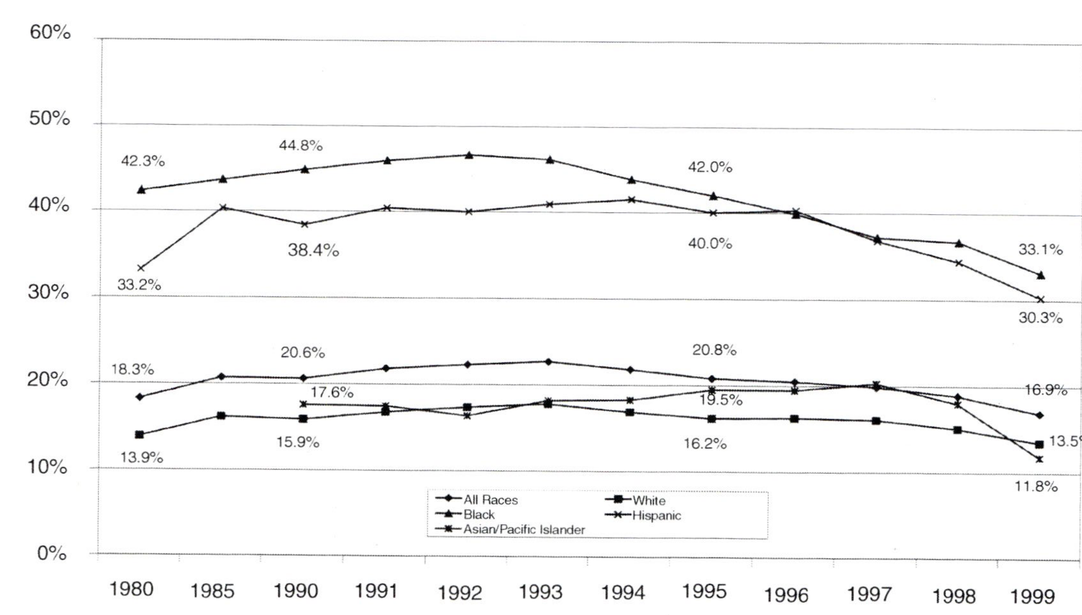

Note: Data collection for Asian/Pacific Islander group started in 1987
Source: Dalaker & Proctor, 2000

Injury

About three quarters of adolescent mortality are the result of some form of injury indicated by the following breakdown for 15-19 year-olds: motor vehicle accidents (36.9%), other unintentional injuries (11.7%), homicide (15.2%), and suicide (11.7%) (NCIPC, 2002). While not the most prevalent of negative health outcomes, mortality is the most severe and reduction of mortality remains an important public health goal. Overall, adolescent mortality rates have decreased and are now at or near historical lows for all ethnic/racial groups–a decrease due in part to substantial salutary changes in injury-related behavior. However, there remain significant disparities in mortality by gender and ethnicity/race, described below (see Figure 3) (Hoyert, Arias, Smith, Murphy, & Kochanek, 2001). A number of ecological factors, including social and economic factors contribute to these disparities, but their causal relationships have often been difficult to disentangle. For example, as shown in the following section, males for all ethnic/racial groups are at greater risk of negative outcomes for injury. Factors, such as differential alcohol and drug use among males as compared to females may help explain some of the contributing factors to the prevalence of injury, but does not fully explain the broader social interactions that result in males being placed at greater risk of adverse outcomes. Economic factors, such as access to a car, appear to place non-Hispanic males at a far greater risk of motor vehicle accidents (MVAs) (as shown in the following section), but economic factors do not account for the higher incidence of deaths among non-Hispanic American Indian/Alaska Native males, whose higher alcohol use may place them at greater risk for MVAs. These complex patterns clearly point to the need for the adoption of an Ecological Risk and Resiliency Approach (Bogenschneider, 1996) to collecting data in order to help explain some of these complex patterns of behaviors observed among youth.

Unintentional Injury

Unintentional injury, in particular motor vehicle accidents (MVAs), is the leading cause of mortality for adolescents. Although still the major cause of adolescent mortality, significant decreases in MVA mortality have been observed over the past two decades, from 38.7/100,000 in 1981 to 26.3/100,000[1] in 1999 for 15-19 year-olds (NCIPC, 2002). This is due in part to changes in behaviors linked to motor vehicle accidents

FIGURE 3. Mortality Trends by Ethnicity/Race, Ages 15-24, 1988-1999

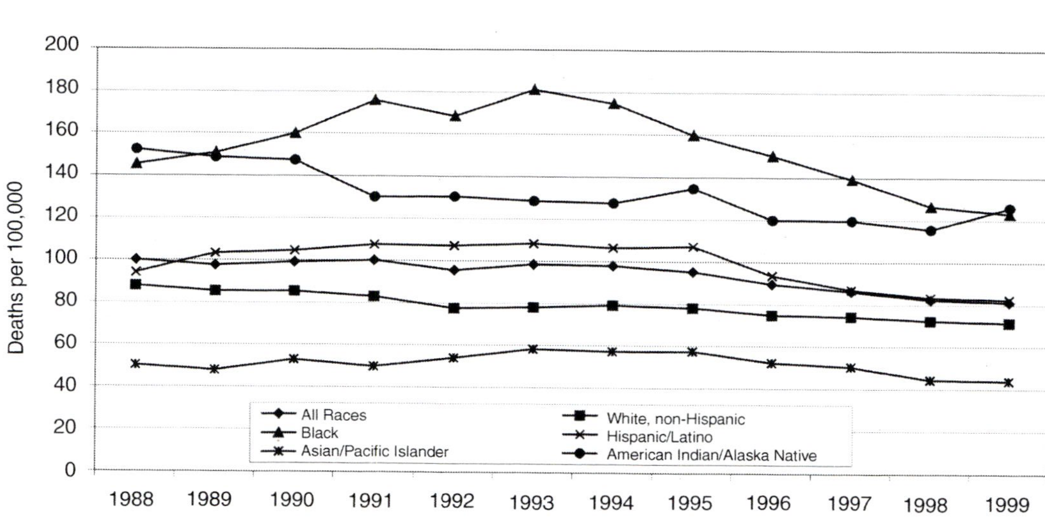

Source: NVSS, 2002

(MVAs)–e.g., drinking and driving (or riding with a driver who has been drinking) and wearing a seat belt.

Although these declines in mortality are welcome news, significant disparities in MVA mortality warrant concern. Gender is the largest risk factor, with males ages 15-19 about 2 times more likely than same-age females to die from MVA-related injury (33.6 vs. 18.6 in 1999). Males have higher rates than females for all ethnic/racial groups (NCIPC, 2002).

Analysis by ethnicity/race and gender for adolescents ages 15-19 shows that, in 1999, non-Hispanic American Indian/Alaska Native males had the highest MVA mortality rates per 100,000 (69.5). This mortality rate is two times higher than the rate for non-Hispanic White males (36.5), and two to four times that of Hispanic/Latino males (29.8), non-Hispanic Black males (25.8) and non-Hispanic Asian and Pacific Islander males (15.3). Mortality rates have declined for all males since 1990, except for non-Hispanic Black males. Among adolescent females ages 15-19 in 1999, non-Hispanic American Indians/Alaska Natives also had the highest rate of MVA mortality (28.7), followed by non-Hispanic Whites (21.9), Hispanics/Latinas (11.7), non-Hispanic Blacks (11.6) and non-Hispanic Asian/Pacific Islanders (9.3) (NCIPC, 2002).

Violence

Violence affects the lives of many youths. Overall, the prevalence of violence in adolescents' lives has decreased in the last decade. In addition to a dramatic decline in homicide rates, data show that youth are perpetrating fewer violent crimes and fighting less, and are less likely to carry a weapon. As shown in this section, a continuing concern, however, is the extent to which violence disproportionately affects the lives of young African-American males. The complex social, economic, and other contextual factors that place African-American youth at greater risk is beyond the scope of this paper, but clearly it is important to note that simply noting ethnic membership does not provide an ecological understanding of the factors contributing to this disparity.

In contrast to the incidence of homicide, the violence victimization rate (the occurrence of violent crimes committed against a person/group, per 1,000 residents or households) has experienced an overall increase from 1980-1996, with rates of 26/1,000 (ages 12-17) for serious violent crimes and 65/1,000 for simple assaults (Snyder & Sickmund, 1999). Average annual victimization rates from 1993-1997 were highest among American Indian adolescents and young adults ages 12-24 (ranging from 141 to 208 per 1,000), were similar for White (85 to 109 per 1,000) and Black (92 to 112 per 1,000) youth, and were lowest for Asian (41 to 55 per 1,000) youth in the same age group (data not available for Hispanic/Latino adolescents) (Rennison, 2001).

Arrest rates for violent crimes peak at age 18, and decline thereafter. Even though there has been a substantial increase in female juvenile arrest rates between 1981 and 1997, male juveniles are five times more likely to be arrested. From 1985 to 1993, arrests of young people ages 10-17 for murder rose by 154%, from 5.7 to 14.5 per 100,000. However, by 1997 this upward trend had reversed, and the arrest rate declined to 8.2 (Snyder & Sickmund, 1999). Particularly striking is the decrease in the homicide offending rate among young Black males–which dropped from 226.7 in 1994 to 67.3 in 1999. For White youth, the corresponding figures were 22.4 and 10.2 (no data available for other ethnicities/races) (Fox & Zawitz, 2001).

While there has been a decrease in reports of physical fighting over the past decade, this issue affects the health of many adolescents. In 2001, 33.2% of high school students reported having been in at least one physical fight in the last 12 months, a decrease from 42.5% in 1991; 4.0% of all students reported sustaining a serious injury in a fight in 2001. Males (43.1%) were much more likely than females (23.9%) to have been in a fight. Differences among ethnic/racial groups in the incidence of fighting were minor, with 36.5% of non-Hispanic Black youth reporting that they had been in a fight during the past 12 months, compared to Hispanic/Latino (35.8%) and non-Hispanic White adolescents (32.2%). In addition, in 2001, 17.4% of high school students reported carrying some type of weapon in the past 30 days, with males (29.3%) more than four times as likely to report this behavior than females (6.2%). Weapon carrying rates were very similar across ethnic/racial groups, with 17.9% of non-Hispanic White youth reporting weapon carrying, compared to 16.5% for Hispanic/Latino and 15.2% for non-Hispanic Black youth (Grunbaum et al., 2002).

Homicide represents the second leading cause of death in both the 15-19 and 20-24 age groups. However, for adolescents ages 15-19, homicide rates per 100,000 dropped to a record low in 1985 (8.4) and increased dramatically until 1993 (20.4), when the rate started to fall again (10.6 in 1999). However, these data mask significant disparities in ethnicity/race and gender. Homicide affects Black males more than any other group. While the 1999 rate of 66.0 for non-Hispanic Black youth ages 15-19 represents a dramatic decline from the 1993 peak of

143.4, homicide is the leading cause of death for Black, non-Hispanic males of this age. In 1999, Black, non-Hispanic males ages 15-19 were over fifteen times more likely to die from homicide than White, non-Hispanic males and more than twice as likely as Hispanic/Latino males. Hispanic/Latino males had the second highest homicide rate in 1999 (29.4), followed by non-Hispanic White males (4.2). These figures also represent significant decreases from the high homicide rates in the early 1990s–60.4 in 1992 for Hispanic/Latino males and 15.0 in 1994 for White, non-Hispanic males (NCIPC, 2002).

Among adolescent females ages 15-19, non-Hispanic Black adolescents also have homicide rates much higher than those of their female peers. The 1999 rate of 10.4 for Black, non-Hispanic females represents a significant decline from the 1993 high of 18.6, but it is still more than twice that of Hispanic/Latina females (4.3 in 1999) and 5 times that of non-Hispanic White females (2.0) (NCIPC, 2002).

Suicide

Suicide represents the third leading cause of death for adolescents and young adults. Non-lethal suicidal behavior and ideation also affect large numbers of adolescents. In 2001, 19.0% of high school students reported seriously considering suicide over the previous 12 months, a decrease from 29.0% in 1991. Suicide ideation among females (23.6%) is much more likely than among males (14.2%). This gender difference was identified for all grades and racial and ethnic groups (Grunbaum et al., 2002).

Suicidal behavior has been related to mental health problems including depression and adjustment or stress reactions (DHHS, 1999). Currently, there are no national surveys that monitor trends in the mental health status of adolescents. However, the prevalence of mental health conditions can be estimated through national surveys, as well as data from smaller studies. In addition, some national surveys on adolescent well-being include questions that reflect their mental health status, such as suicidal ideation and attempts. The Surgeon General's Report on Mental Health estimates that nearly 21% of youth ages 9-17 have a diagnosable mental or addictive disorder associated with at least minimum impairment, while 11%, or 4 million adolescents have a disorder that results in significant impairment (Shaffer et al., 1996, cited in DHHS, 1999). Other studies indicate that mental heath disorders among adolescents are under-diagnosed. In one study of 1,710 adolescents, 30% had at least one current symptom of major depression, but only 2.6% had received a diagnosis (Roberts, Lewinsohn, & Seeley, 1995).

Epidemiological surveys indicate that about 20% of adolescents use mental health services (Leaf et al., 1996).

Actual suicide attempts were reported among 8.8% of high school students, an increase from 7.3% in 1991. Female students (11.2%) were significantly more likely than male students (6.2%) to have attempted suicide one or more times during the previous 12 months. This gender difference holds true across all ethnic/racial groups. Hispanic/Latina females were more likely than non-Hispanic White and non-Hispanic Black females to attempt suicide (15.9% vs. 10.3% and 9.8%, respectively). Among male high school students, Hispanic/Latino and non-Hispanic Black youth were slightly more likely than their non-Hispanic White peers to report having attempted suicide (8.0% & 7.5%, respectively vs. 5.3%). While suicide attempts among female high school students have decreased in recent years, they have risen for males. Overall, 2.6% of high school students required medical attention due to a suicide attempt committed within the previous 12 months (See Figure 4) (Grunbaum et al., 2002).

Overall, suicide rates have remained relatively stable, fluctuating slightly for some ethnic/racial groups. While females attempt suicide more than males, males commit suicide at a rate per 100,000 more than five times higher than the rate for females (12 vs. 2.2). It is again critical to examine data by ethnicity/race and gender. Among 15-19 year-old

FIGURE 4. Non-Lethal Suicidal Behavior by Gender, High School Students, 2001

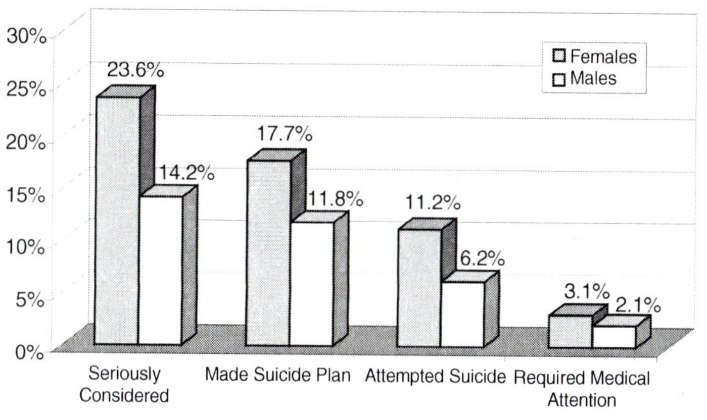

Source: Grunbaum et al., 2002

males, non-Hispanic American Indian/Alaska Native youth have the highest suicide rate, 41.9 in 1999–a rate almost three times that of White, non-Hispanic males (14.5) and more than four times that of Hispanic/Latino (10.1), non-Hispanic Black (10.0), and non-Hispanic Asian and Pacific Islander (7.0) males. Black adolescents have shown the largest increase over a decade, almost doubling from 5.5 in 1981 to 10.0 in 1999, a decrease from the peak of 16.6 reached in 1994 (NCIPC, 2002).

Among females ages 15-19, non-Hispanic American Indians/Alaska Natives also had the highest rate of suicide at 8.2 in 1999–a rate more than twice that for Non-Hispanic Asian/Pacific Islander (3.4), Hispanic/Latina (2.2) and Black, non-Hispanic females (1.7). It should be noted that suicide data for American Indians/Alaska Natives and Asians/Pacific Islanders are unreliable, due to the low number of cases (NCIPC, 2002).

REPRODUCTIVE HEALTH

In the area of reproductive health, most of the trends are positive. For the first time in two decades, fewer adolescents are having sex. Those adolescents who are having sex are using condoms more often, and fewer are contracting Sexually Transmitted Infections (STIs). In addition, fewer adolescents are getting pregnant or giving birth. Major concerns include increases in some STIs, including chlamydia and HIV/AIDS, and the disproportionate burden of STI morbidity borne by females and Black youth.

Sexual Behavior and Condom Use

In 2001, 45.6% of high school students reported ever having had sexual intercourse, a decrease from 53.0% in 1993. Males (48.5%) were more likely than females (42.9%) to have had sex. This number increases with age, with 60.5% of seniors (61.0% of males and 60.1% of females) in high school reporting that they have had sexual intercourse at least once compared to 34.4% of 9th graders (40.5% of males and 29.1% of females) (Grunbaum et al., 2002).

Initiation of sexual activity varies considerably by ethnicity/race within the high school population. Black, non-Hispanic high school students (60.8%) are most likely to have had sex, followed by Hispanic/Latino (48.4%) and non-Hispanic White (43.21%) students. Condom use has increased, with 57.9% of sexually active high school students reporting having used a condom at last intercourse in 2001, compared to 46.2% in 1991. Black, non-Hispanic students (67.1%) are most likely to have used condoms, followed by non-Hispanic White (56.8%) and Hispanic/Latino (53.5%) students. However, White, non-Hispanic students (23.4%) are much more likely to use birth control pills than their Hispanic/Latino (9.6%) and non-Hispanic Black (7.9%) peers (Grunbaum et al., 2002).

Adolescent Pregnancy and Births

The positive trends in sexual and contraceptive behavior described above are reflected in the recent declines in adolescent pregnancy and birth rates. The adolescent pregnancy rate is now at the lowest level since data collection began in 1976. After peaking at 116.5/1,000 in 1991, the pregnancy rate among 15-19 year-olds fell to 94.3/1,000 in 1997. The pregnancy rate for 15-17 year-olds is 63.7/1,000, and doubles to 141.7/1,000 among 18-19 year-olds. About sixty percent of adolescent pregnancies are to 18-19 year olds. This decline was more pronounced among non-Hispanic Black and non-Hispanic White youth than among their Hispanic/Latino cohorts. Black, non-Hispanic (170.4/1,000) and Hispanic/Latina (148.7/1,000) adolescents continue to have pregnancy rates 2 to 3 times that of non-Hispanic Whites (65.1/1,000) (Ventura, Mosher, Curtin, Abma, & Henshaw, 2001).

The decrease in pregnancy rates reflects reductions in abortion and birth rates–both of which have decreased among adolescents ages 15-19. In 2000, the rate of births to adolescents ages 15-19 was 48.5/1,000 females, the lowest rate since 1988. Birth rates have decreased for all racial and ethnic groups, with Black youth experiencing the steepest decline. Between 1991 and 2000, the decrease in the birth rate was highest for non-Hispanic Black adolescents (23%), followed by non-Hispanic White (19%), American Indian (16%), Asian/Pacific Islander (14%), and Hispanic/Latina females (9%) (Martin, Hamilton, Ventura, Menacker, & Park, 2002). Abortion rates have also fallen significantly, from 40.3/1,000 in 1990 to 27.5/1,000 in 1997. Between 1988 and 1997, the percentage of adolescent pregnancies ending in abortion decreased from 40% to 21% (Ventura et al., 2001). Thus, overall these trends hold promise that fewer adolescents will experience the negative repercussions of too-early childbearing, including school dropout, poverty, and the negative health consequences on their and their children's health. Futhermore, it clearly points to the need to consider a variety of strategies to impact a health issue that has long been treated as intractable. In relation to the an ecological model, it calls for additional efforts to consider antecedent factors, such as poverty, sexual abuse, academic opportunities, and viable social and economic alternatives, as well as a wide variety of contextual factors, such as gender-relationship issues, comprehensive sex education, access to health services, economic opportunities, as well as the impact of media on adolescent behavior.

Sexually Transmitted Infections

Estimates indicate that there are 15 million new sexually transmitted infection (STI) cases in the United States each year, and one-fourth of these new infections are in teenagers (CDC, 2000). Compared to older adults, adolescents and young adults ages 10-24 are at high risk for acquiring STIs, because they may be more likely to have multiple sexual partners, engage in unprotected intercourse, and may have higher risk partners. Infection rates for most STIs among adolescents have decreased in recent years. This holds true for all age, racial, and ethnic groups. Trends in chlamydia, however, represent a significant exception to promising STI trends–with chlamydia infection rates among adolescents and young adults ages 10-24 increasing between 15%-50% from 1996 to 2000 (CDC, 2001).

Forty percent of chlamydia cases are reported among adolescents ages 15-19, with reported prevalence among female adolescents exceeding ten percent and male prevalence over five percent (CDC, 2000). Non-Hispanic, Black adolescents (ages 15-19) are disproportionately affected by STDs. In 2000, this population had a chlamydia rate per 100,000 of 4631.2 among 15-19 year-olds–a rate almost twice that of American Indian/Alaska Native (2527.6), three times that for Hispanic/Latino (1584.9), and more than seven times the rates for non-Hispanic White (643.0) and Asian/Pacific Islander (569.0) adolescents (CDC, 2001). Thus, while there have been significant inroads in decreasing the number of sexually active adolescents and improvements in condom use among sexually active adolescents, many adolescents continue to engage in risk-behaviors (e.g. multiple partners, concurrent drug and alcohol use that hampers effective use of condoms) that place them at risk of chlamydia. These trends in part also reflect improvements in access to clinical diagnostic tests, including diagnoses of asymptomatic cases of chlamydia, especially among women. Additional urine-based vs. more invasive screening tests also assure that young men at risk are more likely to be screened and documented earlier as a result of improvements in technology. However, this profile does not help explain what additional contextual and contributing factors continue to place certain groups of youth at greater risk of diseases that threaten their fertility and their health status.

The overall number of cases of gonorrhea among adolescents ages 15-19 decreased by 5% from 1996 to 2000. Although the incidence of gonorrhea among Black adolescents declined in the 1990s, they account for more than three-quarters of all reported cases. Black, non-Hispanic adolescents (ages 15-19) experience gonorrhea at a rate of 2739.1 per 100,000, which is over eight times that of American Indian/Alaska Native (329.7), eleven times the rate for Hispanic/Latino (247.1), and over 25 times the rates for non-Hispanic White (111.3) and Asian/Pacific Islander youth (87.5) (CDC, 2001).

AIDS is relatively rare among adolescents and young adults (360 cases between July 2000-June 2001 reported for ages 13-19, and 1368 cases reported for ages 20-24), but is increasing in prevalence (CDC, 2002). Issues such as confidentiality, insurance coverage, and social stigma continue to make accurate data on HIV/AIDS difficult to obtain. Surveillance data from states which do report HIV/AIDS cases indicate that youth account for a higher proportion of HIV cases (13%) than AIDS cases (3%). Black adolescents and young adults (ages 13-24) account for over half of all HIV cases ever reported among youth (CDC, n.d.). Among adolescents ages 13-19, females are more likely to become infected with HIV than males, comprising 61% of new HIV infections. Females in this age group account for just under half of new AIDS cases reported between July 2000 and June 2001 (CDC, 2002). The reversal in trends along gender lines indicates the increasing predominance of heterosexual transmission of the disease within the adolescent population. Unlike other STIs, the morbidity and mortality associated with HIV/AIDS represents one of the deadliest health risks confronting young people. It will likely continue to increase dramatically over the next decade unless far greater efforts are made to adopt additional health, educational, economic, and social, rather than moralistic, strategies aimed at preventing exposing youth to the HIV virus.

SUBSTANCE USE

Although adolescence is characterized as a time of experimentation, the negative health consequences of using alcohol, tobacco, and other drugs can have a life-long impact. Many substances, including alcohol and tobacco, are highly addictive, and habits developed in the formative years are some of the most difficult to break (W. K. Kellogg Foundation, 1998).

Attitudes and beliefs about drugs have been shown to be important determinants of their use by adolescents. Researchers conducting the Monitoring the Future Survey noted that a change in these attitudes is usually a precursor to a change in actual use, with adolescents being less likely to use a drug if they perceive it as being dangerous. For many substances, including tobacco, the perception of risk among adolescents fell during the 1990s. After three decades of data about the dangers of smoking and tobacco use, only three out of five (57.1%) eighth graders sampled in a national survey thought that a person smoking one or more packs of cigarettes a day puts himself or herself at great risk of harm. In 2001, only 46.3% of 8th graders and 23.5% of 12th graders reported that smoking marijuana occasionally posed a "great risk." While data have fluctuated in the past decade, overall, the percentage of 12th graders reporting that their close friends would disapprove of their using drugs increased over the last three years. Similarly, the proportion of students seeing daily drinking or "binge" drinking as dangerous or reporting that close friends would disapprove of these behaviors has increased (Johnston, O'Malley, & Bachman, 2002).

Tobacco

Tobacco use can have serious negative health effects for adolescents; however, the most severe consequences, such as cancer and lung disease, often do not occur until adulthood. The most common form of tobacco use, cigarette smoking, often begins between grades six and nine, or between the ages of 11 and 15. Among 8th graders, 16% reported that they had tried a cigarette by the fifth grade. Cigarette smoking among all adolescents peaked in the late 1970s and declined throughout the 1980s until the early 1990s, when it rose again until another decline in the late 1990s (Johnston et al., 2002). Among high school students, frequent cigarette use has risen from 12.7% in 1991 to 13.8% in 2001 (Grunbaum et al., 2002).

In 2001, 28.5% of high school students reported having smoked within the past 30 days. Prevalence of use increases with age, with 23.9% of 9th graders reporting use, versus 35.2% of students in 12th grade. White, non-Hispanic high school students (31.9%) were more likely than Hispanic/Latino (26.6%) or non-Hispanic Black (14.7%) students to report smoking in the last 30 days. Male and female high school students were about equally likely to use cigarettes (29.2% vs. 27.7%, respectively) (Grunbaum et al., 2002).

Alcohol

Following dramatic declines during the 1980s, the prevalence of alcohol use among adolescents and young adults has remained largely stable throughout the 1990s, with the exception of recent increases in "binge" drinking. Past month alcohol use is now at all-time lows for adolescents and young adults: Among adolescents ages 12-17, use fell from 49.6% in 1979 to 17.3% in 2001. While adolescents are impacted by this behavior, it is important to note that these patterns also affect young adults. For example, young adult alcohol usage decreased from 75.1% in 1979 to 58.8% in 2001 (SAMHSA, 2002).

The prevalence of binge drinking (i.e., consuming 5 or more drinks on the same occasion), however, has recently increased among young adults. Among adolescents ages 12-17, the prevalence of past month binge drinking fell sharply from 21.9% in 1985 to 10.6% in 2001. For young adults ages 18-25, however, "binge" use increased from 34.4% in 1985 to 38.7% in 2001. Males were slightly more likely to report binge drinking than females; in 2001, 11.2% of 12-17 year old males versus 9.9% of females reported at least one binge drinking episode during the past month. There were also significant differences in binge drinking among ethnic/racial groups. Among 12-17 year-olds, non-Hispanic American Indian/Alaska Native youth had the highest prevalence (12.8% as reported in 2000, the most recent data available). In 2001, the prevalence of binge drinking in other ethnic/racial groups were: 12.1% among non-Hispanic White, 9.8% among Hispanic/Latino, 5.5% among non-Hispanic Black, and 4.6 % among non-Hispanic Asian youth (SAMHSA, 2002).

Illicit Drugs

Although the use of illicit drugs by adolescents and young adults remains well below levels seen in the late 1970s and 1980s, it has increased significantly from the lows reached in the early 1990s, especially among adolescents ages 12-17. In 2001, 10.8% of adolescents reported past-month use of any illicit drug, representing both an increase from 5.3% in 1992, and a substantial decrease from 16.3% in 1979. Adolescent males were slightly more likely than same-age females to report illicit drug use (11.4% vs. 10.2%). Patterns among adolescents clearly influence the behaviors of adolescents transitioning to young adulthood. Among young adults ages 18-25, 18.8% had used an illicit drug within the past month, up from 13.1% in 1992, but well below 38.0% in 1979 (SAMHSA, 2002).

In addition to gender and age disparities, there are significant differences in illicit drug use by ethnicity/race: in 2001, 12-17 year-old non-Hispanic American Indian/Alaska Native youth (22.1%) were most likely to report past-month use of illicit drugs, followed by non-Hispanic White (11.3%), Hispanic/Latino (10.1%), non-Hispanic Black (9.1%), and non-Hispanic Asian (8.0%) youth. Again, patterns among adolescents transitioning into young adulthood mirror behaviors that are shaped during the earlier adolescent years and have implications for earlier points of intervention. Data for ages 18-25 in 2001 show that non-Hispanic White young adults (20.8%) were most likely to report past-month illicit drug use, followed by American Indian/Alaska Native (17.0% as reported in 2000, the most recent data available), non-Hispanic Black (17.1%), Hispanic/Latino (13.4%), and non-Hispanic Asian young adults (10.6%). Trends in use of marijuana, the most widely used illicit drug, by adolescents and young adults follow a pattern similar to that of other illicit drugs. Among youth ages 12-17, past-month marijuana use fell from 14.2% in 1979 to 8.0% in 2001, and among young adults ages 18-25, use fell from 35.6% in 1979 to 16.0% in 2001 (SAMHSA, 2002). Earlier, longitudinal, and ecological interventions (e.g., two generation approaches that recognize the relationship between parental and adolescent use of alcohol and drugs) are needed to decrease alcohol and illicit drug use given the trends among adolescents and young adults.

CHRONIC CONDITIONS

Chronic conditions and disabilities are measured according to activity limitations or long-term reductions in activity resulting from a chronic disease or impairment. Although relatively few adolescents have chronic conditions or disabilities, these young people have complex health care needs, which often require a constellation of services to ensure optimal health and development. Between 1980 and 1998, the percentage of youth ages 5-17 with an activity-limiting chronic condition rose from 6.1 to 7.3%. Males (9.0%) are more likely than females (5.6%) to be affected. In addition, minor differences are found according to race and ethnicity, as well as socioeconomic status. Black adolescents (8.9%) are most likely to have activity limitations resulting from chronic conditions, followed by Hispanic/Latino (7.5%) and White adolescents (7.2%). Among poor youth, 11.8% have a chronic condition, compared with 6.5% of those not living in poverty (NHIS, 2002). The higher incidence of chronic conditions among African American youth may reflect their higher incidence of poverty. However, a variety of additional social and other contextual factors likely contribute to these patterns, including access and utilization of prenatal and perinatal care, the prevalence of early childbearing, and environmental factors.

DISEASE PREVENTION AND HEALTH PROMOTION

This profile of adolescent health ends by addressing health behaviors which, for the most part, have a greater impact on the long-term health of adults. Many of the health problems that develop in adulthood, such as heart disease and cancer, are linked to behaviors established during adolescence. Regular exercise and balanced eating patterns are known to promote health and a sense of well-being. As outlined in this section, obesity–which is linked to poor eating habits and lack of regular physical activity during childhood and adolescence–can have severe health consequences later in life. Focusing on these behaviors in adolescence represents an important strategy for improving the health of the entire population.

Diet, Eating Disorders and Obesity

Diet is an important factor in health throughout the lifespan. A diet high in fruits and vegetables and low in fat content is considered to promote good health. Although the majority of adolescents in the YRBS survey reported eating a diet low in fat (62.3% in 1997), females (70.6%) were significantly more likely than males (55.5%) to report a low fat diet (Kann et al., 1998). Less than one quarter (21.4% in 2001) of students reported eating five or more servings of fruits and vegetables in the day preceding, a decrease from 29.3% in 1997. There is some disparity in these eating patterns between males and females (23.3% vs. 19.7%). A higher percentage of Black, non-Hispanic students (24.5%) reported eating five or more servings of fruits and vegetables in the day preceding than Hispanic/Latino (23.2%) and non-Hispanic White students (20.2%) (Grunbaum et al., 2002).

Overweight and obese adolescents are at greater risk of being overweight as adults, and adults who are overweight are more likely to experience serious long-term morbidity including coronary heart disease, gallbladder disease, diabetes, hypertension, and some cancers (Troiano, Flegal, Kuczmarksi, Campbell, & Johnson, 1995). The percentage of adolescents ages 12-19 who are overweight has increased considerably in the last 25 years from 5% during the 1976-1980 survey period, to 11% during the 1988-94 survey period, and to an all-time high of 14% in 1999 (NHANES, 2002). Data from the 1988-91 survey suggest little difference between the percentage of males and females ages 12-17 who were overweight (22% vs. 21%). Analysis by race shows that Black and White males had roughly the same overweight prevalence, while 29.9% of Black females and 20.3% of White females were overweight (Troiano et al., 1995).

Analyses of NHANES data for females also suggest ethnic/race disparities in risk for cardiovascular disease among children and young adults. Black and Mexican-American young females had a significantly higher body mass index than young White females, with percentages of dietary fat paralleling these findings. Blood pressure levels were higher for Black females than for any other group (Winkleby, Robinson, Sundquist, & Kraemer, 1999). These figures indicate that some ethnic/racial groups face additional risks for chronic health problems in adulthood.

Youth engage in both healthy and unhealthy behaviors for losing weight. In 2001, 59.9% of students (68.4% of females and 51.0% of males) exercised to lose weight or avoid gaining weight over the month prior to the survey; 43.8% (58.6% of females and 28.2% of males) ate less food, fewer calories, or foods low in fat to lose weight or avoid gaining weight. The extent of diet pill use and laxative use or vomiting is discouraging. Among females in particular, 12.6% report diet pill use and 7.8% report taking laxatives or vomiting. Additionally, non-Hispanic White youth were more likely to engage in exercise and eat less food than Hispanic/Latina and non-Hispanic Black females, but Hispanic/Latina youth were more likely to use diet pills and laxatives than their peers (Grunbaum et al., 2002).

Physical Activity

Significant health benefits can be obtained by engaging in physical activity on a regular basis. In 2001, 64.6% of high school students reported engaging in vigorous physical activity three or more days per week. Physical activity decreased with age: 71.9% of 9th graders reported engaging in this level of physical activity compared to 55.5% of 12th graders. Males (72.6%) reported this level of physical activity more often than females (57.0%). There are also differences by ethnicity/race. For example, 66.5% of non-Hispanic White students reported engaging in vigorous physical activity three or more days a week, followed by 60.5% of Hispanic/Latino students and 59.7% of non-Hispanic Black students (Grunbaum et al., 2002).

DISCUSSION

The health profile presented in this article shows many promising trends for adolescents, including a decrease in mortality rates and a decline in injury related behavior, motor vehicle related mortality, homicide, and suicide. Furthermore, fewer adolescents are placing themselves at risk of early childbearing as a result of fewer adolescents engaging in sexual activity and more contraceptive use among sexually active adolescents. However, the data also indicate that there remain many important health concerns, as many of the rates for the aforementioned health issues remain exceedingly high. Furthermore, increases in suicide ideation, sexually transmitted infections, such as chlamydia and HIV/AIDS, and youth victimization remain areas of poor health outcomes for many adolescents. Even more importantly, substantial differences exist across ethnic and racial groups, as well as gender, in the majority of adolescent health indicators. Although the authors have examined data in terms of trends over time and the impact of age, gender, and ethnicity/race, it is worth emphasizing again that data are still lacking on socioeconomic status. This may prove to be one of the most important elements in understanding which young people are at most risk and will also likely explain many of the ethnic and racial differences noted in this article. As the nation's adolescent population grows more diverse, it becomes more important that efforts to improve adolescent health address these economic and social disparities.

In addition, there are limited national data using youth development and ecological approaches. Further research examining both protective and negative antecedents (both individual and contextual) of risk-taking behaviors could yield important information explaining why these disparities exist–information that could inform efforts to develop effective adolescent health programs and policies. Such research would be most useful if it included adolescents representing different ethnic/racial groups, as well as special populations of adolescents, such as immigrants, foster care and homeless youth, and adolescents with disabilities. In addition, there exists little research linking interventions based on these approaches to better health outcomes. In advancing this kind of research, it is important to assess the influence of poverty on the environment in which adolescents live. For example, an important research question is the extent to which poverty limits the types of opportunities available to young people. Certainly, poverty has been clearly documented to have an impact on adolescents' access to health care and information, particularly the lack of health insurance and the disparities in the types and quality of services available (Newacheck, Brindis, Cart, Marchi, & Irwin, 1999).

A complex array of factors–including individual, family, community, and socio-economic influences–affect adolescent health. Efforts to improve adolescent health must reflect this complexity. Findings from Add Health and other studies using ecological approaches suggest that comprehensive strategies that aim to create supportive home, school and after-school environments are needed to reduce the prevalence of risk-taking behaviors and promote healthy adolescent development.

Addressing these issues requires changes at multiple levels–from service delivery, to community environments, resource allocation at the local, state and national levels, and more fundamentally, to the behavior and attitudes of adults who are responsible for raising and nurturing youth. Adolescents across all racial and ethnic groups need access to diverse preventive, diagnostic, and treatment services to address the medical and psychosocial health problems that affect their age group. Furthermore, attention must be focused on providing culturally sensitive and tailored services that focus more directly upon their unique needs. Eliminating economic disparities that are often reflected in the ethnic and racial profiles of youth must also be addressed. While the data presented here provide guidance for policy makers and program managers in identifying the most important health issues and which populations need to be reached with more effective strategies, it continues to be limited by a lack of socioeconomic and other contextual factors that influence individual behavior. In addition, national data on the prevalence of mental health problems are also lacking. Given the importance of mental health in the lives of young people, this data gap is especially noteworthy.

As the field of adolescent health continues to evolve, it will be necessary to integrate risk reduction, youth development, and holistic approaches in order to assure a more comprehensive and affirming approach to adolescence. The changing demographics of this population also require greater awareness, understanding, and integration of cultural competency within societal institutions. Building on the important lessons learned about preventing risk-taking behaviors among adolescents, the field is broadening to better understand how to build assets and to create healthier environments for young people with the aim of reducing the prevalence of risk-taking behaviors. In a nation that highly values individualism, it is critical to acknowledge that complex interactions between the environment and the individual affect adolescent behavior and development through adulthood. Doing so places the responsibility of helping today's youth where it belongs–on society as a collective. It is important to recognize the value of clearly defining potential roles, activities, and joint actions and work collectively to have a substantial impact on adolescent health (Brindis et al., 1998). Developing a comprehensive framework from which to identify health and social problems and associated factors allows improved planning and program and policy implementation to address these problems. Despite the limitations noted here, these data can serve to mobilize communities to take action to address the problems of the country's young people and promote adolescent development.

NOTE

1. All rates are per 100,000 unless otherwise indicated.

REFERENCES

Bloom, B., & Tonthat, L. (2002). *Summary health statistics for U.S. children: National Health Interview Survey, 1997* (DHHS Publication No. PHS 2002-1531). Washington, D.C.: U.S. Government Printing Office.

Bogenscheneider, K. (1966). An ecological risk/protective theory for building prevention programs, policies, and community capacity to support youth. *Family Relations, 45*, 127-138.

Brindis, C. D., Ozer, E. M., Handley, M., Knopf, D. K., Millstein, S. G., & Irwin, C. E., Jr. (1998). *Improving adolescent health: An analysis and synthesis of health policy recommendations, full report.* San Francisco, CA: University of California, San Francisco, National Adolescent Health Information Center.

Brindis, C. D., VanLandeghem, K., Kirkpatrick, R., Lee, S., & Macdonald, T. (1999). *Adolescents and the State Children's Health Insurance Program (CHIP): Health options for meeting the needs of adolescents.* Washington, D.C.: Association of

Maternal and Child Health Programs; and San Francisco: University of California, San Francisco, Policy Information and Analysis Center for Middle Childhood and Adolescence and the National Adolescent Health Information Center.

Census Bureau. (2000). *Projections of the resident population by age, sex, race, and Hispanic origin: 1999-2100* (NP-D1-A). Washington, D.C.: U.S. Bureau of the Census. Retrieved February 4, 2002, from (http://www.census.gov/population/www/projections/natdet-D1A.html).

Census Bureau. (2001). *Current population survey, March 2001: Table 1. General mobility, by region, sex, and age.* Washington, D.C.: U.S. Bureau of the Census. Retrieved, from (http://www.census.gov/population/www/socdemo/migrate/p20-538.html).

Centers for Disease Control and Prevention [CDC]. (2000). *Tracking the hidden epidemics: Trends in STDs in the United States, 2000.* Atlanta, GA: Centers for Disease Control and Prevention, National Center for HIV, STD and TB Prevention, Division of Sexually Transmitted Diseases. Retrieved May 3, 2002, from (http://www.cdc.gov/nchstp/dstd/Stats_ Trends/Trends2000.pdf).

Centers for Disease Control and Prevention [CDC]. (2001). *STD surveillance, 2000.* Atlanta, GA: Centers for Disease Control and Prevention, National Center for HIV, STD and TB Prevention, Division of Sexually Transmitted Diseases. Retrieved May 3, 2002, from (http://www.cdc.gov/std/stats/TOC2000.htm).

Centers for Disease Control and Prevention [CDC]. (2002). *HIV/AIDS surveillance report, 2001*. Atlanta, GA: Centers for Disease Control and Prevention, National Center for HIV, STD, and TB Prevention, Division of HIV/AIDS Prevention. Retrieved May 3, 2002, from (http://www.cdc.gov/hiv/stats/hasrlink.htm).

Centers for Disease Control and Prevention. (n.d.). *Young people at risk: HIV/AIDS among America's youth.* Atlanta, GA: Centers for Disease Control and Prevention, National Center for HIV, STD and TB Prevention, Division of HIV/AIDS Prevention. Retrieved May 3, 2002, from (http://www.cdc.gov/hiv/stat-trends.htm).

Clayton, S. L., Brindis, C. D., Hamor, J. A., Raiden-Wright, H., & Fong, C. (2000). *Investing in adolescent health: A social imperative for California's future.* San Francisco, CA: University of California, San Francisco. National Adolescent Health Information Center.

Dalaker, J., & Proctor, B. D. (2000). *Poverty in the United States: 1999.* Washington, DC: U.S. Government Printing Office.

Dryfoos, J.G. (1998). *Full-Service schools: A revolution in health and social services for children, youth, and families.* San Francisco, CA: Jossey-Bass, Inc.

Fox, J. A., & Zawitz, M. W. (2001). *Homicide trends in the United States.* Retrieved March 22, 2002, from (http://www.ojp.usdoj.gov/bjs/homicide/homtrnd.htm).

Grunbaum, J.A., Kann, L., Kinchen, S. A., Williams, B., Ross, J.G., & Lowry, R. et al. (2002). Youth Risk Behavior Surveillance–United States, 2001. *Morbidity and Mortality Weekly Report, 51* (No. SS-4).

Hoyert, D. L., Arias, E., Smith, B. L., Murphy, S. L., & Kochanek, K. D. (2001). Deaths: Final data for 1999. *National Vital Statistics Reports, 49*(8). Retrieved March 15, 2001, from (http://www.cdc.gov/nchs/about/major/dvs/mortdata.htm).

Irwin, C. E., Jr., Brindis, C., Holt, K. A., & Langlykke, K. (Eds). (1994). *Health care reform: Opportunities for improving adolescent health.* Arlington, VA: National Center for Education in Maternal and Child Health.

Johnston, L. D., O'Malley, P. M., & Bachman, J. G. (2002). *Monitoring the Future: National survey results on drug use, 1975-2001. Volume I: Secondary school students* (NIH Publication No. 02-5106). Bethesda, MD: National Institute on Drug Abuse.

Kann, L., Kinchen, S. A., Williams, B. I., Ross, J. G., Lowry, R., & Brunbaum, J.A. et al. (2000). Youth Risk Behavior Surveillance–United States, 1999. *Morbidity and Mortality Weekly Report, 49* (No. SS-5).

Kann, L., Kinchen, S.A., Williams, B.I., Ross, J.G., Warren, C., & Harris, W. et al. (1998). Youth Risk Behavior Surveillance–United States, 1997. *Morbidity and Mortality Weekly Report, 47* (No.SS-3).

Leaf, P. J., Alegria, M., Cohen, P., Goodman, S. H., Horwitz, S. M., & Hoven, C. W. et al. (1996). Mental health service use in the community and schools: Results from the four-community MECA study. *Journal of the American Academy of Child & Adolescent Psychiatry, 35*(7), 889-897.

Mackay, A. P., Fingerhut, L. A., & Duran, C. R. (2000). *Adolescent health chartbook, Health, United States, 2000.* Hyattsville, MD: National Center for Health Statistics, Centers for Disease Control and Prevention.

Martin, J. A., Hamilton, B. E., Ventura, S. A., Menacker, F., & Park, M. M. (2002). Births: Final data for 2000. *National Vital Statistics Reports, 50*(5).

Montgomery, L. E., Kiely, J. L, & Papas, G. (1996). The effects of poverty, race, and family structure on U.S. children's health: Data from the NHIS, 1978 through 1980 and 1989 through 1991. *American Journal of Public Health, 86*(10), 1401-5.

Newacheck, P., Brindis, C. D., Cart, C. U., Marchi, K., & Irwin, Jr., C. (1999). Adolescent health insurance coverage: Recent changes and access to care. *Pediatrics, 104*(2),195-202.

National Center for Injury Prevention and Control [NCIPC]. (2002). *United States Injury Mortality Statistics* (Private data run). Atlanta, GA: Centers for Disease Control and Prevention. Available from NCIPC Web site (http://www.cdc.gov/ncipc).

National Health Interview Survey [NHIS]. (2002). *Health Statistics* (Private data run). Atlanta, GA: Centers for Disease Control and Prevention. Available from NHIS Web site (http://www.cdc.gov/nchs/nhis.htm).

National Health and Nutrition Examination Survey [NHANES], Centers for Disease Control and Prevention. (2002). *Prevalence of Overweight Among Children and Adolescents: United States, 1999.* Retrieved February 4, 2002, from (http://www.cdc.gov/nchs/products/pubs/pubd/hestats/overwght99.htm).

National Research Council, Panel on High Risk Youth. (1993). *Losing Generations: Adolescents in High-Risk Settings.* Washington, DC: National Academy Press.

National Vital Statistics System [NVSS], Centers for Disease Control and Prevention. (2002). *Mortality Data.* Available from NVSS Web site, (http://www.cdc.gov/nchs/nvss.htm).

Ozer, E.M., Brindis, C. D., Millstein, S. G., Knopf, D. K., & Irwin, C. E., Jr. (1998). *America's adolescents: Are they healthy?* San Francisco, CA: University of California, San Francisco, National Adolescent Health Information Center.

Rennison, C. (2001). *Violent victimization and race, 1993-1998* (NCJ 176354). Retrieved March 4, 2002, from (http://www.ojp.usdoj.gov/bjs/pub/pdf/vvr98.pdf).

Resnick, M. D., Bearman, P. S., Blum, R. W., Bauman, K. E., Harris, K. M., & Jones, J. et al. (1997). Protecting adolescents from harm: Findings from the National Longitudinal Study on Adolescent Health. *Journal of the American Medical Association, 278*(10), 823-832.

Rickel, A., & Becker, E. (1997). *Keeping children from harm's way: How national policy affects psychological development.* Washington, DC: American Psychological Association.

Roberts, R. E., Lewinsohn, P. M., & Seeley, J. R. (1995). Symptoms of DSM-II-R major depression in adolescence: Evidence from an epidemiological survey. *Journal of the American Academy of Child and Adolescent Psychiatry, 34*(7), 1608-1617.

Substance Abuse and Mental Health Services Administration [SAMHSA]. (2002). *Results from the 2001 National Household Survey on Drug Abuse: Volume 1. Summary of national findings* (DHHS Publication No. SMA 02-3758). Rockville, MD: Substance Abuse and Mental Health Services Administration, Office of Applied Studies.

Shaffer, D., Fisher, P., Dulcan, M. K., Davies, M., Piacentini, J., & Schwab-Stone, M. E. et al. (1996). The NIMH Diagnostic Interview Schedule for Children Version 2.3 (DISC-2.3): Description, acceptability, prevalence rates, and performance in the MECA study. *Journal of the American Academy of Child and Adolescent Psychiatry, 35*(7), 865-877.

Snyder, H. N., & Sickmund, M. (1999). *Juvenile offenders and victims: 1999 national report.* Washington, D.C.: Office of Juvenile Justice and Delinquency Prevention.

Taylor-Gibbs, J. (1999). The California crucible: Towards a new paradigm of race and ethnic relations. *Journal of Multicultural Social Work*, 7(1/2), 1-18.

Troiano, R. P., Flegal, K. M., Kuczmarksi, R. J., Campbell, S. M., & Johnson, C. L. (1995). Overweight prevalence and trends for children and adolescents. The National Health and Nutrition Examination Surveys, 1963 to 1991. *Archives of Pediatric and Adolescent Medicine, 149*(10), 1085-91.

U.S. Department of Health and Human Services. (1999). *Mental Health: A Report of the Surgeon General.* Rockville, MD: U.S. Department of Health and Human Services.

Ventura, S. J., Mosher, W. D., Curtin, M. A., Abma, J. C., & Henshaw, S. (2001). Trends in Pregnancy Rates for the United States, 1976-97: An Update. *National Vital Statistics Reports, 49*(4).

Winkleby, M., Robinson, T., Sundquist, J., & Kraemer, H. (1999). Ethnic variation in cardiovascular disease risk factors among children and young adults: Findings from the Third National Health and Nutrition Examination Survey, 1988-1994. *JAMA, 281*, 1006-1013.

W. K. Kellogg Foundation. (1998). *Safe passages through adolescence: Communities protecting the health and hopes of youth.* Battlecreek, MI: W. K. Kellogg Foundation.

Zill, N., & Nord, C. W. (1994). *Running in Place: How American Families Are Faring in a Changing Economy and an Individualistic Society.* Washington, DC: Child Trends, Inc.

Latina Students: Translating Cultural Wealth into Social Capital to Improve Academic Success

Ruth Enid Zambrana
Irene M. Zoppi

SUMMARY. Latina students have the highest high school dropout rate of all racial and ethnic groups. This article has three objectives: provide a brief overview of educational trends for Latina students, discuss factors associated with their educational trajectory and suggest strategies for change based on best practice wisdom. Results show that academic disparities between Latina students and other racial/ethnic female students begin as early as kindergarten and remain through age 17; achievement is compromised by a variety of factors, including family responsibilities, family poverty, lack of participation in preschool, attendance at poor quality elementary and high schools, placement into lower-track classes, poor self-image, limited neighborhood resources, lack of presence of role models and gender role attitudes. These disparities contribute to psychosocial issues and are not directly associated with Latino cultural

Ruth Enid Zambrana, PhD, is Professor and Graduate Director, Women's Studies Department, University of Maryland, College Park and Adjunct Professor of Family Medicine, University of Maryland Baltimore, School of Medicine, Department of Family Medicine. Irene M. Zoppi is a Doctoral Student and Graduate Assistant, College of Education, University of Maryland, College Park.

[Haworth co-indexing entry note]: "Latina Students: Translating Cultural Wealth into Social Capital to Improve Academic Success." Zambrana, Ruth Enid, and Irene M. Zoppi. Co-published simultaneously in *Journal of Ethnic & Cultural Diversity in Social Work* (The Haworth Social Work Practice Press, an imprint of The Haworth Press, Inc.) Vol. 11, No. 1/2, 2002, pp. 33-53; and: *Social Work with Multicultural Youth* (ed: Diane de Anda) The Haworth Social Work Practice Press, an imprint of The Haworth Press, Inc., 2002, pp. 33-53. Single or multiple copies of this article are available for a fee from The Haworth Document Delivery Service [1-800-HAWORTH, 9:00 a.m. - 5:00 p.m. (EST). E-mail address: docdelivery@haworthpress.com].

http://www.haworthpress.com/store/product.asp?sku=J051

10.1300/J051v11n01_02

assets, as Latino cultural capital has not been easily translated into social capital in U.S. society. Economic and social change must precede educational change if academic disparities between Latinas and other racial and ethnic girls are to be decreased.

KEYWORDS. Latina, Latina students, cultural wealth, social capital, academic success, achievement gap, underachievement, improvement

INTRODUCTION

> If culture is what sets one country apart from another, then educate women and you shall have a school in every home, for it is she who shapes the family and stamps upon society the seal of her culture.
>
> *Ana Roque de Duprey, Puerto Rico, 1899*

This article provides a brief overview of educational trends for Latina students, discusses factors associated with their educational trajectory, and suggests strategies for change. Strategies for change can be based on best practice wisdom, which is derived from a perspective of how to translate cultural wealth into social capital. Social capital refers to family and community networks, norms and trust that facilitate coordination and cooperation for mutual benefit. These family and community resources provide access to benefits and investment in individuals' human capital (Bourdieu, 1985; Putnam, 1993, 1995; Portes, 2000).

This article focuses on historically underrepresented and educationally disadvantaged groups in the United States. It departs from the premise that economic disadvantaged status is a central barrier to educational achievement in the U.S. for Latinos.

BACKGROUND

Limitations of Data Sources

Despite the rapid growth of the Latino[1] population in the U.S. and the large percentage of Latinas (51.5%) within the greater Latino population, data on this population are still limited (Hajat, Lucas & Kingston, 2000). Data on Latinos/as were not available until 1975, since until then only four race categories were used: Black, White, Asian and "Other." In 1974, Latinos were placed under the category of "Spanish-surnamed American" (Department of Education 1976). In 1980, the census began to collect Hispanic data, and major educational and health research surveys included Latino-specific data for the first time (National Council of La Raza, 1998; Zambrana & Carter-Pokras, 2001).

A review of literature reveals limited information on the experience of Latinas in education (Zambrana, 1987; Meier & Stewart, 1991; Arellano & Padilla, 1996; Marcano, 1997; Romo, 1998; Bass, 1990; Trueba et al., 1993; Gándara, 1995; Trueba, 1999; Garcia, 2000; Garza, 2001; Alejandro, 2002). Empirical studies rarely focus on how Latino students differ by country of origin, immigration status, socioeconomic status, geographic region, or, more relevant for this article, gender. Because national data are seldom disaggregated by gender, race and ethnicity, little knowledge exists about how the educational needs, achievements, or problems for Latinas from different subethnic groups differ from each other and from those of males (Ginorio & Huston, 2001). Below the authors provide a brief profile of Latino families and youth.

Sociodemographic Profile of Latino Families and Youth

Latino children are one of the fastest growing population groups in the nation. In 2000, 64% of U.S. children were non-Hispanic White (herein after referred to as White); 16% were Latino; 15% were African American; 4% were Asian/Pacific Islander; and 1% were American Indian/Alaska Native (U.S. Census Bureau, 2001). The number of Latino children has increased faster than that of any other racial and ethnic group, growing from 9% of the child population in 1980 to 16% in 2000. Poverty rates vary by race and ethnicity. In 1998, 36.4% of African American children and 33.6% of Latino children lived in poverty, compared to 10% of White children. Puerto Rican and Mexican origin children represent the poorest subgroups among Latinos. The increase in Latino poverty is associated with three factors: historically lower academic achievement of Latinos and lower educational and economic attainment of immigrants (especially Mexican immigrants), combined with higher fertility among Latino women (for a review, see Flores et al., 2002). The percentage of children who are foreign-born varies substantially by racial and ethnic background. In 1990, 98% of the White, African American and American Indian populations were U.S. citizens, compared to 67% of the Asian and 84% of the Hispanic populations. Although language and citizenship have been associated with Latino educational achievement, 1999 data from the U.S. Census Bureau show that the majority of Latino children are U.S. citizens and 77% of children of Hispanic origin did not have difficulty speaking English (Federal Interagency Forum on Child and Family Statistics, 2002).

Briefly examining data on Latinas provides a profile of their educational, economic and family status. In 1990, there were 7 million Latinas age 16 years and over in the U.S., and that number rose to 11 million by the end of 1999. Overall, the Latina population increased by 52% during this time period, compared with 17% for African American women and 7% for White women (U.S. Census Bureau, 2001). Not unexpectedly, 54% of Latinas are poor or near poor and have the lowest percentage of high school graduates (57.5%) compared to all other racial and ethnic groups. The lack of educational attainment is closely associated with high levels of poverty that hinders opportunities for their social mobility and intergenerational mobility. Over the next several decades, Latinas will constitute more than 40% of new labor force entrants (National Council of La Raza (NCLR), 1998). These data are compelling because education is often a prerequisite for entering higher-paying occupations, and Latinas' earnings are greatly affected by the education they have attained. Among Latinas age 25 years and over who were participants of the labor force in 1999, those with less than a high school diploma were the largest group. Data show that 30% of Latinas in the labor force were high school graduates with no college; 17% had some college, but no degree; 7% had associate degrees; and 15% were college graduates (U.S. Census Bureau, 2001). Higher educational attainment generally results in higher labor force participation, lower unemployment rates and resources for investment in the future of one's children. Thus, current low-income Latinas who are the mothers of young Latino girls have limited economic resources to invest in their daughters.

These education and labor force profiles of Latinas signal a need to examine why the education of Latino girls has been neglected (Ginorio & Huston, 2001; National Alliance for Hispanic Health, 2000). Only recently have several reports focused on the plight of Latino girls and educational attainment (Ginorio & Huston, 2001; The State of Hispanic Girls, 2001). Although some work has been conducted on resiliency and Latinos, these studies focus on the rare instances rather than the overwhelming majority of young low-income Latinas who do not complete their education (So, 1987; Arellano & Padilla, 1996). In contrast, the prior focus of research was on ethnic specific educational deficits and failure, with limited attention to institutional factors such as poor quality of public educational systems in low-income Latino communities, low teacher expectations and other forms of racism and discrimination that plague Latino students (Meier & Stewart, 1989; Abi Nader, 1990; NCLR, 1998).

TRENDS IN EDUCATION

Although the number of Latino children and youth in elementary and secondary public schools in the U.S. is 15% of K-12 students overall (The White House Initiative on Educational Excellence for Hispanic Americans, 2000), it is projected to increase to 25% by 2025. Three major trends are associated with sub-optimal educational achievement: concentration and segregation in resource-poor, low quality schools; non-participation in early preschools; and high school non-completion. Latino children are concentrated in ten states with close to 50% of the Latino (Mexican origin subgroup) population residing in California and Texas. Moreover, Latino children account for a large and growing population of the nation's student population (13.5%), with high elementary and secondary enrollment in the top 10 states where Latino children reside. The percent of student enrollment by state for Latino children are: New Mexico, (46.6%); California, (38.7%); Texas, (36.7%); Arizona, (30%); Colorado, (18.4%); New York, (17.4%); Florida, (15.3%); New Jersey, (13.5%); Illinois, (12.2%); and Massachusetts, (9.3%) (U.S. Department of Education, 2001).

Overall these states tend to have low ranking with respect to quality education (dollars spent on education per child, number of students per teacher in the classroom) and are more likely to serve low-income populations who are not encouraged or do not know how to actively engage the schools for more resources and responsiveness to their children (U.S. Department of Education, 1995, 2001; NCLR, 1998). In examining early childhood education trends (see Figure 1), one observes that Latino students are significantly less likely to attend pre-school (Early Start and Head Start) than White or African American children and thus, less likely to be adequately prepared for entry into kindergarten. While 36% of Latino children live in poverty, only 26% attend Head Start programs that are designed to prepare students to enter elementary school ready to learn (Federal Interagency Forum on Child and Family Statistics, 2002). A number of factors may account for lower enrollment

FIGURE 1. Early Childhood Education

Children Ages 3 to 4 Who Are Enrolled in Preschool

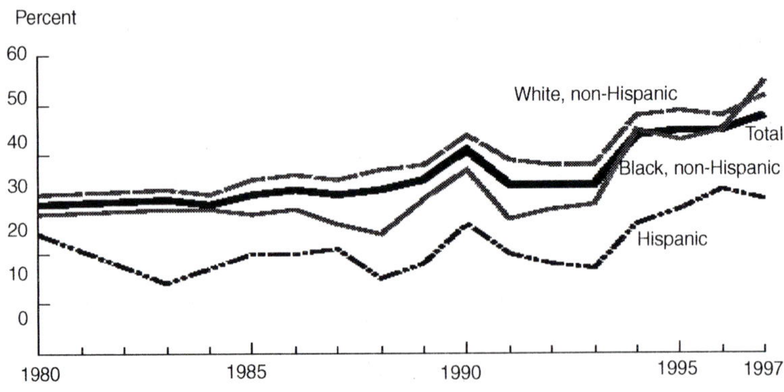

Source: U.S. Department of Education. National Center for Education Statistics. (2001). *Dropout Rates in the United States*, NCES 2002-114, Washington, DC: Kaufman, Phillip; Alt, Martha Naomi; Chapman, Christopher.

in preschools: institutional lack of outreach, teacher attitudes, parental attitudes and lack of knowledge, and language.

The majority of preschool teachers do not perceive themselves to be fully prepared to meet the needs of students with limited English-language proficiency or from diverse cultural backgrounds (Alejandro, 2002). This lack of preparedness or willingness to assist Latino students seriously impedes the quality of their education and, perhaps also, their access to the necessary cognitive and social skills required to compete academically. As the Latino population increases, the need for educators to ensure these students' access to the same educational opportunities as other ethnic groups is critical to the academic success of Latino youth. In 1999, 23% of Latino children had difficulty speaking English compared to 12% of other racial and ethnic groups (Federal Interagency Forum on Child and Family Statistics, 2002). Since low-income Mexican American and Puerto Rican youth have disproportionately higher high school dropout rates that in some regions of the country rise close to 50%, these data suggest that language alone is not the major barrier in achieving academically.

One of the most commonly cited measures of a group's educational progress is its high school graduation rate (Ginorio & Huston, 2001).

Hispanic youth have the highest national dropout rate. However, data fail to capture the loss of students prior to high school graduation. The metaphor of the pipeline for Latino students begins as early as the 7th grade when illiterate students begin to fall behind, young Latino boys and girls enter juvenile detention systems, and/or others assume familial economic provider roles. The last decade has not witnessed considerable improvement in high school completion rates for Latino youth. Dropout rates ranged from 34.8% in 1972 to 32.8% in 1982, 26.6% in 1992 and 26% in 2000 (U.S. Department of Education, National Center for Education Statistics, June 2002). In October 1989, 33% of the Latino population ages 16-24 had not completed high school (Kaufman & Frase, 1990). In 1998, the 30% dropout rate, which represented 1.5 million Latino students ages 16-24, continued to be higher than the rates in other groups–14% for African American youth and 8% for White youth (see Figure 2). According to the data, Latino youth have a high school dropout rate almost four times the rate of White youth (U.S. Census, 2001). The percentage of Latino young adults who were out of school without a high school diploma has remained higher than that of African American and White youth in every year throughout the recent 29-year period (U.S. Department of Education, 2002).

FIGURE 2. High School Dropout Rates for 16 Through 24-Year-Olds, by Race/Ethnicity (October 1972-October 2000)

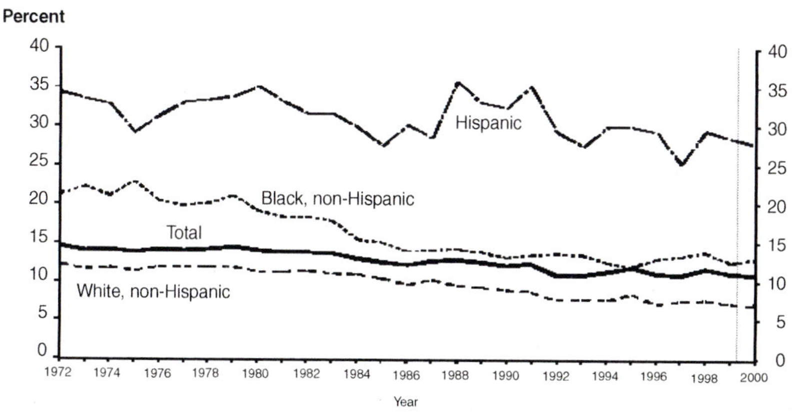

Source: Federal Interagency Forum on Chld and Family Statistics. (2002). *America's Children: Key National Indicators of Well-Being.* Washington, DC: U.S. Government Printing Office.

The graduation rate for Latinas remains lower than any other female racial and ethnic group. In 1993, 8% of Latina students dropped out of school, compared with 5% of African American and 4% of White girls (Ginorio & Huston, 2001). Figure 3 depicts a decrease in the dropout rate of Latino girls from 1972-2000. Despite this decrease, a recent review found that Latinas are lagging behind other racial and ethnic groups of girls in several key measures of educational achievement and have not benefited from gender equity to the extent that other groups have. In comparison to their White or Asian counterparts, Latinas are less likely to take the SAT, and those who do score lower on average than the former. Compared with their female peers, Latinas are under-enrolled in gifted and talented education courses and underrepresented in Advanced Placement (AP) courses (Ginorio & Huston, 2001).

Interestingly, Latino girls overall perform better that Latino boys in multiple areas. In the fourth grade, Latinas score higher than Latinos in reading and history; by the eighth grade, they score higher in mathematics and reading. Finally, by the 12th grade, they score higher in science and reading. However, while Latinas outnumber Latinos in taking the SAT (58% to 42% in 1999), they score lower than Latinos who do take the exam on both the math and verbal sections, and this gender gap between Latinos is greater in comparison to any other group (U.S. Department of Education, 2001; NCLR, 1998, White House Initiative for Hispanic Education, 2000a, b). Although Latinas take the same number or more AP exams than Latinos, they score lower in AP math and science exams. Interestingly, Latinas are almost three times less likely to be suspended and less likely to be referred for special education than Latinos (Federal Interagency Forum on Child and Family Statistics,

FIGURE 3. Latinas Dropout Rates

Source: National Center for Education Statistics, Department of Education, Office of Eduational Research and Improvement (2000). *Dropout Rates in the United States* (NCES 2001-034). Washington, DC.

2002). Examining institutional and familial factors may explain these gaps in achievement.

FAMILY AND INSTITUTIONAL FACTORS ASSOCIATED WITH LATINA EDUCATIONAL ACHIEVEMENT

Because academic disparities between Latina students and other racial and ethnic students begin as early as kindergarten and remain through age 17, newer empirical work has focused on articulating the multiple individual, familial, and institutional factors associated with Latina educational achievement (Arellano & Padilla, 1996; Gándara, 1995, 1999; Alejandro, 2002). Although Latinos have high aspirations for themselves, Latino achievement is compromised by a variety of factors, including poverty, lack of participation in preschool, attendance at poor quality elementary and high schools, placement into lower-track classes, poor self-image, limited neighborhood resources, and the presence of few role models, and gender role attitudes (Zambrana, Dorrington & Bell, 1997; National Council La Raza, 1998; Evelyn, 2000; Niemann, Romero & Arbona, 2000; Nieto, 2000; Ginorio & Huston, 2001).

Institutional resources are highly linked with geographic region and place of residence of students. For Latino children, close to 40% live in poverty and attend inner city or rural schools where both schools and home environments lack educational materials such as computers and books. Despite the fact that computers are essential tools, fewer Latinas than other female students from other ethnic groups have access to a computer at home or school. Latina students use a computer at school 68% of the time (compared with 70% of African American and 84% of White students), and only 18% of Latina students (compared with 19% of African American and 52% of White students) use a computer at home (David & Lucile Packard Foundation, 2000). Limited access to these educational resources compromises Latinas' access to resources required to compete successfully in high school.

Attitudes of instructional personnel in the schools and limited access to mentors and positive role models in the home, school or community are factors that greatly hinder educational achievement among Latinas (So, 1987; Trueba, 1999). Only about 4% of public school teachers and 4.1% principals (3,269 out of 79,618 nationwide) are Latinos whereas Latinos constitute 15% of the student body (Digest of Education Statistics 2000, Table 85, p. 93). Not surprisingly, in 1993-94, the base salary of Latino/a teachers was the lowest nationwide as compared to other racial/ethnic teachers (Digest of Education Statistics 2000, Table 74, p. 82). The limited representation of Latino personnel, such as teachers and principals, undoubtedly makes the representation of Latino issues less likely in the school system. Additionally, factors such as lack of available after-school educational and recreational programs and lack of encouragement to participate in school programs and activities are issues affecting Latinas in their educational attainment. School factors seem to be a major issue in contributing to the dropout rate of Latinas. Issues such as poor academic performance, lack of school counseling, and advice steering students into vocational education for jobs with little career or income potential are known to affect Latino achievement (Romo & Falbo, 1996). Thus, the lack of acknowledgment that educational achievement is highly associated with access to social capital in the form of translators, bridges to information, guidance, role models, and respect for culture and language strongly supports the notion of benign neglect of Latino girls in schools (deAnda, 1984; Abi-Nader, 1990; NCLR, 1998).

Culture-specific family responsibilities in low-income Latino families such as sibling care and economic contributions have been linked to less time and emphasis on educational goals (Gándara, 1995, 1999; Zambrana, Dorrington, & Bell, 1997). Closely related are more traditional gender role attitudes and behaviors that may not promote assertiveness and independence in pursuing one's individual goals, such as education (Gonzalez-Ramos et al., 1998). Gender-role attitudes in U.S. society, schools, and families contribute to Latinas' poor educational performance (Romo, 1998). Oftentimes, low-income Latinas do not foresee their possibilities for doing well in school and pursuing postsecondary education or careers, and so leave school and start a family. One study reported that one-third of Latinas, ages 9-15, left school due to pregnancy or marriage. Compared to other racial/ethnic groups, Latinas had the highest decline in self-esteem: 38% in high school, 59% in middle school, and 79% in elementary school (AAUW Educational Foundation, 1995). Gender roles and stereotypes of Latinas as submissive, underachievers, and caretakers of elder/younger family members are often reinforced by family, school personnel and media (De León, 1996; Ginorio & Huston, 2001).

Parents play an important role in advocating for their children in the school system. Yet, Latino parents tend to be poor and less educated than other groups and reside in areas where there is less parent leadership and civic engagement around improving schools. Furthermore, resource-poor schools are less likely to engage parents. Although Latino mothers are more likely to engage in social activities with their children, such as eating dinner together and daily outings, than White and African American mothers, they are less likely to report helping children with homework or reading to them (Federal Interagency Forum on Child and Family Statistics, 2002). Latino parents need to be encouraged to take a more active role, both at home and in their community, in improving the educational system for their daughters.

NEW FINDINGS ON LATINA STUDENTS: FACTORS LINKED TO POVERTY, SCHOOL ACHIEVEMENT, AND EDUCATIONAL DISPARITIES

Recent data show a cluster of risk behaviors for Latino children and adolescents that may have important associations with patterns of low educational attainment. Data on risk behaviors show that almost one-fourth of 10th-grade Latino adolescents report heavy drinking and illicit drug use in the past thirty days (Johnson et al., 1998). Although these rates are comparable to White youth, they are significantly higher than the rates for African American adolescents. A 1997 Survey of the Health of Adolescent Girls found that more than half of all girls who engage in risk behaviors such as using cigarettes, alcohol and illegal drugs, binging and purging food, and/or not exercising are also more likely to engage in other or more damaging behaviors. In the study, White and Latino girls were more likely to engage in risk behaviors than African American or Asian American girls (Schoen et al., 1997). Rates of smoking differ substantially across groups with White students more likely to smoke, followed by Latino and African American students. Use of any substance places a youth at risk of intentional and unintentional injury as well as risk of legal intervention. Both of these outcomes decrease the likelihood of academic achievement.

Latino adolescents are at risk of experiencing and witnessing violence and are at higher risk of attempting or committing suicide at a younger age than either African American or White youth (Hovey & King, 1996). Persistent worries by the adolescent, coupled with high rates of poverty and poor resources, including poor community and school environments, contribute to feelings of limited hope and depression. Depression is highly linked with suicide and attempted suicide (Hovey & King, 1996; National Alliance of Hispanic Health, 1999). Latino girls are more likely to report depression, attempt suicide, and use substances than White or African American girls (National Alliance for Hispanic Health, 1999).

Suicide attempts and ideations have been linked with gender. Females are more likely to attempt suicide than males. However, in the Latino population, the suicide rate for males and females are comparable, and suicides occur at younger ages than in the White population, with almost one-third occurring under age 25 (Hovey & King, 1996). Suicidal attempts and suicide may also reflect the effects of other stressful life events such as physical and sexual abuse, family conflicts and intergenerational conflicts (Zambrana & Silva Palacios, 1989; Schoen et al., 1997; National Alliance for Hispanic Health, 1999) (see Figure 4). As Rodríguez and Ramírez de Arellano (1994) noted in reference to Latino youth, especially female, "the fact that suicidal behavior is so prevalent in the face of deterrents such as religious values suggests that a significant proportion of Latino youth are in deep despair and unable to get the help they need" (p. 127).

In summary, recent data show that Latinas are at higher risk of depression, suicide attempts, use of alcohol, cigarettes and illegal drugs than African Americans girls. In addition, they are more likely to be overweight, engage in less physical activity, and are less likely to use condoms during sexual activity than White girls (National Alliance of Hispanic Health, 1999; Abma & Sonenstein, 2001; Centers for Disease Control and Prevention, 2002). These factors, in conjunction with low family socio-economic status, immigrant status, inadequate negotiating skills, low value concordance with U.S. dominant culture, and institu-

FIGURE 4. Suicide Attempts Among Latina Students by Race/Ethnicity: Grades 9-12, 1999

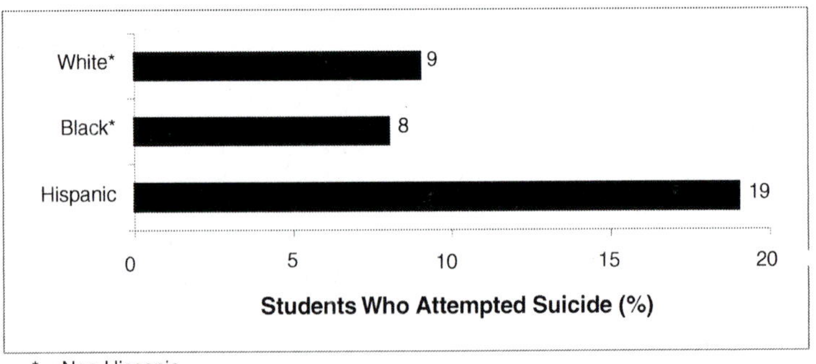

* = Non-Hispanic
Source: National Center for Health Statistics, 1999

tional racism and discrimination, may push Latinas into early exits from school due to uncertain futures (Tinajero, Gonzales, & Dick, 1991; Gonzalez-Ramos, Zayas & Cohen, 1998; Flores et al., 2002; Alejandro, 2002).

CULTURAL WEALTH OF LATINO FAMILIES

Latino families and their daughters confront special challenges as an outcome of the intersection of ethnicity, race, socioeconomic status and receptivity by the host society (Romo & Fablo, 1996; Romo, 1998; Walsh, 1991; Alejandro, 2002). These challenges are not directly associated with Latino cultural assets, as Latino cultural capital has not been easily translated into social capital in U.S. society. Cultural wealth can be defined as a set of values and norms that guide behavior. The resilience literature identifies three domains that are associated with resilient individuals: internal resources, family climate, and social environment (Arellano & Padilla, 1996; Brooke, 1994; The National Alliance for Hispanic Health, 2000). The cultural assets of Latino families are consistent with defined resilient characteristics and include: having religious faith, emphasizing a collective orientation, valuing children and engaging in multiple affective gestures from early on, teaching children values which include responsibility to others, collective responsibility, respecting elders and authority figures, and sibling responsibility, and valuing civility such as the expression of politeness and helpful behaviors (Trueba, 1993; Gonzalez-Ramos, 1998; Sotomayor, 1991; Rodríguez, 1999). Yet anchors or role models that encourage development of self-discipline through positive feedback, problem-solving skills, and access to resources are not readily available to Latinas in their community and school environment. Resiliency is a transactional process that shapes one's sense of self-esteem and sense of mastery, and requires self-discipline to be sustained. Inherent to the continued development of resiliency, the environment in which a Latina functions, schools in this case, must value the cultural assets and strengths she brings as social capital on which to build her academic success.

Social capital has been conceptualized in many different forms to include family and community resources and social networks of civic engagement (voting, participation in boards, advocacy work) (Bourdieu, 1985; Putnam, 1993, 1995; Portes, 2000). Through social capital, Latino families can translate and transmit their cultural assets intergenerationally. Family benefits and resources, if mediated by non-family networks such as teachers and principals in schools, can be used as a means for upper mobility (Portes, 2000). Schools have an important effect on the development of human capital, combined with the social and political environments that enable norms to develop and shape social structure (Bourdieu, 1985; North, 1990; The World Bank, 1998). For example, the support of bilingual schools and the use of Latino cultural representations, such as family stories, would contribute to promoting an educational structure that is more receptive and valuing of Latino culture. According to Gándara (1995), family stories were examples of cultural capital that helped students achieve academically.

The concept of social capital, as noted by Portes (2000) and others, provides some explanatory power for understanding the historical and contemporary underachievement of low-income historically underrepresented Latinos. The Latino culture and the host society have discordant value bases for individual achievement and social interactions that contribute to exclusionary and discriminatory practices in the educational system. For Latinos, "culture is the center of individual self-value" (Alejandro, 2002). Yet, education is transformational and schools reproduce and transmit social capital with little acknowledgement of difference. Hence, students are consumers of the host culture in their efforts to survive (Coleman, 1988; Bourdieu, 1977, 1985). For low-income Latinas, the conflict of familial values with host culture values of independence, assertiveness, and competitiveness combined with stereotypic, negative and unwelcoming attitudes of school personnel, hinder their learning process and achievement (Trueba, 1999; Alejandro, 2002). Cultural assets need to be valued within the societal structure in which they operate so as to strengthen Latino family and child infrastructure; if cultural assets do not produce economic wealth, the assets erode in their interaction with a devaluing society. The process of erosion is most highly associated with the consequences of poverty and the consequent lack of value placed on all the lost potential experienced by that community. Poverty erodes cultural assets as it depletes the sense of self-identity and cultural identity.

Thus, Latino girls' educational disadvantage is more directly associated with family economic disadvantage than cultural disadvantage or lack of aspirations of parents. Economic factors intersect with parental and institutional factors that contribute to high rates of educational failure among Latino girls: (1) poverty due to the low hourly earning rates of parents; and the greater likelihood of parents not having completed high school, which makes them more vulnerable to changes in the economy; (2) increased dual worker families with insufficient income to meet the basic necessities of life including adequate childcare and supervision; (3) a growing proportion of Latino families with children headed by women; and (4) widespread and persistent social and economic discrimination as evidenced by resource poor school systems in Latino communities (NCLR, 1998; Siles & Perez, 2000; Garcia, 2001). Because low educational attainment is associated with limited financial resources, barriers to improved employment opportunities and low rates of intergenerational upward mobility, Latino children, especially Latino girls, continue to have low educational attainment, which has not changed considerably over the last three decades.

The authors' basic argument is that to improve academic success, school personnel need awareness and knowledge of how to translate cultural wealth–ethnic values, customs, traditions and language–into social capital for Latino girls. Investments in both Latino girls and their families include providing informational resources to the parents on the importance of education in this society, the process of entering college and mechanisms for financial assistance, and, as an intergenerational approach, the identification of ethnic specific and appropriate mentors for Latino girls and their families, for example, via university-high school partnerships (Williams, 2002). In acknowledging and encouraging a strong ethnic identity and providing students with academic skills, especially in math and science, as well as the knowledge to negotiate educational systems in the U.S., educational personnel would assume a major role in translating academic aspirations into social capital (Williams, 2002). Translating cultural wealth into social capital will foster resilience and hope among young Latinas and increase their opportunities to develop cognitively, emotionally and behaviorally.

CONCLUSION AND RECOMMENDATIONS

This paper inevitably concludes with a series of questions: What has happened to all the efforts on behalf of Latinos in education? What happened to the work of the White House Hispanic Educational Excellence Initiative on behalf of Latina students? What are the best practices for effective educational systems for Latina students? What partnerships are required to push for change in their educational achievement gap? In attempting to answer these questions, several conclusions can be drawn from the literature. The schools that low-income Latino girls attend do not have the economic or personnel resources to provide an optimal education. This is coupled with the fact that school personnel are not prepared to effectively nurture and develop the academic skills of Latinas and less able to engage their parents. All too frequently, school personnel are not competent in engaging the cultural values and strengths of Latinas and thus their cultural capital erodes, as evidenced by disproportionate rates of suicide and high stressors related to their resource-poor environments (Zambrana & Silva-Palacios, 1989; National Alliance for Hispanic Health, 1999; Ginorio & Huston, 2001). Lastly, representation of the interests of Latino children and girls in the school system, at boards of education and at the policy level, is hampered by the severe under representation of Latinos in these positions (Meier & Stewart, 1991; Trueba, 1993; Marcano, 1997; Garza, 2001; Alejandro, 2002; Wortham et al., 2002).

Recommendations based on the review of the literature clearly suggest that economic and social structural prerequisites must precede educational reform if this society is to effectively decrease academic disparities by promoting Latinas' ability to translate their cultural assets into academic achievement (NCLR, 2001; Garcia, 2001; White House Initiative on Educational Excellence for Hispanic Americans, 1996, 1999, 2000 a-d). Economic and social prerequisites include: (a) Increase family economic security by providing a living wage for low-income working poor families and comprehensive family support services to include health, day care and job development; (b) Expand educational opportunities for children and their families by increasing enrollment and utilization of early childhood educational programs (e.g., Early Start, Head Start); (c) Increase access and availability of community-based programs for parents to complete their high school degree or GED, to obtain job literacy training, to improve their literacy, to study English as a second language, and to participate in civic engagements that promote economic and social integration and self-sufficiency within U.S. society (Zambrana, 1997).

The second set of recommendations are associated with increasing the quality of public school education to reflect the importance of education in this society and equity in access to resources (e.g., better pay for teachers, financial resources for textbooks and other classroom supplies, reduction of class size and the increased involvement of parents). Two overall recommendations that have been repeatedly emphasized are the provision of school based health and mental services for Latinas and increased funding for the retention and mentoring of low and moderate-income Latino students during high school.

In effect, the voice of good educational practice suggests beginning with adequately identifying the best practices that are strongly associated with academic achievement for both girls and their parents. This begins with promoting academic success through such strategies as after-school tutoring programs and Saturday Academy for Latinas that enhance educational skills, build self-esteem, and provide role models. Mother-daughter retreats and support groups that teach negotiation and assertiveness skills and address intergenerational conflicts are critical to the academic success of Latino girls. Equally important, parents must be equal partners with students in the effort. Thus, school personnel should involve students and their families in the process of their daughters' high school completion and college preparation. Latino parents view education as important and want their children to be educated to assure a better life than they had. Intergenerational programs to improve their own education (for example, ESL, GED and occupational training) and inform them of college and financial aid options for their daughters represent the translation of their interests and cultural value on education into social capital for their daughters. School systems should recruit and retain teachers from the Latino community who are aware and knowledgeable of Latino culture, history and literature. This will prove a great asset, as well-resourced schools with diverse and culturally competent personnel in Latino communities are more equipped to meaningfully address stereotypes and societal issues, such as teen pregnancy, that impact on school performance. Moreover, they are better prepared to build on the cultural strengths and assets of Latinas and their parents. These practices are important investments for strengthening Latinas' educational achievement.

Education is the key path to economic and political integration of Latinos into U.S. society. The incorporation of a student's language, culture, and experiences is a central principle of good education practice (Trueba, 1999) and at odds with the historic inequity of dismissing and ignoring the low achievement of Latino children and youth. Equity calls for a humanizing and rigorous pedagogy for all. Educational institutions, joined by Latino educators, students and parents, must seek ways to assure the civil rights of Latinas to educational equity. Latino culture holds the keys to the educational future of Latina youth if efforts are made to translate their cultural wealth into social capital to improve academic success.

NOTE

1. Use of "Hispanic" or "Latino/a"–The term Hispanic is used primarily in the context of population. Most government data are reported under this umbrella term. The term Latino/a is used when referring to a heterogeneous population of Mexican Americans, Puerto Ricans, Cuban Americans, Central Americans and South Americans who inhabit regional communities.

REFERENCES

Abma, J.C., & Sonenstein, F.L. (2001). Sexual Activity and Contraceptive Practices among Teenagers in the United States, 1988 and 1995. National Center for Health Statistics. *Vital Health Statistics, 23*, (21).

Abi-Nader, J. (1990). "A house for my mother": Motivating Hispanic high school students. *Anthropology & Education Quarterly, 21*, 41-58.

Alejandro, B. (2002). *The Hispanic child: Speech, language, culture and education.* MA: Allyn & Bacon.

American Association of University Women Educational Foundation. (1995). How Schools Shortchange Girls. Washington, D.C.: Author.

Arellano, A.R., & Padilla, A.M. (1996). Academic Invulnerability among a select group of Latino university students. *Hispanic Journal of Behavioral Sciences, 18* (4), 485-507.

Bass, B.M. (1990). *Bass & Stogdill's handbook of leadership: Theory, research and managerial applications.* (3rd ed). NY: The Free Press.

Bourdieu, P., & Passeron, J.C. (1977). *Reproduction in education, society and culture.* Beverly Hills: Sage.

Bourdieu, P. (1985). The forms of capital. In J.G. Richardson (ed.), *Handbook of Theory and Research for the Sociology of Education.* NY: Greenwood Press.

Brooke, R. (1994, October). Children at risk: Fostering resilience and hope. *American Journal of Orthopsychiatry, 64* (4), 545-553.

Centers for Disease Control and Prevention. (2002, June 28). Surveillance Summaries, *Mortality and Morbidity Weekly Review, 51* (No. SS-4).

Coleman, J. (1990). *Foundations of social theory.* Cambridge: Harvard University Press.

Coleman, J. (1988). Social capital in the creation of human capital. *American Journal of Sociology, 94*, supplement S95-S120.

Council of Economic Advisers for the Presidential's Initiative on Race. (1998). *Changing America Indicators of Social and Economic Well-Being by Race and Hispanic Origin.* Washington, DC.

David and Lucile Packard Foundation. (2000, Fall/Winter). *The Future of Children: Children and Computer Technology, 10* (2), 1-192.

de Anda, D. (1984). Bicultural socialization: Factors affecting the minority experience. *Social Work, March-April*, 101-107.

De León, B. (1996). Career development of Hispanic adolescents girls. In R. Leadbeater, J. Bonnie, & N. Way (Eds.), *Urban girls: Resisting stereotypes, creating identities* (pp. 380-398). New York: New York University Press.

Evelyn, J. (2000). Research shows lag in Hispanic Bachelor's attainment. *Black Issues in Higher Education, 17* (3), 1-16.

Federal Interagency Forum on Child and Family Statistics. (2002). *America's Children: Key National Indicators of Well-Being.* Washington, DC: U.S. Government Printing Office.

Flores, G., Fuentes-Afflick, E., Carter-Porkas, O., Claudio, L., Lamberty, G., Lara, M., Parchter, L., Gomez, F.R., Mendoza, F., Valdez, R.B., Zambrana, R.E., Greenberg, R., & Weitzman, M. (2002). The health of Latino children: Urgent priorities, unanswered questions, and a research agenda. *JAMA, 28* (1), 82-90.

Gándara, P. (1995). *Over the ivy walls: The educational mobility of low-income Chicanos.* NY: SUNY, NY Press.

Gándara, P. (1999). Telling stories of success: Cultural capital and the educational mobility of Chicano students. *Latino Studies Journal, 10* (1), 38-55.

Garcia, E. (2001). *Hispanic in the United States education: Raíces y alas.* Lanham, MD: Rowman & Littlefield Publishers, Inc.

Garza, H. (2001). *Latinas: Hispanic Women in the United States.* NM: University of New Mexico Press.

Ginorio, A., & Huston, M. (2001). ¡Sí se puede! Yes, we can: Latinas in School. Washington, DC: American Association University Women Educational Foundation.

Gonzalez-Ramos, G., Zayas, L.H., & Cohen, E.V. (1998). Child-rearing values of low-income, urban Puerto Rican mothers of preschool children. *Professional Psychology: Research & Practice, 29* (4), 377-382.

Hajat, A., Lucas, J., & Kingston, R. (2000). *Health outcomes among Hispanic subgroups: United States, 1992-95.* Advance Data from Vital and Health Statistics, No. 310. Hyattsville, MD: National Center for Health Statistics.

Hovey, J.D., & King, C.A. (1996). Acculturative stress, depression, and suicidal ideation among immigrant and second-generation Latino adolescents. *American Academy of Child and Adolescent Psychology, 35,* 1183-1192.

Johnson, L.D., O'Malley, P.M., & Bachman, K.G. (1998). *National survey results on drug use from the Monitoring the Future study, 1975-1997,* (NIH Publication No. 98-4345). Rockville, MD: National Institute on Drug Abuse.

Kaufman, P., & Frase, M. (1990). *Dropout Rates in the United States: 1989.* Washington, DC: National Center for Education Statistics.

Marcano, R. (1997). Gender, Culture and Language in School Administration: Another Glass Ceiling for Hispanic Females. *Advancing Women in Leadership Journal-Online* [Online], 22 paragraphs. Available: *http://advancingwomen.com* [1997, Spring].

Meier, K.J., & Stewart, J. (1989). *The politics of Hispanic education: Un paso pa'lante y dos pa'tras.* NY: State University of New York Press.

National Alliance for Hispanic Health. (2000). *The State of Hispanic Girls* [On-line]. Available: *http://www.hispanichealth.org* [2000, March].

National Council La Raza. (2001). *Beyond the Census–Hispanics and an American Agenda.* Washington, DC.

National Council La Raza. (1998). *State of Hispanic America: Latino Education: Status and Prospects.* Washington, DC.

Niemann, Y., Romero, A., & Arbona, C. (2000). Effects of cultural orientation on the perception of conflict between relationship and educational goals for Mexican American college students. *Hispanic Journal of Behavioral Sciences, 2* (1), 46-63.

Nieto, Sonia. (2000). *Puerto Rican students in U.S. Schools.* NJ: Lawrence Erlbaum Associates, Publishers.

North, D. (1990). *Institutions, institutional change, and economic performance.* NY: Cambridge University Press.

Portes, A. (2000). The Two Meanings of Social Capital. *Sociological Forum, 15* (1), 1-11.

Putnam, R.D. (1993). The prosperous community: Social capital and public life. *The American Prospect Journal-Online* [Online], 22 paragraphs. Available: (http://prospect.org) [1993, March 21].

Putnam, R.D. (1995). Bowling alone–America's declining social capital. *Journal of Democracy, 6*, (1): 65-78.

Rodríguez, C.G. (1999). *Bringing up Latino children in a bicultural world.* NY: Simon & Schuster.

Rodríguez-Trias, H., & Ramírez de Arellano, A. (1994). The Health of Children and Youth. In C.A. Molina and Maquirre-Molina (Eds.) *Latino Heath in the U.S.: A Growing Challenge.* Washington, DC: APHA.

Romo, H. (1998). *Racial and ethnic relations in America.* Boston: Allyn and Bacon.

Romo, H.D., & Fablo, T. (1996). *Latino high school graduation: Defying the odds.* TX: University of Texas Press.

Siles, M., & Perez, S. (2000). What Latino workers bring to the labor market: How human capital affects employment outcomes. *Moving Up the Economic Ladder: Latino Workers and the Nation's Future Prosperity.* Washington, DC: National Council of La Raza, p. 1-34.

Schoen, C.K., Davis, K.S., Collins, L., Des Roches, C., & Abrams, M. (1997). *The Commonwealth Fund Survey of the Health of Adolescent Girls.* NY: Commonwealth Fund.

So, A.Y. (1987). High-Achieving Disadvantaged Students: A Study of Low SES Hispanic Language Minority Youth. *Urban Education, 22* (1), 19-35.

Sotomayor, M. (1991). *Empowering Hispanic Families: A Critical Issue for the '90s.* WI: Family Service America.

The World Bank. (1998). Social Development Family, Environmentally and Socially Sustainable Development Network. *Social capital: The missing link?* Washington, DC: Christiaan Grootaert.

Tinajero, J. V., Gonzales, M.L., & Dick, F. (1991). *Raising career aspirations of Hispanic girls: Fastback 320.* Bloomington, IN: Phi Delta Kappa Educational Foundation.

Trueba, H.T. (1999). *Latinos Unidos.* Lanham, Maryland: Rowman and Littlefield.

Trueba, H.T., Rodríguez, C., Zou, Y., & Cintrón, J. (1993). *Healing multicultural America.* PA: Falmer Press.

U.S. Census Bureau. (2001). Current Population Survey, March 2000, Ethnic and Hispanic Statistics Branch, Population Division. Internet Release Date: March 6. Available at http://www.census.gov/population/www/socdemo/hispanic/ho00-01.html.

U.S. Department of Education. National Center for Education Statistics. (2000). *Dropout Rates in the United States, NCES 2002-114.* Washington, DC: Kaufman, Phillip; Alt, Martha Naomi; Chapman, Christopher.

U.S. Department of Health and Human Services Centers for Disease Control and Prevention. (2000). *CDC-Fact Book 2000/2001.* Atlanta, GA.

U.S. National Center for Education Statistics, Department of Education, Office of Educational Research and Improvement. (2001). *Digest of Education Statistics 2000* (NCES 2001-034). Washington, DC.

U.S. National Center for Education Statistics, Department of Education, Office of Educational Research and Improvement. (1995). *The Condition of Education: The Educational Progress of Hispanic Students* (NCES 95-767). Washington, DC.

Walsh, C.E. (1991). *Pedagogy and the struggle for voice: Issues of language, power, and schooling for Puerto Ricans.* NY: Bergin & Garvey Press.

White House Initiative on Educational Excellence for Hispanic Americans. (1996). *Our Nation on the Fault Line*. Washington, DC: President's Advisory Committee on Educational Excellence for Hispanic Americans.

White House Initiative on Educational Excellence for Hispanic Americans. (1999). *Hispanic Education Plan (HEAP)*. Washington, DC: President's Advisory Committee on Educational Excellence for Hispanic Americans.

White House Initiative on Educational Excellence for Hispanic Americans. (2000a). *Report on the White House Strategy Session on Improving Hispanic Student Achievement*. Washington, DC: President's Advisory Committee on Educational Excellence for Hispanic Americans.

White House Initiative on Educational Excellence for Hispanic Americans. (2000b). *Creating the Will: Hispanic Achieving Educational Excellence*. Washington, DC: President's Advisory Committee on Educational Excellence for Hispanic Americans.

White House Initiative on Educational Excellence for Hispanic Americans. (2000c). *No Child Left Behind*. Washington, DC: President's Advisory Committee on Educational Excellence for Hispanic Americans.

White House Initiative on Educational Excellence for Hispanic Americans. (2000d). *Report on the White House Strategy Session on Improving Hispanic Student Achievement*. Washington, DC: President's Advisory Committee on Educational Excellence for Hispanic Americans.

Williams, V.L. (2002). *Merging University Students Into K-12 Science Education Reform*. Santa Monica, CA: RAND.

Wortham, S., Murillo, E.G., Jr., & Hamann, E. (2002). *Education in the New Latino Diaspora: Policy and the Politics of Identity*. CT: Ablex Publishing.

Zambrana, R.E. (1987). Toward understanding the educational trajectory and socialization of Latina women. *The Broken Web: The Educational Experience of Hispanic American Women*. Encino, California: Thomas Rivera Center and Floricanto Press, 61-77 (reprinted in L. Stone (ed), The Education Feminism Reader, Rout ledge, 1994).

Zambrana, R.E., & Silva-Palacios, V.S. (1989). Gender differences in stress among Mexican immigrant adolescents in Los Angeles, California. *Journal of Adolescent Research, 4* (4), 426-442.

Zambrana, R.E. (1997). Strengthening Latino communities through family support programs: Building on guidelines for family support practice. In *Companion Guide to Guidelines for Family Support Practice, Family Resource Coalition: Special Report, 15* (3&4), 29-34.

Zambrana, R.E., Dorrington, C., & Bell, S.A. (1997). Mexican American women in higher education: A comparative study. *Race, Gender & Class, 4* (2), 127-149.

Zambrana, R.E., & Carter-Pokras, O. (2001). Health Data issues for Hispanics: Implications for Public Health Research. *Journal of Health Care for the Poor and Underserved, 12* (1), 20-34.

From Problems to Personal Resilience: Challenges and Opportunities in Practice with African American Youth

June Gary Hopps
Robbie Welch Christler Tourse
Ollie Christian

SUMMARY. This paper reviews data on select areas relevant to the status, functioning, and general well-being of African American Youth. Practitioners in both policy and clinical intervention must assert a greater role in helping these adolescents grow, develop, and become prepared to take their rightful place in American Society. Attention is afforded the African American Family, particularly Black youth and the threats, both historical and contemporary, which confront their ability to survive, cope, and sustain a resilient presence. Conflict theory is used to under-

---

June Gary Hopps, PhD, is Parham Professor, School of Social Work, University of Georgia, Athens, GA. Robbie Welch Christler Tourse, PhD, is Director of Field Education and Adjunct Associate Professor, Graduate School of Social Work, Boston College, Chestnut Hill, MA. Ollie Christian, PhD, is Professor, Department of Sociology, Southern University, Baton Rouge, LA.

Research assistance was provided by Curtis Todd, MSW, a graduate of the Whitney Young School of Social Work, Clark Atlanta University, Atlanta, GA, and Carlise Billings, MSW, a graduate of the School of Social Work, University of Georgia, Athens, GA.

[Haworth co-indexing entry note]: "From Problems to Personal Resilience: Challenges and Opportunities in Practice with African American Youth." Hopps, June Gary, Robbie Welch Christler Tourse, and Ollie Christian. Co-published simultaneously in *Journal of Ethnic & Cultural Diversity in Social Work* (The Haworth Social Work Practice Press, an imprint of The Haworth Press, Inc.) Vol. 11, No. 1/2, 2002, pp. 55-77; and: *Social Work with Multicultural Youth* (ed: Diane de Anda) The Haworth Social Work Practice Press, an imprint of The Haworth Press, Inc., 2002, pp. 55-77. Single or multiple copies of this article are available for a fee from The Haworth Document Delivery Service [1-800-HAWORTH, 9:00 a.m. - 5:00 p.m. (EST). E-mail address: docdelivery@haworthpress.com].

http://www.haworthpress.com/store/product.asp?sku=J051

10.1300/J051v11n01_03

stand how this population interfaces with oppression, and a resilience framework, coupled with group as a method are presented as strategies for working with Black adolescents. The authors proffer that a justice-based model is useful in supporting this resilience framework within a group approach.

KEYWORDS. Black adolescents profiles, Black youth, resilience, groups, conflict theory, intervention, justice-based orientation

INTRODUCTION

African Americans make up over 12% (12.3%) of the nation's population totaling nearly 34.7 million. Over 32% of this racial group are under eighteen years of age, which indicates that the African American cohort is younger than the White population (McKinnon, 2001; U.S. Census Bureau, 2000). This cohort (12 to 18 years, and those a few years older) who are the major focus of attention of this article, will be noted alternately as youth or adolescents. The authors' theoretical premise is drawn from conflict theory, noting how stratification and control by a dominant group leaves many African American youth feeling powerless, alienated, and angry. To assist Black youth with these feelings and to develop positive coping strategies, intervention will be discussed that focuses on a resilience framework within a group approach. The authors suggest also that, overall, a social justice model of practice must undergird all direct interventions. Such practice indicates that practitioners must become advocates for change in the external environment, including reallocation of greater resources to the truly disadvantaged in this population group.

THEORETICAL FRAMEWORK

As a means to understand the struggle of the disadvantaged, social conflict theory is employed as the theoretical framework in this paper. Conflict theory is rooted in the work of Karl Marx (Tischler, 2002). Many contemporary theorists have articulated the importance of social conflict (Coser, 1956; Feagin & Feagin, 1997; Simmel, 1955; Turner, 1991; Turner, Beeghley, & Powers, 1995), and suggest that society is characterized not by a consensus over values, but by a struggle between social classes, and class conflict between powerful and less powerful groups (Clinard & Meier, 1995).

Blackwell (1991) takes the position that it is only through transformation via fundamental changes in how power is distributed that the African American population can improve its status and make overall life changes in American society. He posits as well, that changing power relations becomes inordinately difficult when contending groups are unequal with respect to economic, political, and educational resources, and when groups are competing for extremely scarce rewards (see also Hopps, 2000). Social inequality, which is the uneven distribution of privileges, material rewards, opportunities, power, prestige, and influence among individuals and groups (Tischler, 2002), is the product of and also perpetuates prejudice and discrimination which continue to contribute negatively to the upward social mobility of African American youth.

A PROFILE OF AFRICAN AMERICAN YOUTH

The differential opportunity structure growing out of social stratification and class conflict, as noted above, increases the alienation of African American youth towards the dominant culture. Very obvious social stratification and income disparities, which places many in the bottom tier of the socioeconomic pyramid (Center on Budget and Policy Priorities, 2001), is a breeding ground for risks that compromise the strength and resilience of this group. Acknowledging that youth know about powerlessness, that they feel powerless and recognize the inability to control their destiny, pushes committed practitioners who want to truly help these youth to think of new paradigms, methods, and approaches to alleviate the intrapsychic pain that can lead to individual shortcomings. This pain is often the outgrowth of macro level economic and social policies that are less than supportive of people of color (Hopps, Pinderhughes, Shankar, 1995; Hopps & Pinderhughes, 1999).

In this society the hope is that youth will grow up and become socialized within a traditional family unit, although it is recognized that the family has taken many new forms and structures (Hopps, 2000). No matter what the composition of the African American family, its status, strength, and resilience play a pivotal role in Black adolescent nurturing, socialization, acculturation, social functioning, competence, and successes. It is where Black youth learn coping and survival skills necessary for dealing with the environment external to the family–an environment that the authors describe as hostile and noxious. A brief profile of young African Americans illustrates that there are continuing struggles for adequate economic and social development, a struggle that has existed since slavery. This profile will center on socioeconomic gains and losses of the African American family, as well as education and educational achievement, labor market participation, and health issues related to African American youth. The authors do not address the foster care system per se, but are cognizant of the major impact it has on African American youth. Black youth comprise roughly 40% of the foster care population, and are obviously disproportionately represented in the system (Child Welfare League of America, 2002).

Socioeconomics

There is a modicum of good news. African American families showed improvement in socioeconomic status, and at a faster rate than White families. These families accounted for 60% of the decline in poor families, some 400,000 from 1996 to 1997, and for 50% of this population, this meant moving up and out of poverty (Dalaker, U.S. Census Bureau, 2001).

The 1999-2000 period witnessed a decline in poverty for all populations in America from 32.9 million (11.8%) to 31.1 million (11.3%), nearly matching the 1973 nadir. For African Americans this period of time was even better, moving to an all time low poverty rate, 22.1%; however, this still nearly represents a quarter of the African American population in contrast to 7.5% for the White population. This decline continues a narrowing of the poverty gap from nearly one-third in 1993 to less than a quarter today. Although better than the 25% higher rate than that of the White population in 1993, the current 15% greater poverty rate for the African American population (Dalaker, U.S. Census Bureau, 2001) is still unacceptable, and fuels negative (often destructive) thoughts that are too frequently followed by self-destructive action among the poor, and particularly poor youth (Hopps, Pinderhughes, & Shankar, 1995).

A persistent problem in this country is child poverty, which is influenced by both ethnicity and family structure. Those eighteen and younger experience poverty more than any other age group, 16.2% in 2000–that was 11 million faces. Six percent, five million children and youth, lived in families experiencing extreme poverty, where income is half below the poverty line (Dalaker, U.S. Census Bureau, 2001). Yet, this is the lowest rate since 1979. For Black children, the rate was 30%, for Hispanic children, 28%, and for White children, 9% (The National Center for Children in Poverty, 2002). For very young Black children living only with a mother, the poverty rate was 52%. Another troubling issue is that most poor young children live in working families; only 11% are in families that depend exclusively on welfare benefits. This suggests that working poor families' incomes are not viable means of support (see below) (The National Center for Children in Poverty, 2002).

The over-representation of African American youth in poverty does not bode well for their future, placing at risk their emotional, social, cognitive, and educational development, and their ability to be resilient. The improvements noted came at a time when the economy was more robust and not challenged by a weakening economy, growing unemployment (The Urban Institute, 2002), and corporate scandals (Strouse, 2002). What then portends for the future where a different scenario is projected?

Education and Educational Achievement

There is documentation of overall improvement in the educational achievement of African Americans, but again, improvement does not mean parity with the White population. For example, during the mid 1970s to late 1990s the gap in high school/GED completion rates between African American and White youth closed substantially, owing heavily to greater GED completion by African American (13%) than White youth (7%) (U.S. Department of Education, 2001). In 1997, the dropout rate was 5.0% for the African American and 3.6% for the White population. Parenthetically, many poor single mothers dropped out of high school, and no doubt this contributes to the very high poverty rate of their young offspring. Even when African American youth manage to finish high school, they are still at serious disadvantage. For instance, math and reading tests showed that these youth scored lower than their White cohorts at every grade level; however, as years in school progressed, reading scores improved (U.S. Department of Education, 2001).

Computers and the Internet. Another divide shows up in computer and internet use in homes, with both technologies becoming the mainstay in today's world. Over one-half of the population (54%) had at least one computer in their home in 2000. In households where income was $75,000 or more, nearly 90% had a computer; and for households below $25,000, 28%. Internet access followed along a similar path.

Black children are less likely than non-Hispanic White children to use a home computer or the internet. For those in the 3 to 17 age range, home computer use is as follows: 77%, White non-Hispanic; 43%, African American; and 37%, Hispanic. This pattern is moderated by school computer utilization: 87% from the higher income strata, and 72%, from the lowest (Neuburger, U.S. Census Bureau, 2001). Schools do change the landscape as greater comparability across race, ethnicity, and income is achieved, but inequality is still quite apparent.

Post-Secondary Education. When African American and White youth had comparable "prior educational achievement," meaning equivalent math and reading scores, the level of college matriculation was greater for African American than for White youth; and college completion rates corresponded with or exceeded those of the White cohort. This was not the case when "prior educational achievement," was not determined–the rate of college completion among African American youth was much lower than that of White students. Black college attendance rates, moreover, declined between 1979 and 1992 (U.S. Department of Education, 2001). An explanation is that African American students reacted to changes in financial aid, which was reconfigured through loans rather than grants. From the mid-seventies to mid-eighties, the portion of aid for grants fell from 80% to 46%, while that for loans grew from 17% to 50%. Correlatively, there was also a change showing positive attitude toward the military. Black male seniors expecting to enter the services jumped from 37% to 50% (the rate for White seniors was from 17% to 21%). Unlike White youth, African American youth did not expect sufficient returns on investment in a college education to warrant borrowing money and thus, looked more favorably on opportunities in the military (The National Research Council, 1989 in U.S. Department of Education, 2001). This is an example of how noticeable changes in financial aid discriminate against the poor and near poor (where many Blacks are aggregated), thereby forcing these youth into an alternative stream that is viewed as more accepting.

Education is perceived as the great equalizer in this country. The system is working better, but many youth are still deprived of a decent future, guaranteeing a life of low earnings, unemployment, and poverty. Fewer African American students (about 13%) than White students (25%) are completing college. Arguably, these factors bear heavily on future earnings of African Americans, for education and one's race have a great influence on earning power (Tourse & Collins, 2000).

Labor Market Participation

Disparities in Black-White participation in the labor market, a historical phenomenon, continues and probably increased from 1979 to 1992, especially for women. Blacks were found more likely to experience unemployment and lower annual and hourly wages than the White population. Indeed, Blacks are more than twice as likely to be unemployed (U.S. Department of Education, 2001).

When employed, disparities in annual earnings were considerable, with young African American workers making less than White workers and men not doing as well as women. Gaps in earnings were even greater for Black males in the 1980s to 1992 (32%) than in 1979 (16%) (U.S. Department of Education, 2001). When prior educational achievement was similar, the wage gap was two-fifths to three-fifths smaller for Black males than for all men, and no significant differences for hourly wages was registered. Similarly, African American women earned as much or more than White women annually and per hour when prior education achievement was comparable (U.S. Department of Education, 2001). What this means is that educational achievement is a strong predictor of employment and earnings outcome.

Youth Employment. Some 40% of 16 to 17 year-old youth matriculating in high school work, and 25% of those holding jobs clocked in more than 25 hours per week (Lerman, 2000). A study based on 1997 data from the National Survey of America's Families, and discussed by Lerman (2000) pointed out that although outcomes are varied for adolescents in the workforce, there are some disturbing indicators. First, a significant achievement gap exists for working youth across socioeconomic strata. For youth who receive welfare benefits, more than half demonstrate weak engagement with schools as compared to the 42% whose families received welfare in the past, the 31% from low income families, and the 24% from moderate to high income families. Second, the need for low income youth to work in order to help support themselves and their families pales in comparison to other variables such as inability to locate work, issues related to motivation, and parental support of work.

The body of research available on the value and the relevance of work experience indicates that the majority of working youth are in jobs that are not connected to the classroom curriculum, do not offer instruction in skills development that can propel them towards advancement, and do not provide sufficient opportunity for useful interaction with adults (Panel on Health and Safety Implication of Child Labor for the

National Research Council, 1998 in Lerman, 2000). Some studies suggest that long hours at work correlate with low academic aspiration and attainment. In contrast, other studies suggest that grades improved and post-secondary education was encouraged when youth were afforded employment opportunity in well-structured jobs (Lerman, 2000).

It must be pointed out that for youth working over twenty hours a week, males were dominant, and this was particularly the case for Black males. These youth reportedly avoided homework and were suspended from school at a greater rate than others (Lerman, 2000). The authors argue that it would seem that given the reading and math gaps, youth from poor families need the time in school if they are to have a more promising future.

Health Issues

A number of health issues continue to plague youth, such as smoking, AIDs, adolescent pregnancy, and suicide. These issues do not begin to cover the wealth of social and environmental health risks factors that confront youth, but are representative.

Nicotine Addiction. Although 8th, 10th, and 12th grade African American youth demonstrate the lowest rates of smoking; when they do smoke, they are at greater risk of developing serious long-term consequences than other racial groups, and these illnesses manifest an earlier age of onset (National Institute on Drug Abuse, 2001).

AIDS. Many youth do not consider the consequences of sexual contact, and this lack of cognitive understanding or complacency places them in vulnerable positions for many sexually transmitted diseases. The one with the most deadly outcome is AIDS. Over three thousand (3002) adolescents (13-19 years of age) in 1998 were reported to be infected with AIDS, which is 0.5% of all AIDS cases. Because of the long incubation time for AIDS, many of these youth will not be aware of their health dilemma until they reach young adulthood (McInnis-Dittrich, Neisler, & Tourse, 1999). Young African American women (16-18 years of age) are at greater risk for HIV infection than males, and infection occurs at a younger age. This group has the highest HIV prevalence among all women (Center for Disease Control and Prevention, 1998).

Adolescent Pregnancy. The National Center for Health Statistics, CDC (2002) reports a decline in adolescent births in the decade of the nineties. This trend reverses that of the 1986-1991 period where there was a 24% increase. Black women had the largest decline; for those between 15 and 19 years of age, the birth rate fell 31% during 1991-2000

(National Campaign to Prevent Pregnancy, 2002). This is promising since approximately only one-third of adolescent mothers obtain a high school education, and 80% of adolescent mothers receive welfare benefits. Furthermore, the sons of these mothers are more likely to go to prison, and 22% of the daughters are apt to repeat their mother's experience of becoming an adolescent mother (National Campaign to Prevent Teen Pregnancy, 2002).

Suicide. A dangerous phenomenon, suicide is growing among Black youth, ranking by the mid-nineties as the third leading cause of death among youth 15 to 19 years old, narrowing the gap with White youth. Between 1980 and 1985, the rate for African American youth 10 to 19 years of age grew from 2.1 to 4.5 per 100,000. The greatest increase was among 10 to 14 year olds (233%) compared to 120% for White youth (Center for Disease Control and Prevention, 1998).

Firearms were used in 72% of the suicides among Black males 15 to 19 years and were involved in more than 95% of the growth of the age 10 cohort suicides (Center for Disease Control and Prevention, 1998).

Juvenile Justice System

Although only 15% of youth below 18 were African American in the late 1990s, Building Blocks for Youth (2002) reported that Black adolescents accounted for 26% of juvenile arrests, 31% of referrals to juvenile court, and 34% of those processed in the juvenile court system. In addition, 46% of African American youth were sent to adult court, and 58% of those were sent to adult state prisons. No matter what the offense, African American offenders were at greater risk for detention than White offenders each year of the 1988-1997 decade. At each point, in the juvenile justice system, Black (along with Hispanic) offenders receive harsher punishment than White offenders. The average length of incarceration is 305 days for Latino, 254 days for African American, and 193 days for White offenders. In the case of drug offenses, African American youth are 48 times at greater risk of being put in juvenile prison than similarly situated White youth (Building Blocks for Youth, 2002). Just as there is over-representation of African Americans in the juvenile justice system, there is under-representation in mental health treatment programs for those arrested for drugs–33% were African American, 63% of those arrested were sent to adult court for that offense, but less than 20% were admitted to drug treatment.

Although during the 1993-1999 period the juvenile homicide rate dropped by 68% (the lowest since the mid-sixties, and for youth under

13, the lowest since 1964 when these statistics were first recorded by the FBI), a punitive approach to youth offenders has been and still is sweeping the country. Most states have enacted legislation, making it less difficult for youth to be prosecuted as adults. It is argued that this burden falls disproportionately on Black and Hispanic youth (Building Blocks for Youth, 2002). This new trend has been referred to as adultifying the juvenile justice system (Schiraldi, 2002).

Despite the ongoing criticism and negative image, homicides at schools have declined some 70% since 1992, making them one of the safest environments for young people. Fewer students are carrying weapons to school today, and violence reaches its high point after school hours, during the 3 to 6 p.m. time block (Children's Defense Fund, 2002).

In summary, the areas profiled suggest that most Black youth are at risk. Their ability to cope and adapt speaks to their resilience. At times however, insufficient internal strength for coping, coupled with the negative influence of external factors, chip away at their ability to be resilient and to develop and achieve successfully. To reinforce and sustain African American adolescent resilience requires for some to obtain psychosocial intervention in a therapeutic environment. Professionals must not forget that enhanced coping skills are not sufficient; they must be ever vigilant and advocate for social justice, not just through professional organizations and selected interest groups, but in the presence of their clients who often learn to model them (Hopps, Pinderhughes & Shankar, 1995). Structural changes (see Justice-Model in Hopps, Pinderhughes & Shankar, 1995; Hopps, Tourse & Christian, 1999) are required as noted by Blackwell (1991) and several other contemporary theorists and proponents of conflict theory (Clinard & Meirer, 1995; Coser, 1956; Feagan, & Feagan, 1997; Simmel, 1955; Turner, 1991).

INTERVENTION WITH AFRICAN AMERICAN ADOLESCENTS

Intervention is the *doing* of the therapeutic process. It operationalizes the practitioner/client agreed upon goals and objectives identified through assessment of the client situation (Corcoran, Grinnell, & Briggs, 2001). Intervention is multifaceted and incorporates theories and methods, as well as approaches and models. The integration of these various aspects of treatment provides the crux of intervention. An intervention approach widely discussed, particularly in relation to youth and adolescents, is resilience (e.g., Belgrave et al., 2000; Blum,

1998; Freshman & Leinwand, 2001; Glantz & Johnson, 1999; Hill, 1998; Levy & Wall, 2000; Smith & Carlson, 1997; Williams, Lindsey, Kurtz, & Jarvis, 2001). Furthermore, group methods have been found to be an effective intervention, especially with Black youth (Hopps, Pinderhughes, & Shankar, 1995; Hopps & Pinderhughes, 1999). Resilience as an approach and group as a method will be discussed as the integrative elements for an intervention framework in working with African American adolescents. Tourse (2002a) uses the empirical findings from the research noted above in developing this resilience framework. Resilience posits that emphasis should be placed on the strengths of group members and on factors that strengthen, protect, and support coping capacities, and provide a sense of well-being. The framework was designed to assist African American youth, but can be applied to any ethnic or racial population. At the same time, practitioners must be mindful of and thoughtful about means of addressing interventions in the external environment that trigger risks to resilience.

Youth Resilience

African Americans in the context of their existence in the United States have survived and overcome oppression in the form of legal institutional slavery and segregation, and even today continue to rally against the affronts of institutional racism, poor educational opportunities, stressful environments, economic depression, and other engulfing problems. Lifelong oppression has required the African American population to adapt creative values and ethical positions (Stevens, 2002) to assist with transcending adverse situations–such as poverty, poor housing and schools, improper city services, social isolation and crime riddled streets–which are compounded by racist social structures (Hopps, Pinderhughes, & Shankar, 1995).

Resilience has been equated with strength (Stevens, 2002), a concept that has traditionally been a part of social work practice. Resilience reinforces the strength concept and has been characterized in three ways: (1) as recovery in the face of trauma and adversity, (2) as means of coping, and (3) as the presence of protective factors that mediate stress, risk, coping, and competence (Freshman & Leinwand, 2001; Levy & Wall, 2000; Smith & Carlson, 1997; Stevens, 2002). From a developmental viewpoint, resilience is the ability to effectively negotiate each successive stage of development (Blum, 1998) by means of intrapsychic strengths, internal coping skills, and an external facilitative environment (Grotberg in Blum, 1998). In these definitions, the environment and one's internal capacity are either implicitly or explicitly indicated, and an effective developmental progression is noted in the latter. It is no surprise, therefore, that resilience is also viewed as a continual process and involves the juxtaposition and interaction between environmental and internal factors (Levy & Wall, 2000; Stevens, 2002). These definitions emphasize the need to address cognitive, behavioral and developmental elements in working with adolescents. Oppression and other environmental stressors have profound impact on these elements (Tourse, Hopps, & Christian, May 2002). Elucidating resilience as an agent of change in the intervention process means also understanding risk, protective factors, and stress.

Risk and Protective Factors

Risk factors have been defined as conditions that interfere with the likelihood of successful development (Blum, 1998). They have also been identified as occurrences that increase the chance for disequilibrium to transpire in different systems. Social scientists, as a result of such a definition, have focused risk factor research on the relationship between functioning in an adaptive manner and situations that exemplify high stress (Steven, 2002). Previously discussed areas contain risk for psychosocial development and, in addition, include situations such as family discord, out of home placement, marital dysfunction, separation or divorce, racist ideologies, alcoholic families, chronic illness/disability, and affiliating with drug using peers (Blum, 1998; Freshman & Leinwand, 2001; Stevens, 2002; Smith & Carlson, 1997). Racist ideologies, drug using peers, and incarceration are noted, in particular, as risk factors for African American youth (Hopps, Pinderhughes, & Shankar, 1995; Schiele, 1998). Stevens (2002) suggests that more research needs to be initiated to understand the concerns that are more prevalent for and unique to African American youth since "[g]enerally, scientific investigations [are] of white youth . . . of middle-class status, in two-parent households, and in suburban communities" (p. 16). Based on youth and adolescent research, such risk factors suggests that cumulative effects of risk situations, not just one risk factor, tend to generate negative outcomes on a consistent basis, and that healthy adaptive functioning can occur despite exposure to threatening circumstances (Levy & Wall, 2000; Stevens, 2002; Smith & Carlson, 1997). The areas that have consistently been proven to place youth at risk for future difficulties are poor academic achievement and poor social relationships (Levy & Wall, 2000), which are supported by the data discussed in the African

American youth profile sections. Adolescents are also more likely to be at risk if they live in low socioeconomic conditions and have people of color status (Levy & Wall, 2000). Such factors can and do place them in vulnerable positions, but many are still able to be resilient–why?

A well accepted definition of protective factors is that they are "influences that modify, ameliorate or alter a person's response to some environmental hazard that predisposes to a maladaptive outcome" (Rutter in Smith & Carlson, 1997, pp. 237-238). In her book on inner city Black female adolescents, Stevens (2002) suggests that such factors compensate for and counterbalance extreme risk effects and support coping processes. Smith and Carlson (1997) suggest that protective factors emerge out of three areas: family, individual, and external supports. They indicate further that research provides validity for positive family support and guidance, a sense of family resilience, fathers being present in children's lives, and basic harmonious parental relationships. Such "factors appear to be the inverse of risk factors" (Freshman & Leinwand, 2001, p. 45). Research also validates other protective factors, such as (1) the adolescents' internal capacities to seek help from adults and believe in themselves, (2) the chance to connect with "conventional opportunities and institutions" (e.g., church and youth organizations), and (3) in external systems, the ability to relate to supportive people (i.e., youth leaders, teachers, neighbors) in the broader society (Levy & Wall, 2000; Smith & Carlson, 1997). Such factors assist with the acquisition of resiliency and promote well-being.

Stress

From a developmental perspective, a certain amount of stress can be a motivator. Stevens (2002) proffers that stress, as an aspect of development, can promote resilience in people over time. When there are multiple and continuous stressors in one's life, however, stress can deter development, as well as positive functioning and adaptation. Stress is the perception and feeling that one is at risk and, therefore, one's life requires adaptation (Blum, 1998; Smith & Carlson, 1997). For youth, situations such as transitioning from middle school to high school, moving to another city or neighborhood, parents divorcing, and an affront to racial and cultural identity can be precipitants for stress; all can be challenges to their usual way of viewing the world and operating in it. For poor and extremely poor youth, other factors (such as daily survival, getting food, shelter, freedom from crime ridden streets, and firearm assaults) also present constant stress to their mental health and emotional and cognitive development. How people mature, their internal capacity to cope, and their ability to seek positive external supports determines their ability to deal with such stress and suggests their capacity to be resilient.

Intervention

Adolescence is a vulnerable time in development. It can be difficult under "normal circumstances" and overwhelming in continuous stressful situations, including environmental stressors such as poverty, lack of employment opportunity, and unavailability of parental support (owing in large part, as already discussed, to many poor children residing in households where both parents work or are over-represented in single parent families). This is a crucial phase in development wherein self-identity is molded in the context of the larger society. It is also a time when youth begin to assert their independence within the confines of family and society. How family, friends, and society perceive adolescents also influence how adolescents perceive themselves, and how they behave. It is a time of paradox, a time for wanting to be independent but craving structure, a time for wanting to establish their own values, but needing moral guidance; and a time for making an identity statement, but needing help to sort out exactly what that identity is. When practitioners begin to think about interventions, they must understand the effect that risk factors have on adolescent development and behavior, and further understand that protective factors that support resilience can change functioning through their interactions with risk factors (Levy & Wall, 2000). "This perspective permits clinicians to design interventions that take progressive as well as dysfunctional elements into account" (pp. 403-404). They must also understand the developmental gender differences that mediate the cognitive and behavioral responses of youth (see for example, Blum, 1998; Freshman & Leinwand, 2001; Hill, 1998; Schiele, 1998; Stevens, 2002). Important to understand as well, is that culture has a great influence on adolescent development through molding self-perception, identity, and public perception (Blum, 1998, p. 369), and, therefore, culture is significant in the advancement of intervention procedures within the method of choice (Hopps & Kilpatrick, 2003; Tourse, 2002b).

Group process is one way to intervene with adolescents, and this method was found in research performed by Hopps, Pinderhughes, and Shankar (1995) to be the most effective with poor, overwhelmed families and youth, among which African Americans are over-represented.

Group process provides a mechanism for identifying and using protective factors, which facilitate positive development and support intrapsychic strengths, and which can also be a catalyst for community and environmental empowerment (Hopps & Pinderhughes, 1999). The use of a resilience framework in working with youth in groups may further increase the effectiveness of this method.

A Resilience Framework for Group Intervention

The framework focuses on four areas: resilience in context, survival elements of ethnic and racial culture(s), values and ethics that support survival, and avenues for positive adaptation. Throughout the course of group processes, practitioner emphasis should be on self-efficacy and personal mastery, and adolescent developmental processes. Inherent in the body of this framework is the eradication of risk factors that cause stress in the lives of Black adolescents.

Resilience in Context. The central theme in this area is strength and survival and the perceptions each member has of these terms vis à vis the self, self in context of peer groups, self and peer groups in relation to society, and the self and peer groups as a resilient body. Embedded in these discussions should be the strengths and positive survival techniques group members have to offer. Discussions in these areas should also assist with self-concept and role identity, from a progression of the self as an individual, to the self relating in the broader society.

In one group, composed of African American adolescents of parents with AIDS, members were engulfed in dealing with the physical trauma and predicted demise of their parent or parents, and the uncertainty they faced for the future. Each member periodically presented thoughts and journeys to the group: singing, writing poetry, and sharing pictures of family members, to name a few. Participation in these creative activities were viewed as strengths, encouraged, and supported by both group members and the group leader. Such activities also provided a focus for discussion in the group. These activities not only assisted the group member/presenter, but gave support, comfort, and means of coping to the other group members as well. The group was able to understand that, as individuals and as a unit, they were an empowering force for one another, as well as for the group as a collective. Members became more empowered and enabled, showing greater resilience as they faced the subtleties and complexities of their personal journeys, family constellations, and home and community environs (Hopps & Pinderhughes, 1999).

For practitioners facilitating this type of group, it must be clearly understood that over the course of one's development, resiliency has to be fostered, and protective factors nurtured and possibly substituted as life changes (Freshman & Leinwand, 2001). This is particularly the case for African American youth who not only have to deal with personal issues and concerns, but have to be constantly vigilant of racial, socioeconomic, class, and cultural affronts that assault their psychic reality (Hopps, Pinderhughes, & Shankar, 1995; Stevens, 2002).

Survival in the Context of Race, Ethnicity, and Culture. Integrating race and ethnicity into the group process will assist group members with understanding the heritage and traditions that provide strength for African American populations. Feeling positive about one's race and ethnicity helps to establish identity. African Americans, males in particular, have long experienced marginalization by society through high unemployment, low status in the societal systems, low academic achievement, poverty and limited resources (see above, as well as Hopps, Pinderhughes, & Shankar, 1995). Stevens (2002) suggests that currently Black youth perceive themselves as outside of American society and not a part of it, which supports the notion that they are marginalized. As part of the group process, it is important to begin to bolster African American adolescents' self-esteem.

Black youth have experienced cultural oppression and, thereby, cultural alienation (Schiele, 1998), as could be predicted from conflict theory. They have been alienated from cultural truths, knowledge about their culture, and their unique contributions to human history (Schiele, 1998). The current theoretical position on culture suggests that it is "those shared meanings of a people that are reflected in personal behavior and social institutions" (Stevens, 2002, p. 185). Discussion, therefore, of cultural heritage is one means to assist in bolstering self-esteem for Black youth vis à vis race, ethnicity, class, and culture. It is important to move youth beyond the traditional athlete, comedian, and rap singer, to foster pride in being an adolescent Black male or female, provide role models, and examples of perseverance and success in the face of adversity, racial and economic oppression, and society's diminution of the Black culture. Identifying and processing the accomplishments of African American men and women who have contributed to society such as Dr. Charles Drew, the developer of the first blood bank and Dr. Mae Jemison, adolescent psychiatrist and first African American woman astronaut, help accomplish this purpose.

In the AIDS group, some had never heard of many notable historical and contemporary African Americans. Knowledge of these models fostered the belief that if these individuals could persevere, overcome obstacles in life, and achieve, so could they. The possibilities for their future began to seem more plausible and real to the youth in the group.

Discussions such as these can help African American adolescents see that they should continue to strive and advocate for equality and justice and create a strong voice for positive affirmation. This will also provide fodder in the establishment of positive values and norms. It will underscore, moreover, the pride as well as the resilience manifest in African Americans as a people.

Values and Ethics That Support Survival. Addressing values supports resilience. According to Hill (1998), studies suggest that people who are resilient are more likely to have positive values than less resilient individuals. Based on these studies, the positive values appear to be "respect for family, high regard for the elderly, strong academic orientation, strong religious orientation, strong work orientation, personal responsibility, and concern about the welfare of others" (p. 52). Discussing this subject area, therefore, will reinforce existing values and assist with positive internalization of values where marginal.

Understanding the core values and ethics of African Americans as a people will undergird their sense of self and support positive means for addressing value discrepancies and ethical dilemmas that exist within the African American population and between the African American population and the broader society (Hill, 1998; Stevens, 2002). Such understanding will assist in looking at changing social values and norms and social structures and policies that effect their well-being.

Significant in the molding of values and ethics perspectives for the African American population has been the Black Church. This social structure has remained independent from ownership by the dominant culture, has a strong history, adaptability, and strength in purpose (Billingsley & Morrison-Rodriguez, 1998). The Black Church is not only a spiritual resource but a social institution as well, with the capacity to touch all facets of family life (Billingsley & Morrison-Rodriguez, 1998). Although some youth may not attend church often, this practice may not negate their strength of religious orientation and sense of spirituality (Hill, 1998; Kamya & Lowery, 1999). The degree of involvement in the Church or the degree to which they express a sense of spirituality can help to identify for practitioners, adolescents' value stance. Spirituality supports a person's inner capacity for resilience (Hopps, Pinderhughes, & Shankar, 1995; Robinson, 2000; Stevens, 2002). The Black Church, long a source of support (Billingsley & Morrison-Rodriguez, 1998), and a resilient institution in and of itself, provides spiritual support and hope for the future.

Another area that seems to correlate with resilience is the "care protective sensibility domain" (Stevens, 2002, p. 90). This domain refers to "the affective and behavioral expressions of care, loyalty, and nurturance in relation to others. Learning to care for others evolves over time during the adolescent period. This evolving sensibility of care and nurturance is central to the adolescent's self-view or social identity. It becomes a self-defining personal-communal view for adaptive living" (Stevens, 2002, p. 90). This domain and other adaptive styles help African American youth to value self and others.

The adolescent group whose parents were either seropositive or had AIDS used their group support in a humanistic spiritual manner that freed them to express their value stance, gain a clearer perspective on what they could do for themselves and their parents, and for some, to embrace the Church for further spiritual support.

Avenues for Positive Adaptation and Change. The group process is a mechanism for multiple levels of change (Hopps & Pinderhughes, 1999). Within this context, group members would examine the self, family, broader environment, and the group as protective factors for learning, planning, and using positive adaptive measures in negotiating self-needs and environmental interaction. Adaptive strategies must also consider bringing about change through community activism directed at policies, attitudes, and practices (Freshman & Leinwand, 2001; Hopps & Pinderhughes, 1999; Hopps, Pinderhughes, & Shankar, 1995) that impede Black adolescent growth (e.g., poor schools and a lack of jobs and meaningful work opportunities as noted earlier). The authors posit that such change comes from a social justice practice orientation which encompasses creative and structured thought and measured implementation (Hopps, Pinderhughes, & Shankar, 1995). Strategies have to be taught and perceived as techniques that can be transferred to other situations and tasks (Spiegel, 1994).

Outside of the therapeutic group are informal and formal groups that are sources of resilience and, thereby, nurture and foster positive adaptation. Informal groups (such as kinship and friendship networks, extended family, and peer groups) and formal groups (such as churches, social service agencies, schools and colleges, and businesses) (Hill, 1998) should be tapped and used when appropriate. An informal or formal group may be one adolescent's risk factor, but another adolescent's protective factor. Assisting African American adolescents in developing adequate coping strategies (such as reaching out for support from positive individuals/mentors and institutions), and good judgement skills (for instance, understanding consequences of actions and thinking through situations) will help them negotiate and determine group affiliations that will support positive coping and adaptation. For example, in the AIDS group, adequate coping strategies and good judgment skills were both objectives and successful outcomes (Hopps & Pinderhughes, 1999).

In summary, intervention involves action, observation, planning and reflection (Stevens, 1997), all of which are integral to this framework and interventive method. Resilience as a concept assists group members to focus on their strengths and underscore the protective factors that support positive adaptation. As indicated by the World Health Organization (in Blum, 1998) "health . . . [is] not merely the absence of illness, but a positive sense of well-being" (p. 372). African American adolescents need to feel that sense of well-being, and a resilience framework for group intervention can help with that acquisition. To sustain this resilience framework, a model for practice should be employed, such as the Justice-Based Model (referred to above) proffered by Hopps, Pinderhughes, & Shankar (1995).

REFLECTIONS: THE FRAMEWORK AND JUSTICE-BASED MODEL

The profile of African American youth is improving; however, the numbers and percentages indicate that these young people remain at risk. They come from a resilient people, but psychosocial risk factors coupled with discriminatory practices can erode intrapsychic strengths, internal coping skills, and the ability to utilize an external facilitative environment. The resilience framework within a group context can provide the support and direction Black youth need. Such work is enhanced by the Justice-Based Model, which was developed as an outgrowth of a study on overwhelmed clients (Hopps, Pinderhughes, & Shankar, 1995). This model centers on helping individuals attain self-efficacy, personal mastery, and competent adaptive behavior. The study found that what is significant for practitioners is the use of eclectic theoretical approaches and intervention strategies (i.e., assessment, advocacy, empowerment, and individual and group treatment), with group methods having the most significance when supported by theory and other interventions. Simultaneously, practitioners and clients focus on self-efficacy, personal mastery, competent adaptive behavior, and also on community building and advocating for justice-based social policy. Justice-based policies call for the elimination of inequality and the expansion of equality.

Noted earlier, this discussion brought attention to youths' lack of accessibility, suitable jobs, competitive education, and the crippling influence of the criminal justice system. Practitioners help clients advocate for change in these conditions as they advocate for individual change. In Hopps and Pinderhughes (1999), a case was noted wherein a group leader working with Black adolescent males focused on the importance of an education, acquisition of employable skills, dating and safe sex, and prevention of drug use. Attention was called to drug prevention activities in the neighborhood, and youth learned how to embrace this as well. This model supports resilience and the group process, and most importantly, encourages justice-based social interventions that will help alleviate individual issues as well as social and class conflicts, promoting a more empowering and harmonious environment.

REFERENCES

Belgrave, F. Z., Chase-Vaughn, G., Gray, F., Addison, J. D., & Cherry, V. R. (2000). The effectiveness of a culture- and gender-specific intervention for increasing resiliency among African American preadolescent females. *The Journal of Black Psychology, 26* (2), 133-147.

Billingsley, A., & Morrison-Rodriguez, B. (1998). The Black family in the 21st century and the church as an action system: A macro perspective. In L. A. See (ed.), *Human behavior in the social environment from an African American perspective* (pp. 31-47). New York: The Haworth Press, Inc.

Blackwell, J. E. (1991). *The black community: Diversity and unity* (3rd ed.). New York: Harper Collins Publishers.

Blum, R. W. (1998). Healthy youth development as a model for youth health promotion. *Journal of Adolescent Health*, 22 (5), 368-375.

Building Blocks for Youth. (2002). Resources for disproportionate minority confinement/over representation of youth of color. *Punitive polices hit youth of color hardest*. Available: http://www.buildingblocksforyouth.org/issues/dmc/factsvoc.html.

Center on Budget and Policy Priority. (2000, Sept. 26). *Poverty rate fell in 2000 as unemployment reached a 31-year low*. Author.

Center for Disease Control and Prevention. (1998, March 28). *Suicide among black youth–United States, 1980 to 1995*. Division of Violence Prevention, National Center for Injury Prevention and Control.

Center for Disease Control and Prevention. (1998). National data on HIV prevalence among disadvantaged youth in the 1990s. Available: (http://www.cdc.gov/hiv/pubs/facts/jobscorps.htm).

Children's Defense Fund. (2002). Key facts: The Uninsured Children's Health Coverage in 2001. Available: (http://www.children'sdefense.orgssydfsviocrime.php).

Child Welfare League of America. (2002). Family Foster Care Fact Sheet. Available: (http://www.cwla.org/program/fostercare/factsheet.htm).

Clinard, M. B., & Meier, R. F. (1995). *Sociology of deviant behavior* (9th ed.). Fort Worth: Harcourt Brace, Inc.

Corcoran, K., Grinnell, Jr., R. M., & Briggs, H. E. (2001). Introduction: Implementing the foundations of change. In H. E. Briggs & K. Corcoran (eds.), *Social work practice: Treating common client problems* (pp. 3-14). Chicago: Lyceum.

Coser, L. (1956). *The functions of social conflict*. New York: The Free Press of Glencoe.

Dalaker, J. U.S. Census Bureau, Current Population Reports, Series P60-214, *Poverty in the United States 2000*, U.S. Printing Office, Washington DC.

Feagin, J. R. & Feagin, C. B. (1997). *Social problems: A critical power-conflict perspective* (5th ed.). Upper Saddle River, NJ: Prentice-Hall.

Freshman, A., & Leinwand, C. (2001). The implications of female risk factors for substance abuse prevention in adolescent girls. *Journal of Prevention & Intervention in the Community*, 21 (1), 29-51.

Glantz, M. D. (Ed.), & Johnson, J. L. (Ed.) (1999). *Resilience and development: Positive life adaptation*. New York, New York: Kluwer Academic/Plenum Publishers.

Hill, R. B. (1998). Enhancing the resilience of African American Families. In L. A. See (ed.), *Human behavior in the social environment from an African American perspective* (pp. 49-61). New York: The Haworth Press, Inc.

Hopps, J. G. (2000). Social Work, a Contextual Profession. In J. G. Hopps & R. Morris (eds.) *Social work at the millennium: Critical reflections on the future of the profession* (pp. 3-17). New York: Free Press.

Hopps, J. G., & Kilpatrick, A. C. (2003). Contexts of helping: Commonalities and human diversities. In A. C. Kilpatrick & T. P. Holland, *Working with families: An integrative model by level of need* (pp. 34-47). Boston: Allyn Bacon.

Hopps, J. G., & Pinderhughes, E. (1999). *Group work with overwhelmed clients*. New York: The Free Press.

Hopps, J. G., Pinderhughes, E., & Shankar, R. (1995). *The power to care*. New York: The Free Press.

Kamya, H., & Lowery, C. (1999). Pastoral counseling: An emerging partner in the field of social service. In R. W. C. Tourse & J. F. Mooney (eds.), *Collaborative practice: School and human service partnerships* (181-200). Westport, CT: Praeger.

Lerman, R. I. (2000, November). Are teens in low income and welfare families working to much? *New Federalism National Survey of American Families*, The Urban Institute, Series B, no. B-25.

Levy, A. J., & Wall, J. C. (2000). Children who have witnessed community homicide: Incorporating risk and resilience in clinical work. *Families in Society: The Journal of Contemporary Human Services, 81* (4), 402-411.

McInnis-Dittrich, K., Neisler, O. J., & Tourse, R. W. C. T. (1999). Socioeducational realities of the twenty-first century: A need for change. In R. W. C. Tourse & J. F. Mooney (eds.), *Collaborative practice: School and human service partnerships* (3-32). Westport, CT: Praeger.

McKinnon, J. (2001). *The Black Population 2000*. U.S. Census Bureau, Department of Commerce. Washington, D C.: U.S. Department of Commerce.

National Campaign to Prevent Teen Pregnancy. (2002). *General Facts and Statistics*. Available: (http://www.teenpregnancy.org/resources/data/genlfact.asp).

National Center for Children in Poverty. (2002). *Reports Low Income Children in the United States: A Brief demographic profile.* Mailman School of Public Health, Columbia University N.Y.

National Institute on Drug Abuse (NIDA). (2001, Jan. 30). *African American teens at Greater risk of tobacco addiction.* Available: (http://www.drugabuse.gov/MedAdv/01/NR1-30.html).

Neuburger, E. (2001). Computers and Internet Use in the United States: August 2000. *Current Population Reports, U.S. Census Bureau.* Washington, D C: U.S. Department of Commerce.

Robinson, H. (2000). Enhancing couple resiliency. In E. Norman (ed.), Resiliency enhancement: Putting the strengths perspective into social work practice (pp. 102-127). New York: Columbia University Press.

Schiele, J. H. (1998). Cultural alignment, African American male youths, and violent crime. In L. A. See (ed.), *Human behavior in the social environment from an African American perspective* (pp. 49-61). New York: The Haworth Press, Inc.

Schiraldi, V. (2002). Available: (http://www.buildingblocksforyouth.org/issues/dec/schiraldi.html).

Simmel, G. (1955). *Conflict and the web of group affiliations.* New York: The Free Press.

Spiegel, D. L. (1994). Promoting Literacy Development. In R. J. Simeonsson (ed.), *Risk, Resilience, and Prevention: Promoting the well-being of all children* (pp. 165-181). Baltimore: Paul H. Brookes Publishing.

Smith, C., & Carlson, B. E. (1997). Stress, coping, and resilience in children and youth. *Social Service Review, 7* (2), 231-256.

Stevens, L. A. (1997). Action research and consultation: Developing collaborative participative relationships with communities. *Maatskaplike Werk/Social Work, 33,* 1, 36-43.

Stevens, J. W. (2002). Smart and sassy: *The strengths of inner city black girls.* New York: Oxford Press.

Strouse, J. (2002, July 7). Capitalism Depends on Character. *New York Times,* p. 9.

Tischler, H. (2002). *Introduction to sociology* (7th ed.). New York: The Harcourt Press.

Tourse, R. W. C. (2002a). The group process and resiliency. Manuscript in preparation.

Tourse, R. W. C. (2002b). Understanding cultural sway: A critical component in Assessment and treatment for practitioners and interns. Manuscript in review.

Tourse, R. W. C. & Collins, P. Marginal women at risk: Working toward economic equity within the context of privatization. In D. S. Iatridis (ed.), *Social justice and the welfare state in central and eastern Europe: The impact of privatization* (pp. 100-117). Westport, CT: Praeger.

Tourse, R. W. C., Hopps, J. G., & Christian, O. (2002, May). *Making field more effective: Applying empirically-based practice strategies.* Paper presented at the 2002 Congress of the Social Sciences & Humanities on Anti-Oppressive Practice and Global Transformation: Challenges for social work and Social Welfare, Toronto, Canada.

Turner, J. (1991). *The structure of sociological theory*. Belmont: Wadsworth Publishing Company.

Turner, J. H., Beeghley, L., & Powers, C. (1995). *The emergence of sociological theory* (3rd ed.). Boston: Wadsworth Publishing Co.

U.S. Census Bureau (2000). *Census 2000. Table DP-1.*

U.S. Department of Education, National Center for Education Statistics. *Educational Achievement and Black-White Inequality*, NCES 20001-061, by Jacobson, J., Olsen, C., Rice, J. K., Sweetland S., & Ralph, J. Project Officer. John Ralph Washington, DC: U.S. Government Printing Office, 2001.

Williams, N. R., Lindsey, E. W., Kurtz, P. D., & Jarvis, S. (2001). From trauma to resiliency: Lessons from former runaway and homeless youth. *Journal of Youth Studies*, *4* (2), 233-253.

Hispanic and African American Youth: Life After Foster Care Emancipation

Alfreda P. Iglehart
Rosina M. Becerra

SUMMARY. This exploratory, qualitative study of 28 (10 Hispanic and 18 African American) former foster care youth attempts to capture the essence of their quest for self-sufficiency. While research on former foster care youth continues to highlight the problems confronting them after they emancipate from care, the depth of their struggles is often lost in the aggregation of statistics. The numbers themselves often fail to capture the hardships, isolation, hope, and despair many of them may face as they attempt to adjust to life after foster care. Furthermore, existing research often regards emancipated youth as a homogeneous population. Interviews with these respondents of color were coded to determine the themes and stories they held. The themes emergent from these interviews were: the importance of people in the independent living programs; vagueness in recalling the content of the independent living programs; family conflict; housing instability; regrets, fears, and lessons learned; and future goals. Im-

---

Alfreda P. Iglehart, PhD, is Associate Professor and Rosina M. Becerra, PhD, is Professor, Department of Social Welfare, School of Public Policy & Social Research, University of California at Los Angeles.

This project is funded by the California Department of Social Services, Research Branch, through a contract to Principal Investigator, Rosina M. Becerra.

[Haworth co-indexing entry note]: "Hispanic and African American Youth: Life After Foster Care Emancipation." Iglehart, Alfreda P., and Rosina M. Becerra. Co-published simultaneously in *Journal of Ethnic & Cultural Diversity in Social Work* (The Haworth Social Work Practice Press, an imprint of The Haworth Press, Inc.) Vol. 11, No. 1/2, 2002, pp. 79-107; and: *Social Work with Multicultural Youth* (ed: Diane de Anda) The Haworth Social Work Practice Press, an imprint of The Haworth Press, Inc., 2002, pp. 79-107. Single or multiple copies of this article are available for a fee from The Haworth Document Delivery Service [1-800-HAWORTH, 9:00 a.m. - 5:00 p.m. (EST). E-mail address: docdelivery@haworthpress.com].

http://www.haworthpress.com/store/product.asp?sku=J051

10.1300/J051v11n01_04

plications for culturally sensitive practice and research are drawn from these data.

KEYWORDS. Foster care, emancipation, youth of color

INTRODUCTION

After an individual reaches adulthood, s/he is no longer expected to require parental support and/or supervision; s/he is emancipated. Legally speaking, emancipation is used to describe that point in time when parents are no longer responsible for their children, and children do not have to answer to their parents (State Bar of California, 1999). Foster care placements of older adolescents often terminate precipitously at the point the adolescents have a birthday signifying the legal age for emancipation and cessation of public support (Lammert & Timberlake, 1986). In California, for example, emancipation automatically occurs under certain circumstances that include reaching the age of 18, at which time an individual becomes an adult and is emancipated (State Bar of California, 1999).

The problems that face adolescents aging out or emancipating from foster care reached the federal legislative agenda with the debate over and subsequent passage of the Foster Care Independence Act of 1999 (P.L. 106-169). The bill amended Part E of Title IV of the Social Security Act to provide States with more funding and greater flexibility in carrying out programs designed to help children make the transition from foster care to self-sufficiency. Section 477 of the bill renamed the Independent Living Program (ILP) to the John H. Chaffee Foster Care Independence Program as a tribute to the late Senator Chaffee's advocacy and commitment to child welfare. Years of advocacy, research, evaluation, hearings, and lobbying finally were instrumental in catapulting the dilemma of former foster care youth to national attention. With this legislation, the public is beginning to accept responsibility for those children who leave public care ill-prepared for self-sufficiency.

States may now use a portion of their independent living funds for older youth who have emancipated from care, but who are not yet 21 years of age. This legislation provides the States flexible funding for financial, housing, counseling, employment, education, and other appropriate services to former foster care recipients to complement their own efforts to achieve self-sufficiency (Foster Care Independence Act of 1999). Furthermore, States may use up to 30% of program funds for room and board for former foster care youth 18 to 21 years of age and may extend Medicaid to this group as well.

The statistics on the adolescent foster care population are daunting. By the end of 1996, there were 530,912 children in out-of-home care, about 30% were teenagers, and over 20,000 were aging out of foster care each year (Child Welfare League of America, 1999). According to the Children's Bureau (1999), on March 31, 1998, there were 520,000 children in foster care and 14% were 16 years of age or older. Because of the growth of the adolescent population, although the proportion of adolescents in foster care has decreased from 45.3% in 1982 to 32% in 1995, the actual number of foster care adolescents has grown from 118,700 in 1982 to 139,434 in 1995 (Child Welfare League of America, 1998). Adolescents, 13 to 18 years of age, make up 12% of the United States' population, but make up about one-third of the foster care population. A large number of these adolescents will make the transition to adulthood not from the supportive care and homes of biological parents, but from the care of surrogate parents in settings supervised by public child welfare agencies.

While the number of adolescents in foster care is changing, the proportion of children of color in the foster care system is also undergoing change. For example, in 1980, 47% of those in foster care were children of color; however, by 1995, that number had grown to 61% (Child Welfare League of America, 1998). According to the Child Welfare League of America (1998), African American and Latino children and youth are disproportionately represented in the system by more than two to one and, in 1990, there were more African American than White children in foster care. Of the 248,000 children who left foster care during fiscal year 1998, 17,360 left through emancipation (U.S. Department of Health and Human Services, 2001), which means that adolescents of color comprise a large proportion of the emancipating group.

EMANCIPATION: ISSUES AND PROBLEMS

Research on emancipation and transition to adulthood for foster care adolescents consistently highlights the numerous issues and struggles of these young people as they adjust to life after foster care. McDonald et al. (1993), in *Assessing the Long-Term Effects of Foster Care: A Research Synthesis*, report the results of a comprehensive synthesis of 27 studies of adult outcomes of foster care that were completed between 1960 and 1990. The authors note that the primary focus of the review was on outcomes for those children in long-term foster care who age out of the foster care system. The authors, after reviewing all 27 studies, concluded:

> While definitive conclusions cannot be drawn from the review of studies presented here, we believe that they do offer convincing evidence that former foster care subjects are at high risk of "rotten outcomes" as adults. These rotten outcomes are not simply a slightly diminished functioning or a failure to reach full potential, but involve a failure to meet minimal levels of self-sufficiency (homelessness, welfare dependency, etc.) and acceptable behaviors (criminal activity, drug use, etc.). (p. 129)

Follow-up studies conducted since the McDonald et al. (1993) review only serve to reinforce the dire findings of the earlier synthesis. For example, recent studies highlight poor health, homelessness, unemployment, welfare dependency, out of wedlock births, incarceration, and lack of education as problems confronting former foster care youth (Chambers, 1997; Collins, 2001; Courtney & Piliavin, 1998; Lindsey & Ahmed, 1999; Orange County Grand Jury, 2000).

For foster care adolescents who emancipate from foster care rather than from the care of their biological parents, several major developmental issues arise. One issue is the adolescents' need to deal with loss of family and other social support networks (Lambert & Timberlake, 1986). At a time when they are attempting to move toward adulthood, these foster care teens experience the traumatic and developmentally premature separation from family members. The naturally progressive individuation that adolescents typically face as they transition to adulthood is replaced by a forceful separation that is thrust upon the foster care youth. Another issue is the development of self-protection mechanisms that result from multiple placement and inconsistent foster parenting. The uncertainty of the foster care placement and the variations in foster parenting place the adolescent in a vulnerable and insecure position. S/he often develops a façade of social distance, self-confidence, detachment, and defensiveness as a self-protective strategy (Kools, 1999).

Foster care adolescents also need to develop the soft skills (planning, decision-making, communicating) that the foster care system may not have emphasized as much as the hard skills (educational/vocational training, cooking, shopping, money management, etc.). Surveys of programs that prepare foster youth for life after foster care reveal an emphasis on tangible self-sufficiency skills (U.S. General Accounting Office, 1999) even though many of these young individuals also need socio-emotional assistance as they prepare for independence. Foster care emancipation also brings with it a need to negotiate separation from foster care. Emancipation becomes a "departure event" about which the adolescent has feelings that require appropriate management (Lammert & Timberlake, 1986). Emancipation adds another developmental task to those tasks that are already a part of adolescent growth.

While these issues confront foster care adolescents in general, it is not clear whether ethnicity affects the emergence, extent, and/or resolution of developmental tasks that may be unique to the foster care experience. As a matter of fact, in a survey of studies on adolescent separation and individuation, Gnaulati and Heine (2001) found that the samples were typically predominantly white or unidentified. Furthermore, those studies that did address ethnic differences were marked by inconsistent results.

One of the most critical issues facing foster care adolescents is the need to establish and maintain self-sufficiency. Successful transition to adulthood is reflected in an individual's ability to support him/herself, to have responsible family and social relationships, and to be a contributing member of society (Family and Youth Services Bureau, 1997). Success then becomes related to one's ability to: obtain and maintain an income-producing position; maintain some type of reasonably stable housing/living arrangement; manage the daily activities of life; make sound and reasonable decisions; and problem solve in a constructive manner.

Because virtually the entire child protective service population is of low socioeconomic status and is disproportionately made up of minorities, the transition of minority foster care youth from emancipation to self-sufficiency is of paramount concern. While it has been argued that the ethnic and class composition of the public child welfare population may be due to institutional racism, another explanation holds that high poverty rates among ethnic minorities may render them vulnerable to child maltreatment (Jones, 1997). Indeed, an adolescent's future of self-sufficiency may be jeopardized in areas of high joblessness and poverty (Hamburg, 1989). Thus, it becomes imperative that the experiences of ethnic minority adolescents as they transition out of foster care receive more critical attention.

Several researchers have used in-depth interviews and focus groups as tools for allowing foster care children and youth to share their own perspectives on foster care and their post-foster care experiences. For example, Gil and Bogart (1982) interviewed 50 foster care children in foster family homes and 50 living in group homes. These researchers effectively used the respondents' words to underscore the major trends and conclusions found in the data. McMillen et al. (1997) explored what former foster youth thought about the independent living services they received while they were still in care. The authors interspersed quotes from the respondents with the discussion of the emergent themes. Kools (1999) interviewed 17 adolescents to explore the self-protection strategies they used to address feelings of devaluation and uncertainty in foster care. Again, respondent quotes served to illuminate the manner in which they sought to protect themselves from disappointment, devaluation, and stigmatization.

For the studies cited, race and ethnicity were often noted when sample characteristics were presented; yet, they were often absent from analysis and discussion. Because of the over-representation of adolescents of color in foster care and in the emancipation process, issues of diversity can be more effectively addressed when race and ethnicity are vital components of the analysis and discussion.

This study builds on previous research by using qualitative interviews to learn what former foster care individuals of color experienced as they left foster care, what their lives looked like, and what views they have about their lives. The views and stories of these young adults about their struggle to gain self-sufficiency can help practitioners and policy-makers to further identify the specific service modifications that may be required to more effectively serve a diverse population. Thus, the voices of emancipated individuals can illuminate the service needs, service gaps, service expansion, and service development that may be needed to support a successful transition to adulthood for those who age out of the foster care system.

METHODS

Respondents

Twenty-eight former foster youth (10 Hispanics and 18 African Americans) living in Los Angeles County participated in this study and none had been emancipated for longer than five years. Los Angeles becomes an extremely credible site for research on emancipation when the numbers are taken into consideration. In 1998, of the 166,035 children who exited foster care nationally, 11,622 (7%) left because of emancipation and, in California alone, 4,003 adolescents, or a third of the nation's total, emancipated from foster care (U.S. House of Representatives, 2000, pp. 726, 738). In general, Los Angeles County has about 10% of the total children in foster care nationally and a quarter of California's annual emancipation population. For Los Angeles County, 931 (out of 4,003 statewide) adolescents aged out of care in 2000 (Los Angeles County Department of Children and Family Services, 2001). Moreover, in December, 2000, 16% of the children in out-of-home care in Los Angeles County were White while 40% were African American, 39% were Hispanic, and the remainder were other race/ethnic groups. Thus, the overwhelming majority of adolescents who age out of care in Los Angeles County are adolescents of color.

To recruit former foster care youth for the study the researchers contacted social service programs known to serve this population. Some of these programs provided transitional housing and other support services for former foster care individuals who met specific criteria. Program staff informed agency clients about the study and provided a telephone number to call if they were interested in being interviewed. When the potential respondent called the number, project personnel explained the study to him/her, arranged an interview time and location if the caller agreed to be interviewed, and assigned that individual an identification number. In addition, respondents were given flyers about the study to share with other former foster care youth they knew. Those seeing the flyer and wishing to participate in the study could call a telephone number listed on the flyer.

The principal investigators and trained project staff conducted all interviews. Because of the focus of the interview, it was important to have an interview environment that the respondent found to be comfortable, private, familiar, and convenient. Interview locations included agency settings, restaurants, apartments, and meeting areas of apartment complexes.

Before the formal interview started, the purpose of the study was explained to the respondent and an informed consent was read aloud and explained by the interviewer to insure the respondent clearly understood. If the respondent agreed to continue with the interview, s/he was asked to sign the consent form and given a copy of the form. In addition, each respondent was asked for permission to audiotape the interview. All those interviewed agreed to being tape-recorded. The tapes allowed the experiences and views of the respondents to be captured in his/her own words. When the interview was completed, each respondent received $50.

Data Collection

The present study utilizes a qualitative, ethnographic interview approach. With this type of interview, broad questions about the research areas serve as a foundation for the subsequent in-depth interviewing (Green, 1999). The qualitative interview elicits in-depth answers about culture, meanings, processes, and problems to find out what people think and know without the interviewer dominating the interviewee by imposing a world view. Because the topic areas were emancipation preparation and emancipation experiences, a semi-structured, focused format was used that relied on open-ended questions. In this format, the interviewer introduces the topic, then guides the discussion by asking specific questions (Rubin & Rubin, 1995).

These interviews were designed to provide a glimpse of the world of these former foster care individuals from their own perspective. The general areas used to guide the interview included: respondent demographics (age, race/ethnic self-identity); age when first placed and why; experiences while in care (placement history, relationships with adults and peers, school and work history, significant experiences); emancipation preparation (training, skills, service provider, usefulness); experiences right after emancipation (where lived, with whom, school, employment, income sources, supports, challenges); current situation (where living, with whom, employment, school, income sources,) future plans; and recommendations for services/programs for emancipating youth.

Because the goal was to capture the world of the emancipated individual in his or her own words, these qualitative interviews represented a modified version of the ethnographic interview. The ethnographic interview shares some similarities with a friendly conversation in that it encourages the respondent to describe his/her experiences using the same language they would employ when speaking to others in their cultural scene (Fetterman, 1989; Spadley, 1979). Indeed, Rubin and Rubin (1995) refer to the qualitative interview as guided conversations. This interview method was selected to capture the world views and attitudes of those who have gone through the foster care system to emerge on the other side as emancipated youth.

While more recent sources provide approaches to thematic analysis (see, for example, Boyatzis, 1998; Patton, 2002), Spradley (1979) offers a detailed guide for the ethnographic interview and its interpretation. The three most important elements in the ethnographic interview process are explicit purpose, ethnographic explanations, and ethnographic questions. With explicit purpose, the interviewer takes control of the verbal exchange, reminds the respondent of the purpose of the interview, and gently continues to lead the interview in that direction. Because ethnographic interviews involve purpose and direction, they tend to be more formal than a friendly conversation (Fetterman, 1989; Spradley, 1979). In this study, the interviewers' task was to keep the attention focused on foster care, emancipation preparation, and emancipation experiences of the respondents.

Spradley (1979) offers several types of ethnographic explanations. The project explanations are essential to the interview process, because they serve to translate the goals of the research into terms the respondent can understand. Such expressions as, "I am very interested in what happened to you after you left foster care," or "Your emancipation experiences are very important in this study," are examples of the project explanations used in this study. Recording explanations were also used because all interviews were tape-recorded. Recording explanations include those statements explaining the reasons for taping the interviews. Questions were also employed because they enabled the interviewer to move from topic to topic with greater ease. Frequently other explanations used were, "Now I would like to ask a different kind of question," and "Let's change the focus a little now."

Ethnographic questions include descriptive, structural, and contrast questions (Fetterman, 1989; Spradley, 1979). With descriptive questions, the respondent is asked to describe the event, experience, location, attitude, and/or feeling that s/he mentioned. Descriptive questions were used, for example, to gather detail about the respondent's post-foster care life. Structural questions help the interviewer to understand how the respondent has organized his/her knowledge. An example of a structural question used in this study includes, "How did you go about finding a job?" Contrast questions help to reveal the meanings the respondent uses to distinguish or contrast events, locations, and/or people. In this study, contrast questions were particularly helpful in illuminating the respondents' movement between various living situations. Examples of these questions include, "How was emancipation different from foster care?" and "How did that job differ from the previous one you had?"

Data Analysis

The interviews were transcribed and a coding protocol was developed. Where feasible, response categories were generated for the open-ended questions. For example, all respondents were asked to indicate what they thought was the reason for their placement. A careful review of the reasons suggested that categories could be created to capture the range of responses. These categories included: neglect; sexual abuse; parental substance abuse; parental mental illness; and juvenile probation. Categories were created to capture areas such as housing situation, employment situation, sources of financial support, current educational activity, and sources of social support. For the other open-ended questions and narratives provided by the respondents, key words and concepts were noted. For example, views of Independent Living Programs were initially categorized as positive, negative or mixed (both positive and negative comments made). Social support was categorized as present or absent.

After these general categories were coded, the content of the responses were reviewed to determine whether themes and/or stories were present. Themes offer descriptions of how people do or should behave, provide explanations for how or why things happen, and describe whom to trust or not trust (Rubin & Rubin, 1995). According to Rubin and Rubin (1995), themes may be present when the respondent explicitly states it, repeats or emphasizes a major point, makes a dramatic statement, or makes an iconic statement. Themes can also be suggested by the researcher's interview summaries and/or by the similarities in the world view of people in different circumstances.

Stories are refined versions of events that may have been condensed or altered to make a point indirectly. For example, stories may be told as adventures or are frequently marked by symbols that carry a great deal of emotion. They may also be set off by a change in speaking tone and/or they may represent a disjunction between a question and a response, that is, the response is extended and does not appear to address the question that was asked (Rubin & Rubin, 1995).

Each interview code sheet was expanded to include notations for themes and stories. The interviews were read again and a one or two word description of themes, if apparent, was entered on the code sheet. Because of the focus of this study, those themes and stories related to emancipation preparation, transition to independence, work, school, social supports, and self-sufficiency were particularly crucial. For example, if the respondent said that individuals coordinating the Independent

Living Program in which s/he participated were valuable, then "People" was entered on the code sheet next to ILP. If at least a quarter (seven) of the respondents made similar comments about the ILP program, then a theme was identified. Stories were noted by a check next to the "Story" column and a brief description of the story was noted on the back of the code sheet.

According to Rubin and Rubin (1995), in the final stages of analysis, the data are organized in ways that help formulate themes, refine concepts, and link them together to create a clear description or explanation of the topic under investigation. For the analysis used in this study, themes are identified and respondent quotes are used to illustrate the themes. If stories that relate to the themes have been identified, then they, too, are included in the analysis.

FINDINGS

Characteristics of the Respondents

Table 1 summarizes some of the characteristics of the sample. The 28 participants included 13 African-American females, five African American males, eight Hispanic females, and two Hispanic males. The respondents ranged in age from 17 to 25 (mean age for the sample was 20). All the youth had emancipated at age 18 or 19 with the exception of one who had been granted emancipation at age 16.

About two-thirds of the sample (64%) emancipated with a high school diploma or general equivalency diploma (GED). At the time of the interview, only four respondents did not have a high school diploma or GED, indicating that six others had completed their high school schooling since emancipation. At the time of interview, about a third of the interviewees (10) were participating in some type of educational program, such as community college or vocational training. Of the 18 respondents who were not currently continuing their education, 13 indicated that they planned to seek additional education in the future.

> School now? No, I'm just trying to keep my financial stability now. In a couple of weeks, I plan to start school. What school? I don't know. Maybe I'll try junior college. [African-American male, 22]

Five of the 13 indicated conflicts with employment as a factor.

TABLE 1. Characteristics of the Sample of Emancipated Youth

(column % in parenthese, rounded)

	African-America Youth (N = 18)	Hispanic Youth (N = 10)	TOTAL (N = 28)
Mean Age Age Range (17-25)	20.3	20.3	20.3
HS Diploma/GED* at Emancipation (Yes)	15 (83.3)	3 (30)	18 (64)
Employed right after emancipation (Yes)	8 (44.4)	4 (40)	12 (43)
Currently Employed (Yes)	12 (66.7)	6(60)	18 (64)
Currently in School (Yes)	7 (38.9)	3 (30)	10 (36)
Mean Number of Placements	4	4	4
Homeless after Emancipation (Yes)	6 (33.3)	2 (20)	8 (29)
Ever Arrested (Yes)	4 (22.2)	2 (20)	6 (21)
Is a Parent (Yes)	7 (38.9)	3 (30)	10 (36)

GED = General Equivalency Diploma

> I couldn't work my school around my job. [African-American male, 19]

Another five of the 18 who were not in school did not have education as part of their plan, as illustrated in the comments of one 22-year old Hispanic female:

> I went to school, but before I failed at something, I quit. I was going to [Community College], I was taking 12 units. A lot of them were hard like biology and all that stuff. I went to continuation school and that was hard too, but being at a college where it was more hard, I just didn't go back.

A 20-year old African American male, who did not have a high school diploma or a GED, had this to say about school:

> As soon as I turned 18, I was like, yea man, I was like, I'm outta here. I just said forget it, man . . . I was like, yea, I'm cool. I don't need it.

Of these five respondents who did not have plans for additional education, two were Hispanic females, two were African American males, and one was African American female.

Right after emancipation, 12 (about 43%) of the respondents worked in order to support themselves. At the time of the interview, 18 (almost two-thirds) were employed. All the males (7) and 11 of the 21 females in the study were all employed. Many of the respondents had held a number of minimum wage jobs in, for example, fast food restaurants, retail sales, clerical positions, or child care. Those currently employed worked in such varied positions as teaching assistant, bank teller, hair stylist, fast food counter person, recreation worker, student assistant, and clerk. Five of the respondents were employed as youth workers or peer counselors with an independent living program. Those who were not employed (10) said that they were either looking for a job or waiting to enter school.

About half (15) had entered foster care when they were at least 13 years of age. All respondents had a mean of either three or four placements. All of the respondents had participated in some type of Independent Living Program prior to emancipation. The mean time since emancipation was two years and four months.

Slightly more than a quarter (8) had experienced homelessness for some period after leaving foster care. Males were more likely to have been homeless. Slightly less than a quarter of the youth had ever been arrested, and they were primarily the males (5 out of 7 males).

About half (10) of the females had at least one child while in foster care. Seven of these mothers were currently receiving welfare. Four of the ten mothers were those who had not completed their high school education. These four females indicated that they planned to obtain additional education in the future but that working was their first priority.

Social Support

No discernible theme emerged from the interviews about social support. All but two of the respondents identified individuals in their lives to whom they could talk about personal issues. These individuals included boyfriends, girlfriends, relatives, friends, friends' families, former foster parents, and workers in various social programs. No particular individuals were mentioned more than others as a support system by any of the youth. On occasion, these supportive individuals also provided concrete support such as money, housing, and transportation. Examples of social support included:

He [uncle] is very supportive. If I need anything, I can count on him. [African-American female, 18]

I have lots of friends, people I can lean on. [African-American female, 23]

I have my girlfriend. We've been together about three years. [Hispanic male, 19]

My one close friend has remained no matter the changes I've gone through. [African-American female, 19]

If nothing else worked, I could move back and stay with my foster mother. [Hispanic female, 23]

I'm really close to my dad. He lives around the corner from me. I see him every day. [African-American male, 21]

If I'm feeling blue, there are so many people I can talk to–the social worker here [transitional housing], my ILP worker. [Hispanic female, 19]

Living Arrangements

After leaving foster care, almost half of the youth (n = 13, 46%) went to live with a relative. At the time of interview, however, only seven of the respondents were living with a relative. At the time of the interview, close to half (13) of the interviewees were participating and living in transitional housing programs. These programs typically provide housing, counseling, education/employment assistance, and food vouchers. For those residents who work, about one-quarter of their earnings is applied to the rent. The "rent" money is really a forced savings plan so that the residents can have a "nest egg" when they leave transitional housing. Respondents found out about transitional housing from ILP workers, social workers, homeless shelter staff workers, and peers. The significance of transitional housing in the lives of these young people is captured in the following observation made by a 21-year-old African-American male:

The first time I walked in the door, it was so big, dishes in the cupboards, silverware, a gift certificate from [a supermarket]. I just

> felt like getting on my knees, and I almost cried. I called everyone I knew to come over. . . .

Theme: Family Conflict

A little over half (n = 15, 53.6%) of the respondents were experiencing some type of family conflict. The parents' dysfunctional behavior was the source of the problem for some of the respondents. For example, a 17-year-old Hispanic female who emancipated at 16 with her daughter moved in with her mother six months before she emancipated. Three weeks after emancipation she moved into her own apartment and maintains distance from her mother's problems.

> I don't see my mother much. My mother's remarried and that's partly why I moved out once I was emancipated. She visits my sisters and brother. She's doing better now . . . She had a drug problem. So I have this family problem with my mother.

Similar situations were expressed by other respondents:

> She [mother] has to understand that I can't keep going through her ups and downs . . . I don't want to need her. I don't want to need her for anything. She's like a kid, running in and out. I don't need that. I'd rather she go away and leave me alone. I think it's better for parents if they say they don't want their kids, that they go away and never come back. That's the worse, having seen them come in and out all the time. [African-American female, 19]

> The last time I saw my mother was on the street. We got into an argument and I told her she would never see her grandson. I'm ashamed of the life she lives and I don't want my son to know her. [African-American female, 20]

A number of respondents reported an absence of family ties.

> To be perfectly honest, my real family is people who I grew up on the streets with, except for a couple of cousins. Other than that, I don't deal with my family cause when I was taken away and put in group homes, nobody tried to get in touch with me. I was learning and living life on my own. Once I was to the age where I knew they didn't give a damn about me–I've been out here getting shot at,

> getting run over by cars–they didn't worry about me. So now I wanna be with my 'family' now–people that was on the streets looking out for me. [African-American male, 22]

> My mom's never been in the picture. I seen her at a couple of court dates, but other than that, I never talked to her. I'm in contact with my dad, but still don't want to have anything to do with him. It's a respect problem. I don't have a say so, my opinion doesn't matter. I have to do what he says. [African-American male, 19]

For four of the fifteen (27%), family conflict was a factor in their becoming homeless. For example, according to a 21-year-old African-American male who was living with his grandmother when he emancipated:

> My grandmother told me, "You need to start working, go to school, graduate from high school, or you need to get out." It's a long story. At 18, I don't know. Me and my grandmother started having problems. It was like a little clash with us cause she was older and stuff and, like, she wouldn't like let me, like, hang out with my friends or go anywhere. Then we started getting into a lot of different things about rent and all these different things. We got into a argument one day and I just walked out.

He had no place to stay after he left his grandmother's house.

In another example, a 22-year-old Hispanic mother emancipated with a housing plan that called for her to return to her mother's house. She spent only one week with her mother because, according to the respondent, "We could not resolve our past issues." She was homeless after she left her mother's house.

Theme: A Drifting Life

After emancipation, about a third (n = 10) of the respondents described lives in which they appeared to be drifting from one living situation to another. Some of these drifting youth included several who experienced homelessness. For example after walking out of his grandmother's house, the 21-year-old African-American male moved in with a friend's mother who also had four children and her nephew living with her. One day the friends told him, "We rented a truck and we're leaving." He became homeless, but managed to stay with different friends for brief spells. According to this respondent:

> Sleeping from here to there. Everywhere. I used to have, like, I grew a 'fro and then I had got dredlocks. I don't know. I looked kind of crazy. I don't know how I looked to people but I would, like, go to work. Then my grandmother would let me come over there and wash clothes. I never told her I was homeless.

Another 22-year-old African American male reported that when he was homeless:

> I was everywhere, alleys, parks, under buildings, sometimes I was couch surfing. People let me sleep on their couches, sleeping in garages, cars. I've had so many times of being homeless–Alabama, Texas, Seattle, Washington. I got GR [General Relief–welfare]. Got a motel voucher and stayed at a motel in Hollywood. Someone tried to get me to go out of state and sell magazines. Wasn't interested . . . The longest time I was on the streets was months in LA. Walk, find somewhere and pass out. I used to break into a van in a parking lot and hide. Get a sack lunch from wherever and just walk the streets.

Another 23-year-old Hispanic mother who experienced homelessness described her situation this way:

> It was different. I always had a home. I tried to make things as normal as possible. It's just my daughter was used to moving around and so was I. And I made that into, you know, I didn't make a big deal out of it. I just said okay, we, we're moving to a new place and I went about my business. I went to school and I tried to find work, but with child care problems. And so, after that I did find a job. About one month later, I started making money and then I rented a room. It was just basically normal, just moving from one place to another, so I didn't make a big deal about it.

Transiency also seemed to be part of the lives of respondents who had not faced homelessness. For example, a 23-year-old Hispanic mother lived with a roommate when she emancipated. She had a job, was in community college and then became pregnant. Later she moved in with her boyfriend for a brief period, but then returned to her roommate's house. Eight to nine months later, she began living with her sister.

A 20-year-old African American mother had two children when she emancipated. She indicated that she learned of her emancipation through a letter. When she turned 18, she said her social worker visited one last time and told her that she could begin receiving her own aid. When she emancipated, she was homeless. She and her two children managed to stay in a shelter. She left the shelter and moved from motel to motel. She was able to find housing until an opening became available in a 90-day shelter. A worker there referred her to the transitional housing program in which she now lives. This respondent added:

> I never knew foster care can help me by helping me find a place if I was homeless. My social case manager never gave me these options. They should be able to give somebody options. Lists of jobs and stuff like that.

A 25-year-old Hispanic female emancipated with a housing plan of residing with her boyfriend's parents. When the family decided to move, she did not want to move with them. She was able to secure a job and an apartment. She remained in the apartment for about a year. Since then she has "bounced around," living in three different states in a period of eight months. At the time of the interview, she had been back in Los Angeles for two months.

The Independent Living Program (ILP)

Theme: ILP–The People Stand Out

About a third (n = 10) of the respondents recalled their participation in Independent Living Programs (ILP) in terms of the people they met during the programs. A 21-year-old African-American male immediately remembered the name of his ILP coordinator and described him as "super cool, really helpful." Respondents reported positive relationships with the ILP coordinator and peers in the class.

> The most important thing for me in emancipation was my family and [ILP coordinator]. My coordinator has helped me for the last five years with college, money for college, getting a scholarship, and just being there. [Hispanic female, 23]

> The classes were helpful, because we learned about budgeting The [ILP coordinator] was really cool. I'm friends with him. He is like a mentor to me. [African-American female, 21]

> That was one of the greatest events that happened in my life because I met so many people that, to this day, are there for me and have done–I mean, I am so close to a lot of the people in the program. [Hispanic female, 19]

> The [ILP] classes were good because you could see other people also going through the same thing. It wasn't a waste of time. It was a good experience. Met good people. [Outreach advisor] was doing classes . . . That was his first class. We would ride together to Los Angeles and I always wanted to know more about what we were talking about in class. I just want to learn a lot. I was always asking questions. So, after that class, he got me a job working for a class and then I kept working for him. [African-American male, 19]

> It [ILP] does help you, in a way, because you get together in a group. . . It gets you used to being with a bunch of people and doing the same thing. [African-American male, 21]

Theme: ILP–I Really Can't Remember

Another 10 respondents had difficulty recalling the ILPs in which they participated. Most of the 10 seemed to think that the program, in the words of a 22-year-old Hispanic female, "would have been more helpful if they were closer to the time one leaves foster care." Others attested to their own lack of receptivity to the program at the time:

> You don't take it serious enough while you're there and when you go out and really have to face the fact that you have to pay rent, you have to pay bills, you have to manage, know how to cook and how to do laundry and you know you're not prepared . . . When you're in a foster home you know that everything is going to be there. If you need clothes, you're gonna have clothes. You know you're gonna have food, and if you're sick, they're gonna take you to the doctor so you know you're gonna be taken care of. And when you come out, it's like, if I get sick now, who do I call? There's no nurse to go to. All these years you've been taken care of and then you're just out there with nobody to call. [Hispanic female, 23]

> A lot of information but I wasn't open to hearing it because I was busy into the boys and clowning around. I wasn't ready to hear it. [African-American female, 19]

> A person can get a lot more out of something if they really want to. Now me, maybe I didn't get as much out of it as I should have because maybe it just was me not paying attention or listening, but they really do have a lot to offer there. [African-American female, 18]

Theme: ILP–Use Former Foster Care Kids as Teachers

Ten of the 28 respondents suggested that former foster care youth should be used as teachers in the ILPs. A 23-year-old Hispanic female thought people like her and others who have successfully emancipated, could:

> Go talk to the kids who haven't emancipated yet. They could identify with me and I could tell them about how scared they are before they turn 18, and also impress upon them the importance of emancipation type skills and also give them some kind of hope that it can be done successfully.

Others provided similar comments:

> They need to bring in emancipated foster youth to explain things. Don't teach out of a book. Need to get more personal. [African-American female, 22]

> [From a respondent who had been homeless] I would listen to the kids more. Find out what they were thinking about, what they wanted to learn. Like I wanted to know what I was going to do when I emancipated. Like I had no idea about transitional housing. I had no idea they gave you any help after you emancipated. I thought it was just like you were emancipated, you're homeless, you're 18, we don't care. [African-American female, 19]

Thoughts of the Past and of the Future

Theme: Regrets, Fears, and Lessons

As the respondents told their life stories, at least half of them spoke with poignancy about their outlook. These observations can be categorized as regrets, fears, and lessons. For example, regrets can be detected in the following comments:

> It's, like, until I started working at McDonalds, I didn't care much, but, like, since I been paying rent and I got a phone now, it's been,

like, boosting my morale a bit, like, I am really doing something, but now I realize my mistakes from early in the program, like, I don't have any money saved. Now that I have a grasp of what I could do in this program, the opportunities it has, it is kinda late . . . Coming out of the foster care system, you're dealing with so much personal emotional stuff, it don't allow you to think about everything else. [African-American male, 21]

I learned that there is not such thing as a 'dream family' and I was really dumb about my baby's father and single parenting. I have dashed dreams. I had hopes and goals before I got pregnant. I made some mistakes and get a little down sometimes. Then I look at my son's smiling face and I have to get up again. [Hispanic female, 21]

A lot of stuff could have been avoided if I would have listened to what I was told, but then, I wanted to learn the hard way. That's probably why I'm not in college now. I should have went straight from high school to college. I was too busy wanting to be in the 'in crowd,' gang banging on the streets. I missed out on the things I really needed . . . [African-American male, 22]

Fears were expressed in this manner:

I wish I was stronger. I would leave and start over. I don't know how to drive. I don't have money for rent or the bills. I'm turning into, like, my mother. I'm ending up just like her and my dad with me and my boyfriend. But I don't know where to go. [Hispanic female, 22]

I don't want to be like my mother. I don't want to be like her. I'm real good with kids, but how would I be on my own? I don't want children because I'm scared. What if I'm like my mom? I would never want to disappoint or hurt a child like she's hurt me. I don't want to be like her. I wouldn't want to put a child through what she's put me through. The things I've seen. The things I've done. It has been unreal. When I think of what my life has been like, it has been like watching a movie. It has been so unreal. [African-American female, 19]

Lessons learned about life are reflected in these observations:

> It's taken a lot of determination to do what I want to do. I've learned to never let anyone put me down or stop me from what I want to do. Cause I have to live with myself and not them. [African-American male, 19]

> Since I got out of the system, I try to avoid violence. I've been in a lot of situations where I wanted to retaliate, hurt people, and I knew I was capable of doing way more than what they did to me, but I look at what I have now–it's not much, but it's a lot to me, so I bite my tongue. Before I got out, I was ready for whatever. I look like a child but I'm a grown man. I'm trying to accomplish things, so leave me alone . . . [African-American male, 22]

> I hated school and I hated everyone. I was bored. Some classes were too easy except math. And in math, I thought, is everybody getting this except me? I was too embarrassed to ask for help. Because of math, I didn't want to go to school. I fell and fell and finally I asked for extra help. Once I asked for help, I started getting As and Bs in math. I thought, well I can't be good at everything so these are the things that I have to work harder at. [African-American female, 19]

> I don't like to rely on people. But if they're willing to open a door for me or extend a hand to help me, I'll take it if I need it . . . It's not easy, but when you don't have anyone to turn to or anywhere to go, there's only so much that people can do for you. But you can make it and you are just grateful for what you get. You just have to roll with the punches. [Hispanic male, 19]

Theme: The Future

The respondents expressed the hopes and dreams they had for their lives. Eighteen saw a future with a college degree and gainful employment. Future occupations mentioned included nurse, make-up artist, computer graphics designer, welder, fireman, actor, electrician, computer programmer, and probation office. Four of the respondents identified social work as their profession of choice.

> I want to be a social worker, probably because I was in the system. I had some good and some bad workers and both have inspired me–to do like the good ones and do better than the bad ones. I feel

like I can do well because I've had so much experience. [Hispanic female, 23]

I would like to continue on in college so I can have a career in banking. [African-American female, 20]

After I complete my GED, I am going to enroll in [community college] and then become a social worker or a probation officer. [Hispanic female, 19]

You know, I'm the first to graduate from high school in my family. Right now, I think I'd like to study to become a fireman. [Hispanic male, 19]

I am starting [community college] this summer in order to take welding classes. I can be pretty competitive in a male field and be better at it than men. I like working with my hands and being creative. [African-American female, 18]

I'd love to go back to school and learn about teaching and social work. Social work because I could correct the downfall of the system. [African-American female, 20]

I couldn't wait to be grown and start paying taxes than live that crummy life anymore . . . I see myself finishing with my BA and going to get a good job. [African-American male, 19]

DISCUSSION

The emancipation stories of these 28 respondents provide a depth and richness that cannot be captured by statistics alone. As youth of color, their experiences mirror many of the issues and problems documented in existing empirical research on the topic, often compounded by issues of age and race/ethnicity. This qualitative approach serves to detail how many of these emancipated young adults traverse a rocky path to adulthood. From the data presented here, several preliminary implications can be drawn. These conclusions are tentative and preliminary because of the size and non-random nature of the sample and the over-representation of youth residing in transitional housing. Although the sample has limitations, the results presented here do support the findings from other research in this area. Emancipated youth are at risk for unstable lives as reflected in emancipation preparation that can be linked to housing instability, education and work uncertainty, and family dysfunction (Chambers, 1997; Collins, 2001; Courtney & Piliavin, 1998; Lindsey & Ahmed, 1999; McDonald et al., 1993).

This study focused exclusively on the experiences of African American and Hispanic individuals who had emancipated from foster care. Because of the over-representation of children and youth of color in the child welfare system, this focus seems warranted. Emancipating from foster care itself places individuals at risk because many of these youth lack an education or marketable skills and general living skills to assist them to become self-sufficient. In addition, they face the many obstacles that all youth of color encounter in the labor market which serve to exacerbate that risk. For this reason, culturally sensitive and responsive programs cannot afford to treat emancipating youth as one homogeneous group. Reporting the themes emergent from the words of the respondents serves as a beginning step to understanding the needs of a culturally diverse group.

For the respondents in this study, independent living programs were recalled in terms of the people in the programs. Thus, relationships proved to be a cornerstone of the programs and for many of the respondents, the relationships overshadowed the skill development aspects of the programs. McMillan et al. (1997) had similar findings in their study of the views of former foster care youth on the independent living services they received. Their focus group results indicated that, for some youth, the ILP workers "provide important assistance at crucial times" (McMillan et al., 1997, p. 478). The relationships developed between the ILP staff and program participants may support, encourage, and promote the participants' growth and maturity. If this aspect of the program is likely to stand out in the minds of the participants, then the goal is to determine how that relationship can be included as a regular feature of the program for all the participants. For example, if the ILP coordinator, advisor, and/or outreach worker plays such a central role in the lives of the foster youth, then more such qualified staff may need to be added to these programs. Clearly, future research in this area is needed to further study the relational aspects of the program and how they can be used to foster successful transitions to adulthood. A key area to explore is the role of worker and child race/ethnicity in the development of the helping relationship.

Many of the respondents only had vague recollections about their ILP participation. The reasons for this lie with both the ILP staff and with the respondents themselves. For youth participating in the programs at age 16, the period between program involvement and emancipation may be long enough to extinguish much of the learning that took place. Refresher courses, follow-up courses, or opportunities to retake courses may have to be explored as possibilities for making sure that ILP learning is not lost. Respondents did mention that former foster care youth would be good teachers. While some ILPs do use these foster care "graduates," a larger role may be a possibility. Perhaps the peer educator concept has some merit here. Thus, as ILPs are reviewed and evaluated, the timing of the program and role of the former foster youth as trainers should be rigorously examined. Here, again, the role of peer counselor and youth race/ethnicity in the forming of peer helping relationships may need to be explored.

On the other hand, some respondents acknowledged that they were not open to hearing what the ILPs had to offer. As adolescents, they had other things on their minds and did not see the ILP as important. Because of the gravity of their situations, these adolescents did not have the benefit of resourceful family systems to sustain them until they were ready to absorb learning about self-sufficiency. This could suggest that the ILP classes are out of step with the adolescents' developmental progress. Classes at age 16 that emphasize emancipation appear to accelerate the preparation for adulthood before they are ready to either understand or accept that responsibility. Indeed, the preparation and the emancipation itself may serve to truncate the adolescent development process. Collins (2001) in reviewing the literature on adolescent and young adult life transition notes:

> Thus, young people leaving care are generally thought to be at some developmental risk because they are on their own earlier than other people their age and before reaching other key transitions such as completing school or finding stable employment . . . Adolescents aging out of care are more likely to establish independence because they are dissatisfied with foster care or because state support ends rather than for more positive, opportunity reasons, such as attending college. (p. 280)

Housing instability, work and school uncertainty, and family dysfunction may be related to the type of emancipation preparation to which an individual is exposed. If every youth emancipated with a clear housing, work, and educational plan, much of the confusion and uncertainty echoed in this study might be minimized. For some of the respondents in this study, housing instability resulted in the face of an unworkable housing plan. Again, responsibility rests with both the emancipating agencies and with the youth themselves. Although adolescents vary in their degree of receptivity to offers of emancipation assistance and advice, child welfare agencies should strive to be consistent in their emancipation planning for all adolescents. Standards for emancipation plans may have to be reviewed, modified, and expanded so that the effectiveness of those plans can be evaluated. This means that child welfare agencies may have to conduct follow-up visits to obtain feedback on the efficacy of the plans. These follow-up studies should seek to obtain feedback that will enhance the cultural relevance of the programs for diverse groups. For example, it becomes vital to understand the types of tangible and socio-emotional assistance that emancipated adolescents need and the sources to whom they turn to seek this assistance. Help-seeking behaviors and sources of help may vary by ethnicity, and these variations should be more effectively researched and understood so that they can be appropriately acknowledged and integrated into service delivery systems.

A realistic consideration of work and education options should also be part of the emancipation plan. Some respondents were trying to negotiate the tension between school and work with work winning in some cases. These young adults believed that education was important and held education as a future goal, but they were unclear as to how to reach that goal. While after-care, post-emancipation programs proliferate, work and education planning should not wait until after the youth has emancipated.

Family dysfunction may also need to be addressed in independent living programs. Programs, however, may find it easier to address the concrete, hard skills rather than the softer skills. While the dysfunction may not ever dissipate, adolescents can begin to learn how to cope with it in a healthy fashion. The family conflict, fears, regrets, and lessons that emerged in this study are indicative of the socio-emotional aspects of making the transition to adulthood. Kools (1999) noted that foster care adolescents may feel the need to develop self-protection mechanisms. Clearly the respondents in this study were attempting to cope with their lives and situations. Independent living programs that actually focus on the emotional aspects of emancipation provide an invaluable service to its participants, particularly if they are sensitive to the cultural backgrounds of children and their families. For example, many youth are returning to families with whom they have unresolved issues, yet feel a need to maintain these cultural ties regardless of the family situation. Indeed, this desire to return to the family of origin may be rooted in cultural norms that carry expectations of loyalty, obedience, and obligation to parents (Gnaulatti & Heine, 2001). Consequently, culturally sensitive efforts to assist adolescents must then address the tension between the need for the foster care placement and the culturally-based expectation of loyalty to the family.

Studies of former foster care youth may benefit from increased use of a resiliency framework or a strength-based perspective. Resiliency frameworks emphasize the ability to cope with stressors and the critical role of accessing social support as a key coping mechanism (Collins, 2001). The strengths perspective emphasizes that the unique strengths, skills, and abilities of persons can create solutions where none seem possible (Graybeal, 2001). Despite the hardships encountered by the individuals in this study, all were attempting to cope with their situations. While it is often necessary to focus on the deficits or at-risk status of former foster youth, it is still important to learn those factors that promote healthy transition and recognize the coping strategies that support resiliency.

Finally, these implications suggest that a continuum of care/service may be warranted for emancipating youth. The first level of care is found in the foster care system in the preparation for emancipation. This would include the skills classes, the socio-emotional sessions, and the emancipation plan. The next level of care may be found in the actual act of emancipation itself–the movement out of the system into a new living arrangement and the implementing of the work and educational plan. The third level of care would be found in the after-care and post-emancipation services for those who required them. With this continuum of care/service, youth would be less likely to drift from one living situation to another, to struggle alone with feelings about family, and to be confused about how to move ahead in life. Such a continuum requires agency coordination and service integration in a culturally sensitive service environment to smooth out the potholes in the road to adulthood for foster care youth.

REFERENCES

Boyatzis, R. E. (1998). *Transforming qualitative information.* Thousand Oaks, CA: Sage Publication.

Chambers, J. M. (1997). *Evaluation of former Nebraska state wards independent living training and skills.* Lincoln: Center on Children, Families, and the Law, University of Nebraska.

Child Welfare League of America. (1998). *Family foster care fact sheet January, 1998. http://www.cwla.org/cwla/fostercr/familyfcfacts98.html* (Retrieved March 28, 2000).

Child Welfare League of America. (1999). Testimony before the Ways and Means Subcommittee on Human Resources for the hearing on challenges confronting older children leaving care. *http://cwla.org/cwla/publicpolicy.html* (Retrieved March 13, 2000).

Children's Bureau, Youth and Families, Administration on Children, Administration for Children and Families, U.S. Department of Health and Human Services. (1999). *How many children were in foster care on March 31, 1998? http://www.acf.dhhs.gov/programs/cb/stats/* (Retrieved March 6, 2000).

Collins, M. E. (2001). Transition to adulthood for vulnerable youth: A review of research and implications for policy. *Social Service Review*, 75, 271-291.

Courtney, M., & Piliavin, I. (1998). *Foster youth transitions to adulthood: Outcomes 12 to 18 months after leaving out-of-home care*. Madison: University of Wisconsin.

Family and Youth Services Bureau, Administration on Children, Youth and Families, Administration for Children and Families, U.S. Department of Health and Human Services. (1997). *Understanding youth development*. Washington, DC: Family and Youth Services Bureau.

Fetterman, D. M. (1989). *Ethnography: Step by Step*, Applied Social Research Methods Series, Volume 17, Newbury Park, CA: Sage Publications.

Foster Care Independence Act of 1999. H. R. 3443. Amendment to Part E of Title IV of the Social Security Act.

Gil, E., & Bogart, K. (1982). Foster children speak out: A study of children's perceptions of foster care. *Children Today*, 11, 7-9.

Gnaulati, E., & Heine, B. (2001). Separation-individuation in late adolescence: An investigation of gender and ethnic differences. *The Journal of Psychology*, 135, 59-70.

Graybeal, C. (2001). Strengths-based social work assessment: Transforming the dominant paradigm. *Families in Societies: The Journal of Contemporary Human Services*, 82, 233-242.

Green, J. W. (1999). *Cultural awareness in the human services. 3rd Ed.* Englewood Cliffs, NJ: Prentice Hall.

Hamburg, D. (1989). Preparing for life: The critical transition of adolescence. *Crisis*, 10, 4-15.

Jones, L. (1997). Social class, ethnicity, and child welfare. *Journal of Multicultural Social Work*, 6, 123-138.

Kools, S. (1999). Self-protection in adolescents in foster care. *Journal of Child and Adolescent Psychiatric Nursing*, 12, 139-152.

Lammert, M., & Timberlake, E. (1986). Termination of foster care for the older adolescent: Issues of emancipation and individuation. *Child and Adolescent Social Work Journal*, 3, 26-37.

Lindsey, E. W., & Ahmed, F. U. (1999). The North Carolina independent living program: A comparison of outcomes for participants and nonparticipants. *Children and Youth Services Review*, 21, 389-412.

Los Angeles County Department of Children and Family Services. (2001). *End month caseload, calendar year 2000*. Los Angeles: Author.

McDonald, T. P., Allen, R. I., Westerfelt, A., & Piliavin, I. (1993). *Assessing the long-term effects of foster: A research synthesis*. Madison, WI: Institute for Research on Poverty.

McMillen, J. C., Rideout, G. B., Fisher, R. H., & Tucker, J. (1997). Independent living services: The views of former foster youth. *Families in Society: The Journal of Contemporary Human Services*, 78, 471-479.

Orange County (California) Grand Jury. (2000). *Orange County is no Camelot for emancipated youth*. Orange County: Author.

Patton, M. (2002). *Qualitative evaluation and research methods*. 2nd Ed. Thousand Oaks, CA: Sage Publications.

Rubin, H. J., & Rubin, I. R. (1995). *Qualitative interviewing*. Thousand Oaks, CA: Sage Publications.

Spradley, J. P. (1979). *The ethnographic interview*. Chicago: Holt, Rinehart and Winston, Inc.

State Bar of California. (1999). *Emancipation. Kids and the law. http://www.calbar.org/* (Retrieved August 2, 1999).

United States Department of Health and Human Services. Administration for Children and Families. National Clearinghouse on Child Abuse and Neglect Information. (2001.) *Foster Care National Statistics. http://www.calib.com/nccacn/* (Retrieved February 2, 2002).

United States General Accounting Office. (1999). *Foster care: Effectiveness of independent living services unknown.* Washington, DC. USGAO.

Unites States House of Representatives. Committee on Ways and Means. (2000). *2000 Green book*. Washington, D.C.: U.S. Government Printing Office.

Parent Involvement as Parental Monitoring of Student Motivation and Parent Expectations Predicting Later Achievement Among African American and European American Middle School Age Students

Sherri F. Seyfried
Ick-Joong Chung

SUMMARY. Parent involvement and parent expectations are fundamental to academic success. However, much of the research has been with elementary school aged children; consequently, we know less about the influence of parent involvement and parent expectations on the academic achievement of middle school students, and we have even less information for African American (AA) students. Do parent involvement and parent expectations have a similar effect on later Grade Point Average (GPA) for European American (EA) and AA middle school youth?

Sherri F. Seyfried, PhD, is Associate Professor, Department of Social Work, Chicago State University, Chicago, Illinois. Ick-Joong Chung, PhD, is Assistant Professor, Department of Social Welfare, Duksung Women's University, Seoul, Korea.

Portions of this paper were presented at the Turning of the Centuries Conference at Chicago State University, Chicago, Illinois, April 4-5, 2002.

[Haworth co-indexing entry note]: "Parent Involvement as Parental Monitoring of Student Motivation and Parent Expectations Predicting Later Achievement Among African American and European American Middle School Age Students." Seyfried, Sherri F., and Ick-Joong Chung. Co-published simultaneously in *Journal of Ethnic & Cultural Diversity in Social Work* (The Haworth Social Work Practice Press, an imprint of The Haworth Press, Inc.) Vol. 11, No. 1/2, 2002, pp. 109-131; and: *Social Work with Multicultural Youth* (ed: Diane de Anda) The Haworth Social Work Practice Press, an imprint of The Haworth Press, Inc., 2002, pp. 109-131. Single or multiple copies of this article are available for a fee from The Haworth Document Delivery Service [1-800-HAWORTH, 9:00 a.m. - 5:00 p.m. (EST). E-mail address: docdelivery@haworthpress.com].

http://www.haworthpress.com/store/product.asp?sku=J051

10.1300/J051v11n01_05

Data from 567 AA and EA urban youth who participated in a longitudinal study were used in this analysis. Within group hierarchical regression analyses reveal parent involvement and parent expectations are statistically significant for both groups. However, partial correlations indicate parental involvement represents the highest unique contribution to later grade point average for EA students, and for AA students, earlier educational achievement represents the highest unique contribution to later grade point average. Implications for practice suggest that approaches to increase parent involvement may work well with improving academic achievement of EA youth, while approaches to increase early educational achievement may work well with AA students.

KEYWORDS. Parent involvement, parent perceptions, academic achievement, middle-school age students, African American students

INTRODUCTION

Parent involvement in the schooling process and parent expectations for educational achievement are important issues of concern for school social workers, teachers, and school administrators. Parent involvement is associated with student achievement (Comer, 1988; Miedal & Reynolds, 1999; Olmstead & Rubin, 1983; Reynolds, 1992). Parent expectations are also related to student learning (Eccles, Jacobs & Harold, 1990; Entwisle & Baker, 1983; Majoribanks, 1984; Thompson, Alexander & Entwisle, 1988). One of the goals of the U.S. Department of Education's Goals 2000 (U.S. Department of Education, 1994) "states . . . every school will promote partnerships that will increase parental involvement and participation in promoting the social, emotional, and academic growth of children."

Clearly, there is little dispute among researchers and educators that parent involvement and parent expectations are fundamental to academic success. However, much of the research has been with elementary school aged children; consequently, we know less about the influence of parent involvement and parent expectations on the academic achievement of junior high school students (Paulson, 1994;

Trusty, 1996). We have even less information for adolescent minority youth (Patrikakou, 1997).

Using longitudinal data, the authors address the influence of parent involvement and expectations in predicting later grade point average among urban, eighth grade African American (AA) and European American (EA) students. Furthermore, this study controls for SES, gender, and earlier educational achievement. There is need to study the effects of parent involvement during the junior high school years because parent involvement tends to decline during this time (Lucas & Lusthaus, 1978). In addition, socioeconomic status (SES), race, and other background variables are associated with parent expectations (Boocock, 1972) and parent involvement (Eccles & Harold, 1996). Within group analyses were conducted to identify the predictors of academic achievement for AA and EA students, respectively. It has been suggested that within group analyses of parent involvement and parent expectations, yield implications for more effective interventions (Eccles & Harold, 1996). The data from this work will be useful in developing culturally appropriate practice interventions with AA and EA junior high school students and their parents.

LITERATURE REVIEW

Parent Involvement

There is very little consensus in the literature regarding *how* to measure or define parent involvement (Kohl, Lengua & McMahon, 2000; Miedel & Reynolds, 1999; Patrikakou, 1997). However, what is clear is that parent involvement behaviors occur within two social contexts, in the school and at home. There are dimensions of parent involvement that are school driven; that is, parent involvement needs are initiated and determined by schools (see Epstein, 1995). Examples include providing parenting classes or involving parents in policy and decision making activities at school. Parent involvement dimensions that are parent driven include activities initiated by the parent (see Eccles & Harold, 1996) such as monitoring homework and the amount of television watched, and volunteering at school. There are some dimensions of parent involvement that are both parent and school driven such as parent participation in school events and parent-child discussions. For example, teachers may encourage parents to engage their children in discussions regarding homework assignments. Parent expectations are also parent and school driven (Keith et al., 1992; Peng & Lee, 1993). Schools overtly and covertly express traditional values regarding academic expectations. Parents also impart to their children family expectations regarding achievement. The degree to which school expectations and family expectations are similar will determine the quality and experience of the school-family relationship (Valdes, 1996).

While most dimensions of parent involvement include specific, tangible activities performed by the parent, fewer dimensions consider parent perceptions of academic motivation as a measure of parent involvement. For the present study, the authors choose this conceptualization of parent involvement, because it can be inferred that parent involvement begins with the parent's assessment and monitoring of their child's academic motivation. In addition student motivation is a major area of concern for educators and school social workers (Sanders, 1999). Furthermore, the issue of student motivation is of particular concern for African American students who are at greatest risk of school failure (Allen-Meares, 1999; Jenkins, 1995). Most importantly, it has been hypothesized that parental perceptions of their child's schooling behavior are linked to academic outcomes (Clark, 1983).

Parent Involvement and Academic Achievement

In a qualitative study that included 33 families, Scheinfeld (1983) found that parents of high achievers encouraged their children to become actively engaged in their social environment. Scheinfeld reports that among parents of high achievers, the parent's ability to identify the child's academic motivation and interests was positively related to the child's achievement. In the same study, it was further noted that the parent's value for the child to develop intrinsic motivation (internal drive) was related to academic achievement. In the present study, the items chosen for parent involvement measure the parent's perception of the child's intrinsic academic motivation.

In a qualitative study designed to capture resilience and protective factors in 86 urban adolescents, it was found that motivational support from family and teachers was instrumental in promoting healthy development (Smokowski, Reynolds, & Bezruczko, 1999). Conversely, in a study of 114 high school dropouts, it was found that children who have parents who are not involved in their education are at risk for dropping out of school (Rumberger et al., 1990).

The relationship between parent involvement and academic achievement is a particular concern for AA youth that lag far behind their EA counterparts in nearly every educational measure. As mentioned earlier, Clark (1983) hypothesizes that AA parental conceptions of their child's school behavior are related to academic outcomes. The idea here is that the level of parental support is influenced by the parent's conception of their child's school behavior. If this hypothesis is true, then one can infer that parents who perceive their children to have high achievement motivation will be more involved in their child's schooling process. Even if one were to accept this hypothesis as being true, it would still be necessary to consider other environmental factors that may moderate parental conceptions of student behavior and academic outcome.

It has been suggested that middle class and EA parent involvement behavior is fortified by social capital that affords them access to resources and supports that are not readily available to lower income parents and ethnic minority parents (Lareau, 1989). For example, middle class parents who have a certain perception of their child's achievement motivation will convey those perceptions and the needs of their child to teachers and educators. It may very well be that these educators live in their neighborhood. More than likely these parents are familiar with the social politics of the schooling process and are very comfortable advocating for their children. In many instances, minority families and lower income families may not be as comfortable navigating the schooling process. They may not have a neighbor down the street who is a schoolteacher who can provide them with helpful information about the politics of schooling. Minority and low income parents may have negative memories of their own school experience, or they may be first generation immigrants and may not feel as comfortable advocating for their children (Valdes, 1996). In some instances, depending on the cultural background of the parents, they may feel that teachers know what is best for their child, and they should not interfere in business that is not theirs.

Minority and low-income families have as much to contribute to schools and the schooling process, as schools have to contribute to them. School social workers are in a position to work within and between those systems that impact the minority student's educational experience (Seyfried, 2000). School social workers can help to develop school practices that enhance collaborative relationships among minority parents and teachers.

Parent Expectations

As with parent involvement, there does not appear to be general agreement about the dimensions or definition of parent expectations

(Gill & Reynolds, 1999). Gill and Reynolds (1999) go on to state that research regarding parent expectations appears to center around three areas: (1) expectations for ability (Crandall, Dewey, Katkovsky, & Preston, 1964), (2) short term expectations for grades (Entwisle & Hayduk, 1978) and, (3) long term expectations for educational attainment (Kurtz-Costes, Halle, Clarke, & Seidu, 1995).

Parsons, Adler, and Kaczala (1982) found parental beliefs regarding their child's ability had a stronger effect on later achievement than earlier performance. In a study that merged data from two longitudinal studies of approximately 2,100 families, Eccles and colleagues (1990) also found parental expectations to play a major role in adolescent achievement. The link between parent expectations and parent involvement may provide insight to the process in which expectations impact academic achievement (Seginer, 1983). If this were true, it would seem that parent expectations may indirectly impact achievement through parent involvement.

The processes related to the transmission of parental expectations to academic achievement are uncertain. This is especially true for AA students (Gill & Reynolds,1999). School social workers who operate at the interface between parents, students and teachers can play a vital role in helping educators identify the links between parent expectations and academic achievement. For parents of color and parents from lower socioeconomic backgrounds, the structural inequalities that impact their daily lives may dampen the effect of parent expectations. That is, although parents of color may hold high expectations for their child's academic success, the stresses of everyday life may interfere with the transmission of those expectations. Limited access to resources reduces social capital, and it is said that social capital facilitates the transfer of parent expectations (Gill & Reynolds, 1999; Ritter, Mont-Reynaud, & Dornbusch, 1993). It is important that teachers and other educators be sensitive to the life experiences of poor families and families of color and not dismiss them as being uninterested in their children's education.

Early Adolescent Development, Parental Expectations and Parent Involvement

For the present study, parent expectations and parent involvement were hypothesized to predict grade point average in the eighth grade. At the eighth grade students are in the early adolescent stage of development (Erikson, 1950/1963). As noted, very little research has examined the relationship between parent involvement, parent expectations and achievement for this age group. There is further need to explore these relationships with early adolescents, because parent involvement declines when children reach junior high and high school (Lucas & Lusthaus, 1978). At the time parent involvement declines, peer pressure increases, and youth spend more time away from home. Students may begin to experiment with illicit drugs during early adolescence.

The educational structure for early adolescents is organizationally dissonant from the structure with which they were familiar in elementary school. This dissonance creates added stress at a developmental period that is already difficult for most youth (Germain, 1999). In junior high school, the student has a homeroom teacher (with whom they spend very little time) and several teachers for each primary subject. This is in direct contrast to elementary school where the same teacher is responsible for all subjects and thus has the opportunity to establish meaningful relationships with students and their parents.

While there is rapid physical growth during early adolescence, youth are developing at different rates. Youth that lag behind their peers in physical development or are ahead of their peers may receive noted attention from their circle of friends. As boys mature, they may become physically intimidating to teachers (Newman & Newman, 1995). This presents a particular problem for AA adolescent male students (Allen-Meares, 1999).

During early adolescence, students are moving from concrete to abstract levels of thinking. Cognitive psychologists and educational theorists believe that cognitive development and ways of knowing do not occur in a vacuum. Optimal cognitive development is brought to fruition through the dynamic of social and cultural relationships (Vygotsky, 1978). Parents and teachers (and increasingly peers) play an instrumental role in the cognitive development of early adolescents.

PURPOSE

In summary, early adolescence is a difficult period for most youth. Consequently, the level of parent involvement and parent expectations is central to healthy social and academic development during this time. For the present study, the authors focus on parental expectations for future educational attainment and parental involvement as monitoring student academic motivation. Parent expectations and parent involvement are hypothesized to predict later grade point average. Furthermore, parent expectations for future educational attainment are believed to be indicators of the family learning environment (Seginer, 1983).

This study asks the following questions: (a) Controlling for gender and SES, does parent involvement at grade 7 predict later GPA at grade 8 for EA and AA students? (b) Controlling for gender and SES, do parent expectations at grade 7 predict later GPA at grade 8 for EA and AA students? (c) Is parent involvement at grade 7 equally related to GPA at grade 8 for AA and EA students? and, (d) Are parent expectations at grade 7 equally related to GPA at grade 8 for AA and EA students?

METHODS

Sample

This study used prospective data drawn from the Seattle Social Development Project (SSDP), a longitudinal study of the development of prosocial and antisocial behaviors. Data were collected at nine different assessment waves. More than 90% of all subjects were retained for at least seven of the nine data assessment waves.

The original study population included all fifth-grade students (N = 1053) in eighteen Seattle elementary schools that over-represented students from urban, high-crime, and low-income neighborhoods. From this population, 808 students (77%) consented to participate in the longitudinal study and constitute the SSDP sample (Battin, Hill, Abbott, Catalano, & Hawkins, 1998; Hawkins, Lishner, Catalano, & Howard, 1986; Hawkins et al., 1997). For the present study, only data from the AA (n = 195) and EA (n = 372) students are used because these groups comprise the largest sub samples. Within this sub sample, 49% are females (n = 279) and 51% are males (n = 288). When looking at gender by ethnicity, 17% are AA females (n = 95), 32% are EA females (n = 184), 17% are AA males (n = 100), and 33% are EA males (n = 188). With regard to socioeconomic status, 61% of the AA students were from families in poverty, as indicated by eligibility for participation in the federal free lunch program, and 21.8% of the EA students were eligible for free lunch status in 1985.

Data from three waves of the SSDP panel were used in the study, corresponding to assessments carried out when subjects were in the fifth, seventh, and eighth grades. Parents of students completed a parent questionnaire. Teachers completed ratings on students' social and academic performance, the Child Behavior Checklist (Achenbach & Edelbrock, 1983), Teacher's Report Form.

Measures

Dependent Variable

Grade Point Average (GPA)–Grade 8 was an average of fall semester eighth grade, GPA and spring semester eighth grade, GPA. Grade point averages for each semester were taken from school records.

Control Variables

Gender. Male was coded as "1" and female was coded as "0."

Free Lunch Status (Proxy for SES)–Grade 5. For the categorical variable SES, a student received a "1" if s/he were eligible for the Federal School Lunch/School Breakfast Program and a "0" if they were not eligible.

Predictors

Predictors span individual and family domains of the child's development. Predictor variables used in this study were drawn from youth self-reports, parents' reports, teachers' reports, and school records. The predictor variables consist of theoretically grouped items. All the items were coded so that higher scores indicate a greater amount of the predictor.

Aggressive Behavior–Grade 5 (alpha = .96) was rated by teachers on the Child Behavior Checklist (CBC) (Achenbach & Edelbrock, 1983). All items were measured on a 3-point scale in which 0 = not true, 1 = sometimes true, and 2 = often true. To compose the scale, teacher ratings were averaged across 24 aggressive behavior items (e.g., items such as "gets in many fights" and "physically attacks people"). All of these items were reported by Achenbach and Edelbrock (1983) to load on the externalizing scale.

Early Educational Achievement–Grade 5 was obtained from school records. This scale was an average of Reading, Language, and Math scores taken from students' scores on the California Achievement Test.

Illicit Drug Use–Grade 8 (alpha = .70) was reported by respondents. This scale was created from student survey data and measured the total frequency of using illicit hard drugs in the past year, including crack and cocaine.

Parent Involvement–Grade 7 (alpha = .85) required parents to assess the following four items: (1) Your child tries hard in school, (2) It is important to your child to get good grades, (3) Your child tries to do things that will make the teacher proud, and (4) Education is so important to your child that he or she thinks its worth it to put up with things about school that he/she doesn't like. The responses range along a four point scale, from 1 = NO!, 2 = no, 3 = yes, and 4 = YES!. The instructions for the scale state; a Big YES! means the statement is *definitely true* for you, Little yes means the statement is *mostly true* for you, Little no means the statement is *mostly not true* for you, and Big NO! means the statement is *definitely not true* for you.

Parent Expectations of Schooling–Grade 7 (alpha = .69) was reported by parents and comprised of two items: "How much schooling would you like your child to get eventually?" and "How much schooling do you actually expect that your child will complete?" The responses range from 1 (some high school) to 7 (graduate or professional school).

Missing Data Procedures

Overall, there was a very low degree of missing data in the SSDP sample. Across all variables (year by subject by variable), 3.3% of the total number of data points were missing. Missing data are almost exclusively due to nonparticipation at a given wave rather than failure to answer. Missing data due to attrition were relatively few; nearly 96% of the original fifth grade sample were interviewed at age 13. Furthermore, nonparticipation at each of the assessment waves was not related to gender or ethnicity.

Many missing data strategies (e.g., listwise deletion, pairwise deletion, and mean substitution) result in unnecessarily reduced sample sizes and biased parameter estimates (Graham et al., 1994, 1997). In order to avoid these problems, the present study used an alternative missing data technique suggested by Little and Rubin (1987)–using an expectation-maximization (EM) algorithm and multiple imputation–to obtain less biased estimates of parameters and to obtain correctly estimated standard errors (Graham et al., 1994, 1997). Data files used in this study were prepared using the NORM (Version 2.02) program developed by Schafer (1997). Three imputed data sets were then each analyzed using the SPSS for Windows (Version 9.0) program, and the results were combined following Graham et al. (1994, 1997).

Data Analysis

Analyses proceeded in two stages. In the first stage, multiple regression was used to determine the combined effect of the independent variables on grade point average (GPA) and to determine the individual effects of each independent variable on GPA when controlling for the other independent variables. The longitudinal data were used in multiple regression analyses to examine whether parent involvement and expectations of schooling at grade 7 are related to GPA at grade 8. Two separate hierarchical regression equations were conducted for EA and AA youth. The regression equations were constructed in three steps. In the first step, gender and SES were entered in the equation. In the second step, early educational achievement, and aggressive behavior were added. In the final step, illicit drug use, parent involvement and parent expectations were added to the equation.

Next, the ethnicity interaction with parent involvement and then the ethnicity interaction with expectations of schooling were examined in depth. The point of intersection and regions of significance were established for parent involvement and parent expectations of schooling.

FINDINGS

Bivariate Correlations Among Variables and Mean Differences by Ethnicity

Table 1 presents the bivariate correlations among the variables, means, and standard deviations of variables for EA and AA youth. For the EA students, GPA had significant relationships with other predictor variables except illicit drug use. GPA was significantly and negatively related to gender, SES, and aggressive behavior. That is, the boys, poor children, and aggressive children achieved lower GPA scores, whereas girls, non-poor children, and non-aggressive children achieved higher GPAs. GPA was significantly and positively related to early educational achievement, parent involvement and parent expectations.

For the AA students, GPA also had significant relationships with other predictor variables except SES and illicit drug use. GPA was significantly and negatively related to gender and aggressive behavior, and GPA had significant and positive relationships with early educational achievement, parent involvement and parent expectations. The magnitude of the correlations for AA students is smaller than that for EA students.

As shown in Table 1, t-tests indicate EA students have higher GPA and early achievement scores than AA students. AA students have higher aggressive behavior scores, but use fewer illicit drugs (the t-test

TABLE 1. Correlations, Means, Standard Deviations, T-Tests for Variables for European American and African American[a]

Vars	V1	V2	V3	V4	V5	V6	V7	V8
V1	–	−.24**	−.27**	−.47**	.51**	−.06	.53**	.53**
V2	−.23**	–	−.10*	.20**	−.12**	−.14**	−.21**	−.01
V3	−.04	−.15*	–	.11*	−.19**	.18**	.001	−.25**
V4	−.30**	.09	.10	–	−.31**	−.06	−.28**	−.21**
V5	.34**	−.04	−.28**	−.27**	–	.04	.32**	.41**
V6	.004	−.14*	.09	.09	.05	–	.01	−.04
V7	.24**	−.16*	.31**	−.14*	−.08	−.22**	–	.25**
V8	.29**	−.003	−.35**	−.28**	.26**	−.10	.17**	–
European American								
Mean	2.56	0.51	0.22	0.16	522.91	0.30	2.96	5.22
SD	0.84	0.50	0.41	0.33	44.95	1.24	0.61	1.22
African American								
Mean	1.75	0.51	0.65	0.46	477.79	0.14	2.91	4.80
SD	0.81	0.50	0.48	0.57	37.50	0.83	0.62	1.28
t-test								
t	11.11	–	–	−7.86	12.00	1.67	0.96	3.83
Sig. [b]	.000	–	–	.000	.000	.095	.339	.000

Note: V1 = GPA; V2 = Gender; V3 = SES; V4 = Aggressive Behavior; V5 = Early Educational Ability; V6 = Illicit Drug Use; V7 = Parent Involvement of Schooling; V8 = Parent Expectations of Schooling.
a. Correlations of European American children are above the diagonal and correlations of African American children are below the diagonal.
b. Two-tailed.
* $p < .05$; ** $p < .01$.

reaches marginal significance). Parents of EA students have higher expectations of schooling for their children than parents of AA students. There is no statistical difference between the means for parent involvement.

Regression Analyses Predicting GPA (Academic Achievement)

To determine the overall contribution of the variables and then the unique contribution each variable makes towards predicting GPA, regression analyses were conducted. As described above, three regressions were run for each ethnic group in a hierarchical fashion. The results of the analyses for EA are shown in Table 2. This model explained 59% of the variance in GPA for the EA students. In step 1, demographic variables were entered. Gender and SES were significant

TABLE 2. Regression Models: Parent Involvement and Parent Expectations at Grade 7 Predicting GPA at Grade 8 for European American

	β[a]	β	β
	STEP 1	STEP 2	STEP 3
Male	−0.275**	−0.157**	−0.132**
SES	−0.295**	−0.180**	−0.138**
Aggressive Behavior		−0.310**	−0.230**
Early Educational Ability		0.360**	0.180**
Illicit Drug Use			−0.065†
Parent Involvement			0.307**
Parent Expectations			0.290**
R^2	0.15	0.42	0.59
R^2 Change		0.27**	0.17**
Adj. R^2	0.14	0.41	0.58

a. Standardized regression coefficients.
† $p < .10$; *$p < .05$; **$p < .01$ (two-tailed tests).

and remained significant in the final step. Of the variables that were entered into the model in step 2, aggressive behavior and early educational achievement were significant. In the final step, illicit drug use, parent involvement and parent expectations were added. All the variables except illicit drug use were significantly related to GPA. Illicit drug use had a marginally significant relationship. Particularly, parent involvement and parent expectations had a strong effect on GPA after controlling for other variables.

The results for AA students are summarized in Table 3. The model explained 26% of the variance in GPA for the AA students. In step 1, only gender was significant and remained significant in the final step. In step 2, aggressive behavior and early educational achievement were significant. In step 3, all the variables except SES and illicit drug use were significantly related to GPA.

Interaction Effects by Ethnicity

A test of the coefficient for the product term is a test of interaction and is equivalent to a test of the increment in the proportion of variance accounted for by the product term, over and above its constituent vari-

TABLE 3. Regression Models: Parent Involvement and Parent Expectations at Grade 7 Predicting GPA at Grade 8 for African American

	β[a]	β	β
	STEP 1	STEP 2	STEP 3
Male	−0.239**	−0.193**	−0.164*
SES	−0.073	0.034	0.024
Aggressive Behavior		−0.209**	−0.145*
Early Educational Ability		0.284**	0.272**
Illicit Drug Use			0.038
Parent Involvement			0.192**
Parent Expectations			0.163**
R^2	0.06	0.20	0.27
R^2 Change		0.14 **	0.07**
Adj. R^2	0.05	0.18	0.24

a. Standardized regression coefficients.
† $p < .10$; * $p < .05$; ** $p < .01$ (two-tailed tests).

ables (Pedhazur, 1997). As shown in Table 4, the overall regression equation of GPA on parent expectations of schooling with ethnicity interaction term is:

$$Y = .65 + .37\,X_1 + .21D - .18\,X_1D$$

In the analysis, 1 was assigned to AA and 0 to EA. The separate regression equations are obtained plugging in these assigned values in the overall regression equation. Having calculated the separate regression equations, the point the two regression lines intersect can be calculated.

$$Y_{EA} = .65 + .37\,X_1$$
$$Y_{AA} = .86 + .19\,X_1$$

Where Y = GPA; EA = European American; AA = African American; and X_1 = Parent Expectations. Data were plotted in Figure 1 with the two regression lines. This model explained 36% of the variance in GPA. As shown in Figure 1, the point of intersection is $X_1 = 1.17$, $Y = 1.08$. Students with parent expectations above 1.17 are expected to have a higher GPA if they are EA, whereas AA students with parent expectations above 1.17 are expected to have a lower GPA.

TABLE 4. Regression of GPA: Parent Expectations and Interaction Effects by Ethnicity (N = 567)

	b[a]
Parent Expectations	.37**
Ethnicity (African American = 1)	.20
Interaction	−.18**
Constant	.65**
R^2	0.36
Adj. R^2	0.35

[a] Unstandardized regression coefficients.
[†] $p < .10$; * $p < .05$; ** $p < .01$ (two-tailed tests).

FIGURE 1. Regressions of GPA at Grade 8 onto Parent Expectations at Grade 7 for European American and African American

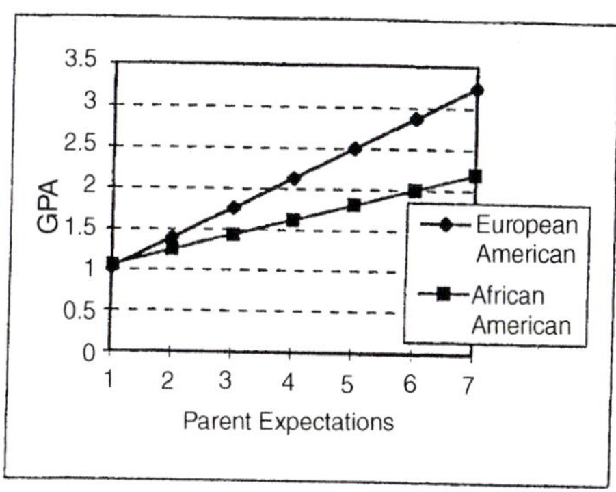

As shown in Table 5, the overall regression equation of GPA on parent involvement of schooling with the ethnicity interaction term is:

$$Y = .37 + .74\ X_2 + .46D\ 2^*.43\ X_2D$$

The separate regression equations are:

$$Y_{EA} = .37 + .74\ X_2$$
$$Y_{AA} = .83 + .31\ X_2$$

TABLE 5. Regressions of GPA: Parent Involvement and Interaction Effects by Ethnicity (N = 567)

	b [a]
Parent Involvement	.74 **
Ethnicity (African American = 1)	.46
Interaction	−.43 **
Constant	.37 †
R^2	0.35
Adj. R^2	0.34

[a] Unstandardized regression coefficients.
† $p < .10$; * $p < .05$; ** $p < .01$ (two-tailed tests).

Where Y = GPA; EA = European American; AA = African American; and X_2 = Parent Involvement. As shown in Figure 2, the point of intersection is $X_2 = 1.07$, $Y = 1.16$. Students with parent involvement of schooling above 1.07 are expected to have a higher GPA if they are EA, whereas AA students with parent involvement above 1.07 are expected to have a lower GPA if they are AA. This interaction model explained 35% of the variance in GPA.

DISCUSSION

Summary of Findings

Bivariate correlations reveal that for EA students, SES and later GPA share a statistically negative relationship. For AA youth, SES and later GPA are not statistically significant. T-tests indicate EA parents have higher expectation mean scores than AA parents do. However, there was no statistical difference between AA and EA parent involvement mean scores.

Hierarchical regression models explain 59% of the variance in later GPA for EA students and 27% of the variance in later GPA for AA students. SES maintains significance at all three steps of the regression for EA students; however, SES fails to reach statistical significance in all three steps for the AA students. Illicit drug use reaches marginal significance ($p < .10$) for EA students, and it is not significant for AA students. For EA students, parent involvement has the strongest impact on later

FIGURE 2. Regressions of GPA at Grade 8 onto Parent Involvement at Grade 7 for European American and African American

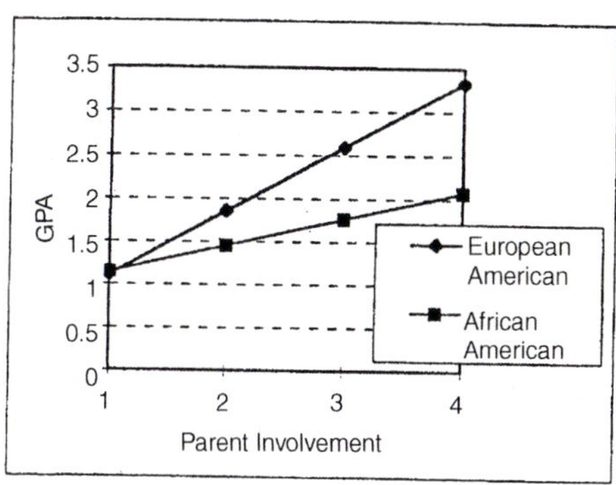

GPA, and for AA students earlier educational achievement has the strongest impact on later GPA.

Finally, two significant negative interaction effects were found. The first interaction model, parent expectations and ethnicity (AA = 1 and EA = 0), explains 36% of the variance in later GPA. The model indicates EA and AA students with equal parent expectation ratings do not receive the same GPA at grade 8; AA youth receive lower GPA scores. The second interaction model, parent involvement and ethnicity, explains 35% of the variance in later GPA. EA and AA students with equal parent involvement ratings do not receive equal GPA scores; AA students receive lower GPA scores. In an earlier study using the same data set, similar negative interaction effects were found for earlier achievement and ethnicity and also teacher perceptions of aggression and ethnicity (Seyfried, 2000). In the former study, the interaction terms were entered separately into the full model.

SES (Socioeconomic Status)

The literature overwhelmingly agrees that SES is an important predictor of academic outcome, particularly for minority youth that are disproportionately represented among the poor. In this study, for AA youth, the association between SES and later GPA is not significant. For AA youth, it may be that SES has an indirect influence on later GPA through earlier educational ability, parental involvement, and parental expectations. Other analytic techniques, such as path analysis, are needed to substantiate this hypothesis.

Parent Involvement

Findings from a t-test indicate that there was no statistical difference between EA and AA parent involvement means, that is EA and AA parents had similar ratings regarding their perceptions of student motivation. Significant positive bivariate correlations and significant positive beta weights indicate highly motivated children receive higher GPAs. This finding is supported in the literature (Clark, 1983; Scheinfeld, 1983; Smokowski, Reynolds, & Bezruczko, 1999).

Negative interaction effects of race and parent involvement suggest that for the AA students, parent involvement is not as strong a predictor of later GPA as it is for the EA students. This finding suggests that the AA parents in this study must not rely on their perceptions of their children's motivation as a way to monitor academic motivation. The AA child that tries to please her teacher, tries to get good grades, and is willing to put up with things she doesn't like about school may not be rewarded (in terms of higher GPA) in the same way her EA classmate would be rewarded.

Perhaps as Lareau (1989) suggests, parent involvement is confounded with the parent's social capital, that is, the EA parents in this study (the majority of whom are *not* eligible for free lunch status) have access to resources within the school and the community which actuate their perceptions of their child's motivation. The teachers in this study may have different expectations for EA students, so that when an EA student tries to please the teacher, the teacher responds by rewarding the student for the behavior. In the parent-teacher conference, the teacher validates the parents' perceptions of their child's behavior, creating a mutually reinforcing dynamic. School social workers are in a position to empower families and communities of color with knowledge and practical skills designed to negotiate the socio-political culture of schools. Clearly, further study is needed to determine the factors that diminish the effect of parent perceptions of student motivation on later GPA for AA students.

Parent Expectations

t-tests indicate that the higher EA parent expectation means are statistically different from the AA parent expectation means. Although

AA families generally have high expectations for their children's education (Jenkins, 1995), the stresses and realities of everyday life may dampen the influence of those expectations. The AA parents in this study may have high expectations for their children; however, the parent's reality of their past school experience and the reality of their child's present experience may discourage hope for their child's educational future.

The negative interactive effects between ethnicity and parent expectations indicate that parent expectations are not as strong a predictor of later GPA for the AA students as they are for the EA students in this study. While the t-test results indicate that the EA parents generally have higher educational expectations for their children, the negative interactive effects suggest that AA parent expectations that are equal to EA parent expectations will not have the same effect on later GPA for the AA students. As mentioned earlier, the effects of parent expectations may be diminished by real life experiences. If this is so, then school and community supports are needed to help sustain parent expectations among ethnic minority populations. More within group research is needed that examines the relationship between AA parent expectations and later achievement.

IMPLICATIONS FOR SOCIAL WORK PRACTICE

Given the same parent expectations for education and parental perceptions of achievement motivation, EA students have better GPAs than AA students. Interventions with EA students and parents are likely to require different approaches from those targeted towards AA youth and their parents. This demonstrates the need to develop intervention strategies to improve academic achievement that is culturally relevant and grounded in social context. Interventions focused on parent expectations and expectations regarding achievement motivation might be more appropriate for EA students. Interventions directed towards early academic achievement might serve AA students well. Kunjufu (1988) reports "fourth-grade syndrome" as one of the theoretical explanations of academic failure among AA youth. This syndrome explains a phenomenon wherein third grade AA students begin to fail academically. The syndrome is full blown by the time the students reach 4th grade, and AA males are disproportionately impacted by this phenomenon.

In addition, AA parents may benefit from interventions designed to empower them in the schooling process. For example, they may profit from information about the influence of early achievement on later GPA. More importantly, ethnic minority parents should be aware of the harmful, long, term effects of academic labeling on later achievement. Also, AA parents should be familiar with educational laws and policies, they should know their legal rights and the rights of their children. Interventions should also be developed to address organizational issues in the school. Teachers may benefit from interventions that are designed to enhance culturally competent practice. Teachers may not be aware of personal attitudes and beliefs that may influence their interactions with students and parents who are different from them and their expectations of students' achievement.

Finally, because school social workers interact within school and community systems, they are in a position to facilitate home-school partnerships. School social workers can help to develop *collaborative* relationships between AA parents and schools. Social workers can help to ensure that the school environment creates a warm and inviting atmosphere for all parents and students, especially ethnic minority parents and parents from lower socioeconomic backgrounds.

REFERENCES

Achenbach, T. M., & Edelbrock, C. S. (1983). *Manual for the child behavior checklist and revised child behavior profile*. Burlington: University of Vermont, Department of Psychology.

Allen-Meares, P. (1999). African American males: Their status, educational plight, and the possibilities for their future. In L. E. Davis (Ed.) *Working with African American males: A guide to practice* (pp. 117-128). Thousand Oaks: Sage Publications.

Battin, S. R., Hawkins, J. D., Thornberry, T. P., & Krohn, M. D. (1998). *Gang membership, delinquent peers, and delinquent behavior. Juvenile Justice Bulletin*, October 1998, 1-10.

Boocock, S. P. (1972). *An introduction to the sociology of learning*. Boston: Houghton Mifflin.

Clark, R. M. (1983). *Family life and school achievement: Why poor black children succeed or fail*. Chicago: The University of Chicago Press.

Comer, J. P. (1988). Educating poor minority children. *Scientific American*, 259, 42-48.

Crandall, V. J., Dewey, R., Katkovsky, W., & Preston, A. (1964). Parents' attitude and behaviors and grade-school children's academic achievement. *Journal of Genetic Psychology*, 104, 53-66.

Eccles, J. S., & Harold, R. D. (1996). Family involvement in children's and adolescents' schooling. In A. Booth & J. F. Dunn (Eds.), *Family school links: How do they affect educational outcomes?* (pp. 3-34). Mahwah, NJ: Erlbaum.

Eccles, J. S., Jacobs, J. E., & Harold, R. D. (1990). Gender role stereotypes, expectancy effects, and parents' socialization of gender differences. *Journal of Social Issues*, 46, 183-210.

Entwisle, D. R., & Baker, D. P. (1983). Gender and young children's expectations for performance in arithmetic. *Developmental Psychology*, 19, 200-209.

Entwisle, D. R., & Hayduk, L. A. (1978). *Too great expectations: The academic outlook of young children.* Baltimore: Johns Hopkins University Press.

Epstein, J. L. (1995). School/family/community partnerships: Caring for the children we share. *Phi Delta Kappan*, (May), 701-712.

Erikson, E. H. (1950/1963). *Childhood and society*. New York: Norton.

Germain, C. B. (1999). An ecological perspective on social work in the schools. In R. Constable, S. McDonald & J. P. Flynn (Eds.) *School social work: Practice, policy, and research perspectives* (pp. 33-44). Chicago: Lyceum Books, Inc.

Gills, S., & Reynolds, A. J. (1999). Educational expectations and school achievement of urban African American children. *Journal of School Psychology*, 37(4), 403-424.

Graham, J. W., Hofer, S. M., & Piccinin, A. M. (1994). Analysis with missing data in drug prevention research. In L. M. Collins and L. Seitz (Eds.), *Advances in data analysis for prevention intervention research.* National Institute on Drug Abuse Research Monograph Series (#142), Washington DC: National Institute on Drug Abuse.

Graham, J. W., Hofer, S. M., Donaldson, S. I., MacKinnon, D. P., & Schafer, J. L. (1997). Analysis with missing data in prevention research. In K. Bryant, M. Windle, & S. West (Eds.), *The science of prevention: Methodological advances from alcohol and substance abuse research* (pp. 325-366). Washington, D.C.: American Psychological Association.

Hawkins, J. D., Lishner, D. M., Catalano, R. F., & Howard, M. O. (1986). Childhood predictors of adolescent substance abuse: Toward an empirically grounded theory. *Journal of Children in Contemporary Society*, 18(1-2), 11-48.

Hawkins, J. D., Graham, J. W., Maguin, E., Abbott, R. D., & Catalano, R. F. (1997). Exploring the effects of age of alcohol use initiation and psychosocial risk factors on subsequent alcohol misuse. *Journal of Studies on Alcohol*, 58(3), 280-290.

Jenkins, A. H. (1995). *Turning corners: The psychology of African Americans.* Needham Heights: Allyn & Bacon.

Keith, T. Z., Keith, P. B., Bickley, P. G., & Singhm K. (1992). *Effects of parental involvement on eighth grade achievement: LISREL analysis of NELS-88 data.* (Eric Document Reproduction Service No. ED 347 640).

Kohl, G. O., Lengua, L. J., & McMahon, R. J. (2000). Parent involvement in school: Conceptualizing multiple dimensions and their relations with family and demographic risk factors. *Journal of School Psychology*, 38(6), 501-523.

Kunjufu, J. (1986). *Countering the conspiracy to destroy black boys* (2 vols.). Chicago: African American Images.

Kurtz-Costes, B., Halle, T., Clarke, A., & Seidu, K. (1995, March). *The influence of parental beliefs and behaviors on school achievement in low-income African American children.* Paper presented at the meeting of the Society for Research and Child Development, Indiannapolis, IN.

Lareau, A. (1989). *Home advantage.* London: Falmer Press.

Little, R.J., & Rubin, D. B. (1987). *Statistical analysis with missing data.* New York: J. Wiley & Sons.

Lucas, B. G., & Lusthaus, C. S. (1978). The decisional participation of parents in elementary and secondary schools. *Journal of High School*, 61(5), 211-220.

Majoribanks, K. (1984). Aspirations: Sibling and family environment correlates. *Genetic Psychology Monographs*, 110, 3-20.

Miedel, W. T., & Reynolds, A. J. (1999). Parent involvement in early intervention for disadvantaged children: Does it matter? *Journal of School Psychology*, 37(4), 379-402.

Newman, B. M., & Newman, P. R. (1995). *Development through life: A psychosocial approach*. Pacific Grove: Brooks/Cole.

Olmstead, P. P., & Rubin, R. I. (1983). Linking parent behaviors to child achievement: Four evaluation studies from the parent education follow-through programs. *Studies in Educational Evaluation*, 8, 317-325.

Parsons, J. E., Adler, T., & Kaczala, C. (1982). Socialization of achievement attitudes and beliefs: Parental influences. *Child Development*, 53, 310-321.

Patrikakou, E. N. (1997). A model of parental attitudes and the academic achievement of adolescents. *Journal of Research and Development in Education*, 31(1), 7-26.

Paulson, S. E. (1994). Relations of parenting style and parental involvement with ninth grade students' achievement. *Journal of Early Adolescence*, 14, 250-267.

Pedhazur, E.J. (1997). *Multiple regression in behavioral research: Explanation and prediction* (3rd ed.). New York: Holt, Rinehart & Winston.

Peng, S. S., & Lee, R. M. (1993). Home variables, parent-child activities, and academic achievement: A study of 1988 eighth graders. In F. Smit, W. Van Esch, & J. J. Walberg, (Eds.), *Parental involvement in education.* Nijmegen: Institute for Applied Social Sciences.

Reynolds, A. J. (1992). Mediated effects of preschool intervention. *Early Education and Development*. 3(2), 139-164.

Ritter, P. L., Mont-Reynaud, R., & Dornbsch, S. M. (1993). Minority parents and their youth: Concern, encouragement, and support for school achievement. In N. F. Chavkin (Ed.), *Families and schools in a pluralistic society* (pp. 107-119). Albany, New York: State University of New York Press.

Rumberger, R. W., Ghatak, R., Poulos, G., Ritter, P. L., & Dornbusch, S. M. (1990). Family influences on dropout behavior in one California high school. *Sociology of Education*, 63, 283-299.

Sanders, D. (1999). Annual goals and short-term objectives for school social workers. In R. Constable, S. McDonald & J. P. Flynn (Eds.) *School social work: Practice, policy, and research perspectives* (pp. 307-317). Chicago: Lyceum Books, Inc.

Schafer, J. L. (1997). *Analysis of Incomplete Multivariate Data.* Chapman & Hall, London.

Scheinfeld, D. R. (1983). Family relationships and school achievement among boys of lower-income urban black families. *American Journal of Orthopsychiatry*, 53, 127-143.

Seginer, R. (1983). Parents' educational expectations and children's academic achievements: A literature review. *Merrill-Palmer Quarterly*, 29, 1-23.

Seyfried, S. (2000). Teacher perceptions, race, ability, and grade point average: What's happening in the classroom? *School Social Work Journal*, 42(2), 1-19.

Smokowski, P. R., Reynolds, A. J., & Bezuczko, N. (1999). Resilience and protective factors in adolescence: An autobiographical perspective from disadvantaged youth. *Journal of School Psychology*, 37(4), 425-448.

Thompson, M. S., Alexander, K. L., & Entwisle, D. R. (1988). Household composition, parental expectations, and school achievement. *Social Forces*, 67(2), 424-451.

Trusty, J. (1996). Relationship of parental involvement in teens' career development to teens' attitudes, perceptions and behavior. *Journal of Research and Development in Education*, 30, 63-69.

U.S. Department of Education. (1994). *Goals 2000 legislation and related items* [On-line]. Available: http://www.ed.gov.G2K/.

Valdes, G. (1996). Con respecto: Bridging the distances between culturally diverse families and schools. New York: Teachers College Press.

Vygotsky, L. S. (1978). *Mind in society*. Cambridge: Harvard University Press.

Adolescent Violence: With Whom They Fight and Where

Todd Michael Franke
Anh-Luu T. Huynh-Hohnbaum
Yunah Chung

SUMMARY. While adolescent violence is a significant societal concern, there has been limited research as to the context of the fighting. In other words, where do adolescents fight the most? With whom are they most likely to fight? Understanding the patterns of adolescent fighting will allow for a more comprehensive grasp of the problem. The data for the present analysis are drawn from the National Longitudinal Study of Adolescent Health (Add Health) (Wave1), and are from the adolescent and matching parent in-home assessment and include only those adolescents who report being in a physical fight (n = 10,450). Adolescents report fighting most often at school and with a friend or someone they know. Differences in terms of sociodemographic variables (e.g., age, ethnicity, gender, parent ed-

Todd Michael Franke, PhD, is Associate Professor, Department of Social Welfare, School of Public Policy and Social Research, University of California at Los Angeles, Los Angeles, CA 90095-1656. Anh-Luu T. Huynh-Hohnbaum, MSW, is a Doctoral Student and Yunah Chung, MSW, is a graduate, Department of Social Welfare, School of Public Policy and Social Research, University of California at Los Angeles.

[Haworth co-indexing entry note]: "Adolescent Violence: With Whom They Fight and Where." Franke, Todd Michael, Anh-Luu T. Huynh-Hohnbaum, and Yunah Chung. Co-published simultaneously in *Journal of Ethnic & Cultural Diversity in Social Work* (The Haworth Social Work Practice Press, an imprint of The Haworth Press, Inc.) Vol. 11, No. 3/4, 2002, pp. 133-158; and: *Social Work with Multicultural Youth* (ed: Diane de Anda) The Haworth Social Work Practice Press, an imprint of The Haworth Press, Inc., 2002, pp. 133-158. Single or multiple copies of this article are available for a fee from The Haworth Document Delivery Service [1-800-HAWORTH, 9:00 a.m. - 5:00 p.m. (EST). E-mail address: docdelivery@haworthpress.com].

http://www.haworthpress.com/store/product.asp?sku=J051

10.1300/J051v11n03_01

ucation level) and family, school, and community attachment are discussed.

KEYWORDS. Race, adolescent violence, fighting, location, victims

INTRODUCTION

Adolescent violence remains a growing problem in the United States and is an issue of concern for the general public and policymakers. According to the Centers for Disease Control and Prevention's 2001 Youth Risk Behavior Surveillance System, about one-third of all high school students said that they had been in one or more physical fights during the past 12 months and of those, approximately 13% fought more than once on school property (Grunbaum et al., 2002). Furthermore, while the recent tragic cases of school shootings show that it is a significant concern in schools, violent incidents involving adolescents occur across settings, such as in their homes and neighborhoods.

Adolescence is a developmental period of heightened violence; compared to all other age groups, adolescents disproportionately engage in violent behaviors (Bracher, 2000; Kosterman, Graham, Hawkins, Catalano, & Herrenkohl, 2001; Osgood, O'Malley, Bachman, & Johnston, 1989; Riner & Saywell, 2002). Physical fighting is a common form of adolescent violence (Everett & Price, 1995; Lowry, Powell, Kann, Collins, & Kolbe, 1998; Malek, Chang, & Davis, 1998a) and can often lead to more serious acts of violence, such as homicide (Moeller, 2001; Services). In fact, The Department of Health and Human Services (2000) has identified adolescent fighting as a leading health indicator, and one of the Healthy People Year 2010 objectives is to reduce fighting among adolescents.

Little is known about the context, such as setting and person, in which fighting involving an adolescent occurs. While it is understandable that researchers studying adolescent fighting would naturally look at the school since it is the most common setting for adolescent violence (Simon, Crosby & Dhalberg, 1999), it is not the only setting in which fighting occurs. Few, if any, studies examine patterns of fighting across settings (Loeber & Dishion, 1984; Malek et al., 1998a; Malek, Chang, & Davis, 1998b). Furthermore, those studies which look only at the school tend to be limited to student interpersonal relationships and neglect to look at adolescent fighting with a family member or a total stranger.

Therefore, by not extending the environment beyond the school, researchers are limited in looking at the person with whom adolescents may be fighting.

The purpose of this study is to begin to fill the gap in the knowledge base of the context of adolescent violence. The study will provide a closer look at the pattern of physical fighting in adolescents by identifying the person and the setting associated with these violent behaviors.

LITERATURE REVIEW

The theoretical framework that guides this study is based on a social ecological theory of development, which is a transactional and multilevel concept of behavior development. Thus, an adolescent's behavior, both violent and non-violent, is neither the function of solely the individual or the experiential context, but rather an interaction of the individual and the social system in which the adolescent is embedded (i.e., individual, family, peer, home, school, neighborhood) (Bronfenbrenner, 1979, 1986; Sameroff, 1983, 1987). The adolescent's environments are interrelated and all serve to influence corresponding levels of adolescent violence (Cicchetti & Lynch, 1993). Therefore, it is important to identify the settings in which adolescents are frequently involved in violent behavior in order to properly look at the characterization of adolescent fighting.

Setting

The majority of studies tend to identify the patterns of fighting in one setting. As noted earlier, the school is the most common setting for adolescent fighting (Simon, Crosby, & Dahlberg, 1999). The school is also a common setting for researchers when looking at adolescents (Feshbach & Feshbach, 1998; Hyman & Snook, 1999; Kingery, Coggeshall, & Alford, 1998; Larson, 1998; Lowry et al., 1999). While the school does expose children to violence, the Departments of Education and Justice (OJJDP) (1998) argue that the risk is minimal compared to the risk that adolescents face outside the school. Furthermore, after analyzing the FBI's national database of all crimes reported to law enforcement agencies, the Office of Juvenile Justice and Delinquency Prevention (1995) claims that students are, in fact, safer at school than away from school; students are at the greatest risk of being victimized at the end of the school day when they are unsupervised.

Other researchers have pointed to the relationship that home and neighborhood factors have with levels of school violence (Everett & Price, 1995; Horton, 2001; Kingery et al., 1998; Loeber & Dishion, 1984; O'Keefe, 1997; Riner & Saywell, 2002). Adolescents who are exposed to fighting in the home and neighborhood are more likely to engage in fighting at school (Loeber & Dishion, 1984; Riner & Saywell, 2002). Moreover, Kingery et al. (1998) found that more extreme forms of school violence, such as carrying a weapon to school, were correlated with a violent neighborhood. The neighborhood provides the most immediate environment outside of the family (Oetting, Donnermeyer, & Deffenbacher, 1998) and is the second most likely setting for adolescent violence to occur (Richters & Martinez, 1993). O'Keefe (1997) found that even after controlling for family violence, males who were exposed to violence at the school and neighborhood were significantly more likely to behave aggressively, including engaging in physical fights.

In a study of 567 7th grade students from three middle schools in Louisiana and Massachusetts, Malek et al. (1998a) found that nearly 30% of fights occurred at the adolescent's home or the home of a friend. Similar to the argument made by the OJJDP that adolescents are more likely to behave violently when unsupervised, Loeber and Dishion (1984) found that adolescents are also more likely to fight at home when left unmonitored.

With Whom?

Research shows that while adolescents fight primarily with friends (Malek et al., 1998b; Richters & Martinez, 1993), fights are not limited to friends. Richters and Martinez (1993) found that adolescents also fight significantly more often with family and acquaintances than strangers. In fact, there is a growing trend in juvenile homicide that adolescents are more likely to be murdered by a friend or acquaintance than a stranger (Fox, 1996).

Generally, the majority of studies simply ask if the adolescent was involved in a fight in the past year (Cotten et al., 1994; Everett & Price, 1995; Fox, 1996; Kingery et al., 1998; Lowry et al., 1998; Paschall, Ennett, & Flewelling, 1996; Services; Simon et al., 1999), but do not go into greater detail about the setting and the person with whom they fought.

Race

Although violence is not a race-inherent problem (Fingerhut & Kleinman, 1990), violence does disproportionately affect American minority youth, both as victims and perpetrators (Arbona, Jackson, McCoy, & Blakely, 1999; Everett & Price, 1995; Lowry et al., 1998; Osgood et al., 1989; Prothrow-Stith & Weissman, 1991). For 15-24 year olds, the rate of death by homicide per 100,000 is significantly higher for African American (54.7) and Hispanic (23.3) youth than for White youth (7.6) (*National Health Statistics Report*, 2000). On the other hand, while minority adolescents are typically more likely to be involved in violent behavior, Kosterman et al. (2001) found that Asian American youth were least likely to be involved in fights. However, Go (1999) and Kim and Goto (2000) found that the more acculturated Asian American adolescents were, the more likely they would be involved in delinquent activities. Acculturation also plays a significant role in predicting the increase of delinquent behaviors for other minority groups (Samaniego & Gonzales, 1999; Vega, Gil, Warheit, Zimmerman et al., 1993).

Generally, research has found that demographic variables demonstrate differences in participation in violent acts. Greater incidence is associated with being African American (Lowry et al., 1998; Pallone & Hennessy, 2000; Paschall et al., 1996), male (Cotten et al., 1994; Everett & Price, 1995; Grunbaum et al., 2002; Kingery et al., 1998; Malek et al., 1998a; Osgood et al., 1989), a younger adolescent (Cotten et al., 1994; Grunbaum et al., 2002; Kingery et al., 1998; Kosterman et al., 2001), and in a family of lower socioeconomic status (Everett & Price, 1995). Not only are prevlance rates of physical fighting higher for males than females, even after controlling for age and race (Synder & Sickmund, 1995), but males are more likely to be involved in more severe forms of fighting (Durant, Getts, Cadenhead, & Woods, 1995). Pallone and Hennessy (2000) found that when controlling for both gender and age, African American male adolescents are significantly at risk to be involved in violence, both as offenders and victims. However, it is important to take income into consideration since adolescents who come from low socioeconomic status families are more likely to be involved in fighting than those from middle to high socioeconomic status families (Durant et al., 1995; Everett & Price, 1995).

METHODS

Survey and Sample

The current study uses data from the National Longitudinal Study of Adolescent Health (Wave 1) gathered in 1994-1995. NLSAH (Add

Health) is a longitudinal study of adolescents in grades 7 through 12. The primary sampling frame included all high schools in the United States that had an 11th grade and at least 30 students in the school. From this, a systematic random sample of 80 high schools was selected proportional to enrollment size and stratified by region, urbanicity, school type and percentage of students who were White. Once a high school was recruited, its feeder schools–that is, those schools that include 7th grade and sent their graduates to that high school–were identified. From among the possible feeder schools, one school was selected with a probability proportional to the number of students it contributed to the high school.

The Add Health survey consisted of two components, an in-home component and an in-school component. Schools provided a roster of all enrolled students from which a random sample of adolescents, stratified by gender and grade, were selected for the in-home interview. A total of 18,924 students were included in the Wave 1 in-home sample with appropriate sampling weights. Data analyzed for the purpose of this paper are from the adolescent and matching parent in-home assessment and include only those adolescents who report being in a physical fight (n = 10,450). This represents approximately 55% of the total sample from the study. Both CAPI (Computer-assisted Personal Interview) and audio CASI (Computer-assisted Self-Interview) techniques were used to assess a respondent's health and health-related behaviors, emotional well-being, and family and educational environment. The more sensitive questions were administered using audio CASI.

Outcome Variables

The outcomes examined in this study measure the person and setting where adolescents report most recently being involved in physical fights. The question that determines with whom adolescents report fighting was "The last time you were in a physical fight, with whom did you fight? The response categories used were: (1) "a total stranger," (2) "a friend or someone you knew," (3) "a parent, brother, sister, or other family member," and (4) "someone not listed above." The question measuring setting was "The last time you were in a physical fight, where did it occur?" The response categories were: (1) "at school," (2) "in your neighborhood," (3) "at home," and (4) "someplace else."

Independent Variables

The analysis included individual and family characteristics as predictors of violent behavior. Unless otherwise noted, the item responses for the variables in the analysis were based on adolescents' self-reports. The socio-demographic variables included gender, age, the race/ethnicity of the adolescent (African American, Asian American, Hispanic, White), grade (7-12), and the highest educational level of the person identified as the mother or father (Did not graduate from HS, HS graduate or equivalent, Some post HS education, College Graduate, Post Graduate).

Three measures of connection or attachment were used in this study: family, school, and community. Family attachment was a measure of the relationship between the adolescent and the family and consisted of the sum of three Likert (Likert, 1932) scale items with response categories ranging from "not at all" (1) to "very much" (5): (a) "How much do you feel the people in your family understand you?" (b) "How much do you feel you and your family have fun together?" (c) "How much do you feel your family pays attention to you?" School attachment was a measure of the relationship between the adolescent and the school. The measure consisted of the sum of three Likert scale items with a response ranging from "strongly agree" (1) to "strongly disagree" (5). The items in the scale were (a) "You feel close to people at your school," (b) "You feel like you are part of your school," and (c) "You are happy to be at your school." Community attachment was a measure of the relationship between the adolescent and neighborhood. The measure consisted of the sum of three dichotomous (Yes, No) items. The items in the scale were (a) "Do you know most people in neighborhood?", (b) "In the past month have you stopped & talked to neighbors?", and (c) "Neighbors lookout for each other."

Data Analysis

Descriptive statistics are presented for the adolescents who report engaging in a physical fight. For categorical variables percentages are reported. For continuous variables means and associated standard errors are reported. The chi-square test of independence and multinomial logistic regressions were used in this study. For the multinomial logistic regression analyses, relative risk ratios and confidence intervals are presented. The relative risk ratio can be interpreted in a manner similar to the odds ratio. The reference group for the multinomial logistic regressions was the category with the highest percentage. Statistical analyses were adjusted for complex sample designs using Stata (StataCorp, 2002). All estimates were calculated using the sampling weights to represent adolescents in the 7th-12th grade in the United States. The alpha level used for all analyses was .05.

FINDINGS

Persons With Whom Adolescents Fought

Adolescents report fighting most often with a friend or someone they know (49.8%). All of the variables in Table 1 are significantly associated with the outcome. Unless otherwise noted, percents in Table 1 are row percents. While males and females report fighting most with a friend (48.8% and 51.7%), the pattern regarding the person with whom they fight is somewhat different. Females report fighting with a family member as the second most common (20.2%) and someone else as last (9.2%). For males, fighting with a total stranger is the second most common (31.3%) with family member representing the least reported (5.7%). While fighting with a friend or a total stranger are the two most frequently reported categories, for race/ethnicity, grade, and parental education, some within group patterns are apparent. For example, changes across grade in the categories of friend and stranger demonstrate exactly the opposite trajectory. The results indicate that adolescents report fighting less with friends across the grades, going from a high of 55.1% in the 7th grade and dropping to 44.7% by 12th grade. Fighting with total strangers changes from a low of 19.6% in 7th grade to a high of 31.5% in 12th grade. As the educational level of the parent increases, there is a notable increase in the percent of adolescents who report fighting with a parent or family member. For parents who did not graduate from high school, it is 7.6%, changing to 16.6% as the educational level of the parent increases to the post graduate level.

As noted in Table 2, family, school, and community attachment and age are all significantly associated with the person with whom the adolescent reports most recently being in a fight. With increasing age, adolescents are significantly more likely to report fighting with a stranger ($RRR = 1.2, p < .001$) or someone other than a friend ($RRR = 1.07, p < .01$). The increases in family, school and community attachment are all associated with a decreased likelihood of the adolescent fighting with others. Compared to fighting with a friend, adolescents are significantly

TABLE 1. Percentages by Socio-Demographic Variables for Person and Setting

		The last time you were in a physical fight, with whom did you fight?				The last time you were in a physical fight, where did it occur?			
		a total stranger	a friend or someone you knew	a parent, brother, sister, or other family member	someone not listed above	at school	in your neighbor-hood	at home	some place else
		%	%	%	%	%	%	%	%
	Overall[1]	26.7	49.8	11.1	12.4	42.8	18.2	13.3	25.7
Gender [a b]	%								
Male	63.2	31.3	48.8	5.7	14.2	44.7	19.8	7.7	27.9
Female	36.8	18.9	51.7	20.2	9.2	39.5	15.5	23.1	21.9
Race/Ethnicity [a b]									
Black or African American	20.8	26.0	54.3	7.9	11.8	47.0	22.0	11.4	19.6
Asian American	3.2	25.3	49.0	14.2	11.5	41.4	13.3	17.6	27.7
Hispanic	13.3	32.8	43.1	9.4	14.7	47.3	14.3	10.0	28.4
White	62.7	25.5	49.9	12.6	12.0	40.4	18.1	14.6	26.9
Grade [a b]									
7	17.3	19.6	55.1	12.8	12.5	50.0	18.6	13.7	17.8
8	17.7	22.3	54.1	12.1	11.5	47.8	19.1	13.9	19.3
9	18.6	25.8	52.3	10.6	11.3	41.4	21.0	13.9	23.7
10	16.2	28.8	47.1	11.1	13.0	40.7	18.3	13.8	27.1
11	14.7	31.9	46.4	9.5	12.2	41.3	16.2	11.9	30.6
12	15.4	31.5	44.7	10.3	13.6	34.7	15.1	12.5	37.7

TABLE 1 (continued)

		The last time you were in a physical fight, with whom did you fight?				The last time you were in a physical fight, where did it occur?			
		a total stranger	a friend or someone you knew	a parent, brother, sister, or other family member	someone not listed above	at school	in your neighbor-hood	at home	some place else
Parental Education[a b]									
Did not graduate from HS	13.9	28.4	51.4	7.6	12.6	45.1	19.2	10.9	24.7
HS graduate or equivalent	35.4	28.0	50.5	9.7	11.7	43.1	20.9	11.7	24.3
Some post HS education	21.7	23.6	50.3	12.9	13.2	41.1	17.9	15.3	25.7
College Graduate	19.8	25.7	48.0	12.6	13.6	41.3	16.2	14.3	28.3
Post Graduate	9.2	22.4	50.5	16.6	10.4	42.3	13.2	18.3	26.2

[1]Column Percents
[a] $p < .001$ With whom did you fight?
[b] $p < .001$ Where did it occur?

TABLE 2. Means and Standard Errors for Person and Setting

	The last time you were in a physical fight, with whom did you fight?					The last time you were in a physical fight, where did it occur?			
		a total stranger	a friend or someone you knew	a parent, brother, sister, or other family member	someone not listed above	at school	in your neighbor-hood	at home	someplace else
	Mean	Mean	Mean	Mean	Mean	Mean	Mean	Mean	Mean
	SE	SE	SE	SE	SE	SE	SE	SE	SE
Adolescent Age [a b]	15.45	15.84	15.29	15.14	15.51	15.27	15.37	15.26	15.90
	0.12	0.12	0.12	0.14	0.15	0.13	0.13	0.14	0.11
Attachment									
Family [a b]	10.95	11.02	11.05	10.61	10.67	11.14	10.94	10.67	10.79
	0.05	0.08	0.06	0.08	0.10	0.07	0.09	0.08	0.08
School [a]	10.97	10.84	11.13	10.93	10.68	11.08	10.95	10.99	10.80
	0.05	0.08	0.06	0.11	0.10	0.06	0.10	0.10	0.09
Community [a b]	2.27	2.28	2.31	2.18	2.21	2.26	2.40	2.21	2.24
	0.02	0.03	0.02	0.04	0.04	0.02	0.03	0.04	0.03

[a] $p < .001$ With whom did you fight?
[b] $p < .001$ Where did it occur?

less likely to report fighting with a family member (RRR = .93, p < .001) or someone else (RRR = .94, p < .001). Moreover, adolescents are significantly less likely to report fighting with a family member (RRR = .96, p < .001) or a stranger (RRR = .94, p < .001) compared to fighting with a friend as their attachment to school increases. Similarly, adolescents who report being more connected to their communities are significantly less likely to report fighting with a family member (RRR = .86, p < .01) or someone else (RRR = .90, p < .05) compared to fighting with a friend.

The results of the multinomial logistic regression analysis for the persons with whom adolescents engage in physical fights are presented in Table 3. The table includes adjusted relative risk ratios (aRRR), 95% confidence intervals and associated probabilities. As indicated earlier, the reference group for this analysis is the friend category. For the predictor variables, the reference group is indicated by a relative risk ratio (RRR) of 1.0.

Socio-Demographic Variables

Males are significantly more likely to report fighting with a stranger or some else and significantly less likely to report fighting with a family member than females. Hispanic adolescents are significantly more likely to report fighting with a stranger or someone else than White adolescents, while African American adolescents are significantly less likely to report fighting with family members. Adolescent age is predictive only for fights with strangers, where increases in age are associated with an increased likelihood of the adolescent fighting with strangers compared to friends. The importance of the educational level of the parent(s) is only significant for fights with family members. Adolescents whose parent(s) have some post high school education are 2.03 times more likely to fight with family members. The relative risk increases steadily as the education level of the parent(s) increases. Adolescents whose parent(s) have a post graduate education are 2.9 times more likely to report fighting with family members.

Family, School, and Community Attachment

While there is no consistent pattern in the measures of attachment, all the relative risk ratios indicate that in comparison to fighting with friends, the increases in these measures are associated with decreased risks (RRR significantly less than 1.0) of fighting. The most consistent

TABLE 3. Multinominal Logistic Regression-Person

Friend is the comparison group	The last time you were in a physical fight, with whom did you fight? Adjusted RRR	P > t	95% CI
A total stranger			
Male	1.75	0.000	1.5-2.04
Female	1.00		
African American	0.95	0.600	0.77-1.16
Asian American	1.01	0.972	0.62-1.63
Hispanic	1.56	0.000	1.25-1.94
White	1.00		
Did not graduate from HS	1.00		
HS graduate	1.06	0.595	0.85-1.34
Some post HS education	0.90	0.443	0.69-1.18
College Graduate	1.02	0.913	0.76-1.35
Post Graduate	0.85	0.365	0.06-1.21
Adolescent Age	1.16	0.000	1.11-1.22
Family	1.02	0.234	0.99-1.05
School	0.96	0.006	0.94-0.99
Community	0.97	0.416	0.89-1.05
A parent, brother, sister, or other family member			
Male	0.27	0.000	0.22-0.33
Female	1.00		
African American	0.55	0.000	0.44-0.68
Asian American	1.05	0.865	0.62-1.77
Hispanic	0.97	0.869	0.7-1.36
White	1.00		
Did not graduate from HS	1.00		
HS graduate	1.43	0.050	1.00-2.05
Some post HS education	2.03	0.001	1.36-3.03
College Graduate	2.32	0.000	1.57-3.44
Post Graduate	2.93	0.000	1.92-4.47
Adolescent Age	0.94	0.057	0.89-1.00
Family	0.96	0.018	0.92-0.99
School	0.99	0.606	0.96-1.03
Community	0.94	0.255	0.84-1.05

TABLE 3 (continued)

Someone not listed above			
Male	1.82	0.000	1.49-2.22
Female	1.00		
African American	0.98	0.835	0.78-1.23
Asian American	0.96	0.872	0.58-1.59
Hispanic	1.50	0.007	1.12-2.01
White	1.00		
Did not graduate from HS	1.00		
HS graduate	1.04	0.808	0.76-1.42
Some post HS education	1.14	0.453	0.8-1.63
College Graduate	1.16	0.384	0.83-1.64
Post Graduate	0.88	0.477	0.61-1.26
Adolescent Age	1.03	0.261	0.97-1.1
Family	0.94	0.002	0.91-0.98
School	0.96	0.008	0.93-0.99
Community	0.90	0.046	0.81-0.99

Note: Friend is the comparison group

pattern of results occurs for the category of fighting with someone else. In this case, increases in family, school and community attachment are all associated with a decreased likelihood of engaging in a fight with someone else compared to fighting with a friend. Adolescents are significantly less likely to report fighting with family members as family attachment increases and significantly less likely to report fighting with strangers as attachment to school increases.

Where Did It Occur?

The reported setting for adolescents fights is most often at school (42.8%), followed by "someplace else." All of the variables in Table 1 (gender, race/ethnicity, grade, and parental education) are significantly associated with this outcome. As indicated above, unless otherwise noted, percents in Table 1 are row percents. While males and females report fighting most often at school (44.7% and 39.5%, respectively), the pattern of the setting in which they report fighting is somewhat different. Females report fighting at home as the second most common setting (23.1%) and in the neighborhood as last (9.2%). For males, fighting "someplace else" is the second most common setting (27.9%) with fighting at home as the least reported (7.7%).

Although fighting at school or in the neighborhood are the two most frequently reported categories for race/ethnicity, grade, and parental education, some within group patterns are apparent. The settings of school, neighborhood, and home demonstrate a decline across grades. The most substantial decline is in fighting at school, which decreases from 50% in 7th grade to 34.7% in 12th grade. Alternatively, fighting "someplace else" displays a striking increase from 17.8% in 7th grade to 37.7% in the 12th grade. A similar pattern, though less pronounced, occurs when the educational level of the parent(s) is examined. Fighting at school and in the neighborhood declines as the educational level of the parent(s) increases, while fighting in the home and "someplace else" increases. Despite the increase in fighting in the home with increasing educational levels, it remains the least common location in which fighting occurs.

All of the variables in Table 2 are significantly associated with the setting of the most recent fight except for attachment to school. Adolescents are significantly more likely to report "someplace else" (RRR = 1.2, $p < .001$) than at home with increasing age. The increases in family attachment result in a decreased likelihood of adolescents fighting across all settings (neighborhood, school, and "someplace else"). Compared to fighting at school, adolescents are significantly less likely to report fighting in the neighborhood (RRR = .97, $p < .05$), at home (RRR = .93, $p < .001$), or "someplace else" (RRR = .95, $p < .001$). Adolescents are significantly less likely to report fighting "someplace else" (RRR = .96, $p < .01$) compared to at school as their attachment to school increases. Increases in the adolescents' attachment to the community is associated with an increased likelihood of fighting in the neighborhood (RRR = 1.2, $p < .001$).

The results of the multinomial logistic regression analysis for setting in which adolescents engage in physical fights are presented in Table 4. The table includes adjusted relative risk ratios (RRR), 95% confidence intervals and associated probabilities. As indicated earlier, the reference group for this analysis is the school setting. For the predictor variables, the reference group is indicated by a relative risk ratio (RRR) of 1.0.

TABLE 4. Multinominal Logistic Regression-Setting

	The last time you were in a physical fight, where did it occur?		
	Adjusted RRR	P > t	95% CI
In your neighborhood			
Male	1.14	0.167	0.95-1.36
Female	1.00		
African American	1.03	0.786	0.84-1.26
Asian American	0.86	0.586	0.5-1.49
Hispanic	0.66	0.003	0.5-0.86
White	1.00		
Did not graduate from HS	1.00		
HS graduate	1.09	0.512	0.83-1.43
Some post HS education	0.97	0.799	0.74-1.27
College Graduate	0.86	0.341	0.64-1.17
Post Graduate	0.70	0.047	0.50-.99
Adolescent Age	1.03	0.389	0.97-1.09
Family	0.96	0.008	0.94-0.99
School	0.98	0.345	0.95-1.02
Community	1.19	0.000	1.09-1.30
At home			
Male	0.26	0.000	0.21-0.32
Female	1.00		
African American	0.64	0.000	0.52-0.78
Asian American	1.22	0.264	0.86-1.74
Hispanic	0.63	0.004	0.46-0.86
White	1.00		
Did not graduate from HS	1.00		
HS graduate	1.18	0.318	0.85-1.62
Some post HS education	1.75	0.002	1.24-2.49
College Graduate	1.79	0.001	1.26-2.55
Post Graduate	2.17	0.000	1.45-3.25

TABLE 4 (continued)

Adolescent Age	1.01	0.658	0.96-1.07
Family	0.95	0.003	0.92-0.98
School	1.01	0.391	0.98-1.05
Community	1.01	0.766	0.93-1.11
Someplace else			
Male	1.01	0.934	0.85-1.19
Female	1.00		
African American	0.61	0.000	0.51-0.74
Asian American	1.03	0.868	0.74-1.43
Hispanic	0.97	0.798	0.74-1.26
White	1.00		
Did not graduate from HS	1.00		
HS graduate	1.09	0.439	0.88-1.35
Some post HS education	1.21	0.102	0.96-1.53
College Graduate	1.33	0.021	1.05-1.70
Post Graduate	1.11	0.529	0.81-1.52
Adolescent Age	1.22	0.000	1.17-1.28
Family	0.97	0.050	0.94-1.00
School	0.98	0.224	0.95-1.01
Community	1.02	0.537	0.95-1.10

Note: School is the comparison group

Socio-Demographic Variables

Males are significantly less likely to report fighting at home than females. Compared to White adolescents, Hispanic adolescents are significantly less likely to report fighting in the neighborhood or at home, while African American adolescents are significantly less likely to report fighting at home or "someplace else." An increase in adolescent age is associated with an increased likelihood of fighting "someplace else" compared to at school. The importance of the educational level of the parent(s) is inconsistent except for the at home category. Adolescents whose parent(s) have some post high school education are 1.7 times more likely to fight at home. The adjusted relative risk increases steadily as the education level of the parent(s) increases. Adolescents whose parent(s) have a post graduate education are 2.2 times more likely to report fighting at home.

Family, School, and Community Attachment

There is no consistent pattern in the measures of attachment. An increase in attachment to family is associated with decreased risk of fighting at home or in the neighborhood. The only other significant result is related to increases in attachment to community which is associated with an increased likelihood of fighting in the neighborhood compared to school.

DISCUSSION

The primary objective of this study was to investigate the context of adolescent fighting by taking a closer look at where and with whom physical fights are likely to occur. This study provides researchers and clinicians with a snapshot of persons with whom and in which settings middle and high school adolescents become involved in physical fights. Data from the National Longitudinal Study of Adolescent Health (NLSAH) provides a rich context in which to explore violent behaviors in early adolescence, as well as providing researchers the opportunity to further explore associations between context and numerous individual and family characteristics. Unlike numerous other studies of violence in adolescence, which often use convenience samples, the NLSAH is a nationally representative sample across a broad age range. The NLSAH data include 7th-12th graders, providing researchers with the opportunity to investigate the role of various protective and risk factors across the span of adolescence. The high prevalence of violence adds further support to the call for services and interventions which aim to reduce and prevent youth violence, particularly in early adolescence. Having a better understanding of the people involved and the setting is essential to preventing and reducing physical violence in the lives of adolescents.

As noted earlier, the research is modest in regards to the circumstances of the fights. However, the results are somewhat consistent with the limited literature. Using a nationally representative study of 9th-12th graders, Simon et al. (1999) found that adolescent fighting is most likely to occur at school. Malek et al. (1998a) found that among 7th graders in three dissimilar U.S. communities, fighting with a friend was not uncommon. While Richters and Martinez (1993) argue that the neighborhood is the second most common setting, the findings in the present study indicate that the neighborhood is not the second most common. However, Richters and Martinez used a sample of children living in a moderately violent inner-city community. Furthermore, they found that adolescents were more likely to fight with family members than a stranger; however, present findings show that this is true for females, but not for males. The data clearly indicate that a greater percentage of male adolescents fight with a total stranger than a family member.

With respect to race/ethnicity, Hispanic and African American adolescents were more likely to fight at school than White adolescents. One possible explanation is that minority students are more likely to feel uncomfortable and unsafe at school than White adolescents (Samaniego & Gonzales, 1999). African American adolescents are significantly less likely to engage in physical fights with their parents or family members, compared to White adolescents. This finding calls into question some of the popular notions about the role and nature of the African American family and is more in keeping with the literature regarding strong kinship ties in the African American extended family. Also, as noted in the literature and found in this study, the Asian American adolescents were overall the least likely group to get involved in a physical fight (Kosterman et al., 2001). At the same time, a higher percentage of Asian American adolescents were involved in fights with parents or family members than the other racial/ethnic groups.

Given this pattern of results, the temptation is to conclude that setting or person is a function of race/ethnicity. However, these results must be interpreted with caution since it is very unlikely that race/ethnicity, in and of itself, is a causal factor for where and with whom adolescents fight. Violence is not a uniquely racial problem (Fingerhut & Kleinman, 1990; Rosenberg, 1996). Previous studies suggest that youth violence could in large part be accounted for by economic and social factors associated with poverty and unemployment (Rosenberg, Carroll, & Powell, 1992; Runyan & Gerkin, 1989). There is a need to closely examine other correlates that have consistently emerged: individual, family, peer, school, and neighborhood/community. Understanding the role of race/ethnicity in youth violence is dependent on a clearer picture of these correlates and their relationship to the economic and social causes of violence.

The parent's level of education plays an interesting predictive role in adolescent fighting. As the parent's level of education increases, adolescents are more likely to fight with a parent or family member compared to a friend. This is clearly related to the parallel finding that as parental education increases, adolescents are more likely to fight at home than school. Conversely, adolescents are increasingly less likely to fight with a friend as their parent's level of education increases. One possible explanation, and one that deserves further study, is that as parent's level of education increases, the style of parenting moves from being more authoritarian to permissive. This may lead to increased conflicts between the parents or other family members (e.g., siblings).

Consistent with the literature, gender was a significant predictor. Males were more likely to be in a fight (Cotten et al., 1994; Everett & Price, 1995; Grunbaum et al., 2002; Malek et al., 1998a; Osgood et al., 1989) and more likely to fight with a stranger, while females were significantly more likely to fight at home with individuals with which they have a relationship, in this case, family members. Although the female juvenile arrest rate remains below that of males, girls are increasingly implicated for certain types of crimes (U.S. Department of Justice, 1998) and based on the results of this study, certain people and settings in deference to others.

As adolescents get older, they are less likely to fight at school and with a friend and more likely to fight someplace else and with a stranger. These findings appear consistent since adolescents are more likely to come into contact with a friend at school and a stranger at a place other than the adolescent's school, neighborhood, and home. This change may also be reflective of the evolving understanding of friendship and the reasons for fighting. As adolescents progress through middle school and into and through high school, the world accessible to them expands. They spend increasing amounts of time without adult supervision, the nature of friendship changes and the strength of their bonds increase. Adolescents may have an increasing repertoire of strategies, and the actions that at an early age lead to a physical fight may now be interpreted through a different set of life experiences. The changing context and available strategies need to be studied in more detail. However, it is interesting to note that many of the prevention/intervention strategies used on school campuses are based on providing adolescents with alternative strategies (Riner & Saywell, 2002). For example, the Peacemakers Program is a school-based intervention for students in grades four through eight (Shapiro, Burgoon, Welker, & Clough, 2002). In addition to the primary prevention component, which is delivered by teachers and to all students, there is a remedial component which is implemented by school psychologists and counselors to referred students. The primary prevention component consists of a curriculum in which values and attitudes about violence and psychosocial skills to avoid violence are discussed. The remedial component then works directly with students with aggressive tendencies.

Attachment is crucial in human development (Bowlby, 1958). Evidence accumulated across domains indicates that the family and school environments are important predictors of the presence, severity, and maintenance of youth violence, drug use, and conduct disorders (Andrews & Trawick-Smith, 1996; Block, Block, & Keys, 1988; Patterson, 1986). As commonly found throughout the literature, attachment to the family (Arbona et al., 1999; Samaniego & Gonzales, 1999), school (Somers & Gizzi, 2001), and community (Scheier, Miller, Ifill-Williams, & Botvin, 2001) all served as protective factors. In these analyses on a nationally representative sample of adolescents, attachment to family, school, and to a lesser extent community, also served as protective factors. One interpretation of these results is that when working with adolescents and families involved or at risk for involvement in violent behaviors, increases in attachment might potentially lead to a decreased level of physical fighting whether in the school, home or community. These results add to the understanding of the roles of risk and resiliency factors in adolescents' lives (Rutter, 1987; Werner, 1990). These results also point to the importance of attachment as one avenue to address the problems related to adolescent violence. As demonstrated in this study, the multiple contexts in which attachment can occur provide varied opportunities to develop prevention and support mechanisms for adolescents and families. The counter intuitive finding regarding the increased likelihood of fighting in the neighborhood with increased levels of attachment to the community deserves further investigation. This may be an artifact related to exposure and opportunity. The more comfortable adolescents feel in their neighborhood may relate to increased time spent there and the increased likelihood of fights occurring. Attachment to community may decrease fights occurring between community members, but may increase their sense of territoriality, making it more likely for them to fight with "outsiders." It appears that attachment to community does not necessarily impact the amount of fighting as does attachment to family and school.

LIMITATIONS

While this study advances knowledge about protective factors for adolescent violence, it has several limitations. Regardless of this nationally representative sample of early adolescents, care must be taken in interpreting the results of this study, because of the cross-sectional nature of the data. This study cannot claim to have identified causal links between the specific risk and resiliency factors and fighting. The usefulness of these findings depends on the validity of the self-reports of fighting by early adolescents. Previous research (Clark & Tifft, 1966; Hindelang, Hischi, & Weiss, 1981) and the use of computer-assisted self-interview techniques suggest that these self-reports are fairly reliable (Turner et al., 1998). One of the other prominent limitations is the absence of any information regarding why these adolescents are fighting, particularly in light of the finding which suggests context matters. Knowing why these adolescents are getting into physical altercations with friends and family might allow prevention and intervention programs to be designed more specifically for the contextual needs of adolescents.

IMPLICATIONS

There are no immediate solutions for the challenge posed by violence among youth, but there are steps that can be taken in the areas of research, practice and policy. Future research should focus on the mediating and moderating effects of gender, race, and family structure and their association to attachment and delinquency patterns of adolescents. Another important issue relates to the different developmental pathways along which males and females proceed. While it is clear that adolescent males engage in interpersonal violence at a higher rate than adolescent females, future studies need to closely examine the risks and protective factors for females as potentially separate and distinct from those of males and examine the interaction between the persons with whom they fight and the setting in which the fights occur.

Future interventions and policies need to focus on the multiple dimensions of youth violence, as well as give consideration to a multipronged approach in addressing the needs of youth. These efforts need to focus on preventing violence, protecting children and adolescents from violence, and promoting strengths in children and adolescents that do not currently exist (Bloom, 1996). Given the fundamental importance of attachment and the importance it had in this study as a protective factor, it seems that providing all children with the skills and opportunities necessary to form secure attachments with parents, families, and schools should be at the forefront of prevention efforts. These efforts should not just target at-risk adolescents, but rather, be provided to all children and strive to focus on the particular context (person and setting). Also, age should be considered a salient factor when interventions are designed specifically to enhance adolescent attachment to families, schools and communities. Interventions designed to undo the effects of deficits in backgrounds may not be successful or may backfire, particularly with older adolescents (McCord, 1996).

Interpersonal violence in adolescence can be prevented if the efforts of social service and health care providers are used in conjunction with schools, whose unique position to assist with this task should not be underestimated. These approaches need to be comprehensive and interdisciplinary in order to address needs across systems in which the youth is experiencing difficulty (e.g., family, school, and neighborhood/community). It is also important to maintain individualized treatments to address the specific strengths and needs of each adolescent and family.

BIBLIOGRAPHY

Andrews, L., & Trawick-Smith, J. (1996). An ecological model for early childhood. In T. P. Gullotta (Ed.), *Preventing Violence in America* (Vol. 4, pp. 233-262). Thousans Oaks: Sage Publications.

Arbona, C., Jackson, R. H., McCoy, A., & Blakely, C. (1999). Ethnic identity as a predictor of attitudes of adolescents toward fighting. *Journal of Early Adolescence, 19*(3), 323-340.

Block, J., Block, J., & Keys, S. (1988). Longitudinal foretelling drug usage in adolescence: Early childhood personality and environmental precursors. *Child Development, 59*, 336-355.

Bloom, M. (1996). Primary prevention and resilience: Changing paradigms and changing lives. In T. P. Gullotta (Ed.), *Preventing Violence in America* (Vol. 4, pp. 87-114). Thousand Oaks: Sage Publishing.

Bowlby, J. (1958). The nature of the child's tie to his mother. *International Journal of Psychoanalysis, 39*, 350-373.

Bracher, M. (2000). Adolescent violence and identity vulnerability. *Journal for the Psychoanalysis of Culture and Society, 5*(2), 189-211.

Bronfenbrenner, U. (1979). *The ecology of human development: Experiments by nature and design*. Cambridge, MA: Harvard University Press.

Bronfenbrenner, U. (1986). Ecology of the family as a context for human development. *Developmental Psychology, 22*, 723-742.

Cicchetti, D., & Lynch, M. (1993). Toward an ecological/transactional model of community violence and child maltreatment: Consequences for children's development. *Psychiatry: Interpersonal & Biological Processes, 56*(1), 96-118.

Clark, J. P., & Tifft, L. L. (1966). Polygraph and interview validation of self-reported deviant behavior. *American Sociological Review, 31*, 516-523.

Cotten, N. U., Resnick, J., Browne, D. C., Martin, S. L., McCarraher, D. R., & Woods, J. (1994). Aggression and fighting behavior among African-American adolescents: Individual and family factors. *American Journal of Public Health, 84*(4), 618-622.

Durant, R. H., Getts, A. G., Cadenhead, C., & Woods, E. R. (1995). The association between weapon carrying and the use of violence among adolescents living in and around public housing. *Journal of Adolescent Health, 17*(6), 376-380.

Everett, S. A., & Price, J. H. (1995). Students' perceptions of violence in the public schools: The Met Life survey. *Journal of Adolescent Health, 17*(6), 345-352.

Feshbach, N. D., & Feshbach, S. (1998). Aggression in the schools: Toward reducing ethnic conflict and enhancing ethnic understanding. In P. K. Trickett & C. J. Schellenbach (Eds.), *Violence against children in the family and the community* (pp. 269-286). Washington, D.C.: American Psychological Association.

Fingerhut, L. A., & Kleinman, J. C. (1990). International and interstate comparisons of homicide among young males. *Journal of American Medical Association, 236*, 3292-3295.

Fox, J. A. (1996). *Trends in juvenile violence: A report to the United States Attorney General on current and future rates of juvenile offending*. Washington, DC: Bureau of Justice Statistics, United States Department of Justice.

Grunbaum, J. A., Kann, L., Kinchen, S. A., Williams, B., Ross, J. G., Lowry, R., & Kolbe, L. (2002). Youth risk behavior surveillance: United States, 2001. *Surveillance Summaries, 51*(SS04), 1-64.

Hindelang, M. J., Hischi, T., & Weiss, J. G. (1981). *Measuring delinquency*. Beverly Hills, CA: Sage Publications.

Horton, A. (2001). The prevention of school violence: New evidence to consider. *Journal of Human Behavior in the Social Environment, 4*(1), 49-59.

Hyman, I. A., & Snook, P. A. (1999). *Dangerous schools: What we can do about the physical and emotional abuse of our children*. San Francisco: Jossey-Bass.

Kingery, P. M., Coggeshall, M. B., & Alford, A. A. (1998). Violence at school: Recent evidence from four national surveys. *Psychology in Schools, 35*(3), 247-258.

Kosterman, R., Graham, J. W., Hawkins, J. D., Catalano, R. F., & Herrenkohl, T. I. (2001). Childhood risk factors for persistence of violence in the transition to adulthood: A social development perspective. *Violence & Victims, 16*(4), 355-369.

Larson, J. (1998). Managing student aggression in high schools: Implications for practice. *Psychology in the Schools, 35*(3), 283-295.

Likert, R. A. (1932). A technique for the measurement of attitudes. *Archives of Psychology, 140.*

Loeber, R., & Dishion, T. J. (1984). Boys who fight at home and school: Family conditions influencing cross-setting consistency. *Journal of Consulting and Clinical Psychology, 52*(5), 759-768.

Lowry, R., Cohen, L. R., Modzeleski, W., Kann, L., Collins, J. L., & Kolbe, L. J. (1999). School violence, substance use, and availability of illegal drugs on school property among US high school students. *Journal of School Health, 69*(9), 347-355.

Lowry, R., Powell, K. E., Kann, L., Collins, J. L., & Kolbe, L. J. (1998). Weapon-carrying, physical fighting, and fighting related injury among U.S. adolescents. *American Journal of Preventive Medicine, 14*(2), 122-129.

Malek, M. K., Chang, B., & Davis, T. (1998a). Fighting and weapon-carrying among seventh-grade students in Massachusetts and Louisiana. *Journal of Adolescent Health, 23*(2), 94-102.

Malek, M. K., Chang, B., & Davis, T. (1998b). Self-reported characterization of seventh-grade students' fights. *Journal of Adolescent Health, 23*(2), 103-109.

McCord, J. (1996). Family as crucible for violence: Comment on Gorman-Smith et al. (1996). *Journal of Family Psychology, 10*(2), 147-152.

Moeller, T. G. (2001). *Youth aggression and violence: A psychological approach.* Mahwah, NJ: Lawrence Erlbaum Associates.

National Health Statistics Report. (48(11))(2000). Washington, DC: National Center for Health Statistics, HHS.

Oetting, E., Donnermeyer, J., & Deffenbacher, J. (1998). Primary socialization theory. The influence of the community on drug use and deviance. III. *Substance use and misuse, 33*(8), 1629-1665.

O'Keefe, M. (1997). Adolescents' exposure to community and school violence: Prevalence and behavioral correlates. *Journal of Adolescent Health, 20*(5), 368-376.

Osgood, D. W., O'Malley, P. M., Bachman, J. G., & Johnston, L. D. (1989). Time trends and age trends in arrests and self-reported illegal behaviors. *Criminology, 27,* 389-417.

Pallone, N. J., & Hennessy, J. J. (2000). Blacks and Whites as victims and offenders in aggressive crime in the U.S.: Myths and realities. In N. J. Pallone (Ed.), *Race, ethnicity, sexual orientation, violent crime: The realities and the myths* (pp. 1-33). Binghamton, NY: The Haworth Press, Inc.

Paschall, M. J., Ennett, S. T., & Flewelling, R. L. (1996). Relationships among family characteristics and violent behavior by black and white male adolescents. *Journal of Youth & Adolescence, 25*(2), 177-197.

Patterson, G. R. (1986). Performance models for antisocial boys. *American Psychologist, 41*, 432-444.

Prothrow-Stith, D., & Weissman, M. (1991). *Deadly consequences.* New York: Harper-Collins.

Richters, J. E., & Martinez, P. (1993). The NIMH Community Violence Project: I. Children as victims of and witnesses to violence. *Psychiatry: Interpersonal & Biological Processes, 56*(1), 7-21.

Riner, M., & Saywell, R. M. (2002). Development of the social ecology model of adolescent interpersonal violence prevention (SEMAIVP). *Journal of School Heath, 72*(2), 65-70.

Rosenberg, M. L. (1996). Violence in America: An integrated approach to understanding and prevention. *Journal of Health Care for the Poor and Underserved, 6*(2), 102-112.

Rosenberg, M. L., Carroll, P. W., & Powell, K. E. (1992). Let's be clear: Violence in America is a public health problem. *Journal of the American Medical Association, 267*, 3076-3077.

Runyan, C. W., & Gerkin, E. A. (1989). Epidemiology and prevention of adolescent injury, a review and research agenda. *Journal of the American Medical Association, 262*, 2273-2279.

Rutter, M. (1987). Psychological resilience and protective mechanisms. *American Journal of Orthopsychiatry, 57*, 316-331.

Samaniego, R. Y., & Gonzales, N. A. (1999). Multiple mediators of the effects of acculturation status on delinquency for Mexican American adolescents (Special Issues: Adolescent Risk Behavior). *American Journal of Community Psychology, 27*(2), 189-194.

Sameroff, A. J. (1983). Developmental systems: Contexts and evolution. In W. Kessen (Ed.), *Handbook of child psychology: Vol. 1 History, theories, and methods* (pp. 238-294). New York: Wiley.

Sameroff, A. J. (1987). The social context of development. In N. Eisenberg (Ed.), *Contemporary topics in developmental psychology* (pp. 273-291). New York: Wiley.

Scheier, L. M., Miller, N. L., Ifill-Williams, M., & Botvin, G. J. (2001). Perceived neighborhood risk as a predictor of drug use among urban ethnic minority adolescents: Moderating influences of psychosocial functioning. *Journal of Child and Adolescent Substance Abuse, 11*(2), 67-106.

Services, U. S. D. o. H. a. H. *Healthy People 2010. 2nd ed. With Understanding and Improving Health and Objectives for Improving Health. 2 vols.* Washington, DC: U.S. Government Printing Office.

Shapiro, J. P., Burgoon, J. D., Welker, C. J., & Clough, J. B. (2002). Evaluation of The Peacemakers Program: School-based violence prevention for students in grades four through eight. *Psychology in the Schools, 39*(1), 87-100.

Simon, T. R., Crosby, A. E., & Dahlberg, L. L. (1999). Students who carry weapons to high school. *Journal of Adolescent Health, 24*(5), 340-348.

Somers, C. L., & Gizzi, T. J. (2001). Predicting adolescents' risky behaviors: The influence of future orientation, school involvement, and school attachment. *Adolescent & Family Health, 2*(1), 3-11.

StataCorp. (2002). Stata Statistical Software (Version Release 6.0). College Station, TX: Stat Corporation.

Synder, H. N., & Sickmund, J. (1995). *Juvenile offenders and victims: A national report.* Washington, D.C.: U.S. Department of Justice, Office of Justice Programs, Office of Juvenile Justice and Delinquency Prevention.

Turner, C. F., Ku, L., Rogers, S. M., Lindberg, L. D., Pleck, J. H., & Sonenstein, F. L. (1998). Technology, experimentation, and the quality of survey data. *Science, 280*, 847.

U.S. Department of Justice. (1998). *OJJDP Fact Sheet: What about girls?* (84). Washington, DC: U.S. Department of Justice.

Vega, W. A., Gil, A. G., Warheit, G. J., Zimmerman, R. S., et al. (1993). Acculturation and delinquent behavior among Cuban American adolescents: Toward an empirical model. *American Journal of Community Psychology, 21*, 113-125.

Werner, E. E. (1990). Protective factors and individual resilience. In J. P. Shonkoff (Ed.), *Handbook of early childhood intervention* (pp. 97-116). Cambridge, MA: Cambridge University Press.

Perception of Substance Use Problems in Asian American Communities by Chinese, Indian, and Vietnamese American Youth

Mo Yee Lee
Fang Mei Law
Eunjoo Eo
Elizabeth Oliver

SUMMARY. The study was a cross-sectional survey using a convenience sample of 87 Asian American youth respondents to examine their perceptions of substance use problems in the Asian American community. The authors examined respondents' perceptions of the severity of substance use problems in the Asian American community, perceived

---

Mo Yee Lee, PhD, is Associate Professor, College of Social Work, The Ohio State University, 1947 College Road, Columbus, OH 43210 (E-mail: lee.355@osu.edu). Fang Mei Law, PhD, is Executive Director of Asian American Community Services, Room 301, 4100 North High Street, Columbus, OH 43214. She is a faculty member at the College of Education, University of Dayton. Eunjoo Eo, PhD, is Director of Family Department, Asian American Community Services. Elizabeth Oliver, MSW, is Administration Specialist, Asian American Community Services.

The study was conducted as part of the "Asian Drug Free Initiatives," a community-based project operated by Asian American Community Services, Columbus, Ohio. The project was funded by The Ohio Commission of Minority Health.

[Haworth co-indexing entry note]: "Perception of Substance Use Problems in Asian American Communities by Chinese, Indian, and Vietnamese American Youth." Lee et al. Co-published simultaneously in *Journal of Ethnic & Cultural Diversity in Social Work* (The Haworth Social Work Practice Press, an imprint of The Haworth Press, Inc.) Vol. 11, No. 3/4, 2002, pp. 159-189; and: *Social Work with Multicultural Youth* (ed: Diane de Anda) The Haworth Social Work Practice Press, an imprint of The Haworth Press, Inc., 2002, pp. 159-189. Single or multiple copies of this article are available for a fee from The Haworth Document Delivery Service [1-800-HAWORTH, 9:00 a.m. - 5:00 p.m. (EST). E-mail address: docdelivery@haworthpress.com].

http://www.haworthpress.com/store/product.asp?sku=J051

10.1300/J051v11n03_02

characteristics of persons with problems of substance use, perceived etiology of substance use problems, beliefs about treatment, perceived help-seeking preferences and helpful services. The youth demonstrated an increased awareness of the severity of substance use problems in the community, although such awareness was more prominent for drinking problems than drug use problems. Respondents showed a positive attitude toward treatment, although such an attitudinal change was not yet accompanied by a change in their behavioral preferences. Findings suggested a tendency for Asian American youth respondents to utilize personal resources rather than professional help or formal treatment programs in response to substance use problems. In addition, respondents shared similar "myths" of Asian problem drinkers and drug users. Implications for developing culturally relevant interventions for prevention and treatment as well as future research are discussed.

KEYWORDS. Alcohol use, drug use, Asian American youth populations, help-seeking

INTRODUCTION

Despite the proliferation of collective knowledge and understanding of substance abuse and its treatment, the experience of Asian American youth populations has been understudied. Helping professionals addressing substance use problems of Asian American youth populations encounter numerous challenges that are usually associated with the "hidden quality" of such problems. The existence of substance abuse problems has largely been minimized or denied by the community and the government because of the stereotype of Asian American populations as a "model minority" (Ja, 1991). Underutilization of substance abuse treatment facilities has been used as an indicator of a lack of problem in the Asian American community (Ja, 1991). Cultural stigma around substance use problems only serves to further encapsulate the problem within the Asian American community (Ja & Aoki, 1998). In addition, understanding of the prevalence, pattern, and perceptions of substance use among Asian American youth populations is extremely limited as Asian/Pacific Islander (AAPI) populations are either being omitted or lumped into an "other" category in major national studies (Dawson, 1998; Harachi, Catalano, Kim, & Choi, 2001).

According to the 2000 U.S. census, Asian Americans make up 4.3% of the total U.S. population. This number represents an increase of 63% from the 1990 census, making Asian Americans the fastest growing of all the major racial/ethnic groups in the U.S. in terms of percentage growth (U.S. Census Bureau, 2000). It is being projected that by the year 2050, Asian/Pacific Islanders will comprise 8.2% of total population (US Department of Commerce, 1998). Knowledge regarding how Asian American youth populations perceive the phenomenon of and respond to substance use problems will have significant implications for providing preventive education and developing culturally competent interventions for them. The earlier the substance use begins, the more likely it is to progress to abuse or dependence (Gerstein & Harwood, 1990). Preventive community intervention targeted at the youth population is imperative to successfully combat substance use problems within the Asian American community.

PURPOSE

The purpose of the present study was to examine the perception of substance use problems and help-seeking responses among three Asian American youth groups: Chinese, Indian, and Vietnamese. These three groups represented youth populations from East Asia, South Asia and Southeast Asia. Substance use was defined as the consumption of alcohol and/or illicit drugs; the latter includes the use of marijuana, ecstasy, LSD, hallucinogens, cocaine, crack, heroin, and other opiates. The definition of drug use was based on criteria developed by the National Technical Center for Substance Abuse Needs Assessment for statewide needs assessment administered under the Center for Substance Abuse Treatment (McAuliffe et al., 1994). Specifically, the authors examined respondents' perceptions of the severity of substance use problems in the Asian American community, perceived characteristics of persons with problems of substance use, perceived etiology of substance use problems, beliefs about treatment, perceived help-seeking preferences and helpful services.

LITERATURE REVIEW

Prevalence of Substance Use Among Asian American Youth Populations

Knowledge regarding substance use among Asian American youth populations is rather limited. For a long time, the focus of most national studies on substance use has been on African American, Hispanic, and White populations. AAPI populations are not currently included in the most extensive surveys of adolescent substance use, such as the National Household Survey on Drug Abuse (NHSDA) sponsored by the Substance Abuse and Mental Health Services Administration and the Monitoring the Future Study (MTF) sponsored by the National Institute on Drug Abuse. In addition, many studies ignore heterogeneity within the AAPI populations (Dawson, 1998) although AAPI populations encompass over 60 separate racial/ethnic groups and subgroups (Sue, 1987).

There are, however, several state and local epidemiological surveys that include Asian American youth populations and provide valuable information about their drug and alcohol use. Examples of these studies are: California Student Substance Use Survey (CSS) that provides data on 586 Asian American 9th and 11th graders (Skager & Austin, 1993; Austin, 1999); 1983 and 1990 New York State surveys of secondary students (Barnes & Welte, 1986; Barnes, Welte, & Dintcheff, 1993); Minority Youth Health Project in Seattle that includes 551 Asian Americans 6th to 8th graders (Harachi et al., 2001); Sasao's study that includes a sample of 953 high school Vietnamese and Chinese students (1994, 1999); Seattle Social Development Project (Gillmore, Catalano, Morrison, Wells, Iritani, & Hawkins, 1990) that examined predictors of substance use initiation among 919 urban 5th graders comparing Asian, European, and African American youth. The focus of these studies was primarily on the prevalence of substance use among adolescents as well as risk and protective factors with regard to their substance use initiation.

The epidemiological data in general suggested that AAPIs are at a relatively lower risk for drug and alcohol use than youth from most other ethnic groups (Skager & Austin, 1993; Bachman, Wallace, O'Malley, Johnston, Kurth, & Neighbors, 1991; Barnes & Welte, 1986; Barnes et al., 1993; Harachi et al., 2001). For instance, based on data from the Minority Youth Health Project, 37.62% of Asian students answered "yes" to the question "Have you ever drunk alcohol?" as compared to 43.78 White students and 49.54 African American students (Harachi et al., 2001). Similarly, 58.6% and 17.4%of non-Asian ninth and eleventh graders reported using alcohol and illicit drugs in the past six months while only 20.7% and 3.9% of Chinese American students reported so (Skager & Austin, 1993).

On the other hand, data also indicated that substance use by AAPI youths may not be as low as generally assumed and that there were variations among different Asian ethnic groups. Data from the California Student Substance Use Survey indicated that Asians equaled or exceeded rates reported by African Americans in the categories of "weekly drinking of any alcohol (11%)," "heavy drinking in last two weeks (14%)," "cocaine (4%)," "LSD (3%)," "amphetamine (4%)," and "inhalant (8%)" use in the past 6 months (Austin, 1999). Data from the Minority Youth Health Project also indicated that Asian middle school students (1.9%) reported a higher rate of using crack or cocaine as compared to White (1.3%) or African American students (.9%). Based on the limited information, Asian American youth may have a lower rate of alcohol use although they may be relatively heavy drinkers if they do drink (Austin, 1999; Chi, Lubben, & Kitano, 1988). Also, there is limited empirical evidence showing that Asian American youth may have a higher rate of using cocaine and crack than the comparison group despite an overall lower rate of drug use (Harachi et al., 2001).

Variations among diverse Asian groups are evident based on data of several studies. Data from the California Student Substance Use Survey indicate a higher prevalence of substance use among Pacific Islander students than most other Asian groups. In general Chinese and Southeast Asian show lower rates of alcohol use (20.7% and 16.8% in the past six months) while Japanese, Korean, Pacific Islander, and Filipino show higher rates of alcohol use (33.9%, 42.2%, 50%, and 42.6% respectively) (Skager & Austin, 1993). Chi and her associates (Chi, Lubben, & Kitano, 1989) also found a higher rate of heavy drinking among those of Japanese descent than among those of Chinese, Filipino or Korean descent. Despite lower rates of alcohol use, Southeast Asian students had higher rates of using cocaine than other Asian groups (Bachman et al., 1991; Harachi et al., 2001; Sasao, 1999; Skager & Austin, 1993). Few studies examined differential substance use between genders. Data from 1983 and 1990 New York State surveys of secondary students suggest that Asian American females generally have among the lowest drug prevalence rates although rates for illicit drug use were similar to those of Asian American males (20% and 20%) (Barnes & Welte, 1986; Barnes et al., 1993).

Risk and Protective Factors of Substance Use Among Asian American Youth Populations

Several studies included AAPI youth populations to examine risk and protective factors for initiation of substance use (Gilmore et al., 1990; Sasao, 1994, 1999; Harachi et al., 2001). The identified factors include factors in the individual and peer domains as well as those in the family domain. Based on data of 919 urban 5th graders, Gilmore and his associates found that availability of and peer use of drug and alcohol were significantly related to substance use (Gilmore et al., 1990). Other identified risk factors in the individual and peer domains are intention to use drugs as adults (Gilmore et al., 1990), being male, lack of subjective well-being, perceived interethnic tensions among ethnic groups at schools (Sasao, 1994, 1999), psychological maladjustment, greater acculturation (Zane, Park, & Aoki, 1999), and perception of peers' antisocial beliefs (Harachi et al., 2001). Family conflict or discord is a commonly cited risk factor in the family domain that is positively associated with substance use (Harachi et al., 2001; Zane et al., 1999). Data from The Minority Youth Health Project in Seattle that included 551 Asian American 6th to 8th graders identified parents' disapproval of substance use, family management, parent-child attachment, parent-child involvement in prosocial activities, and household rules as protective family factors against substance use in adolescents (Harachi et al., 2001). Other identified protective factors included absence of a deviant sibling, and living with both parents (Gilmore et al., 1990). Gender, SES as measured by free lunch eligibility (Gilmore et al., 1990), ethnic identification, self-esteem, sense of not fitting in, and English as a second language status (Sasao, 1994, 1999) are not related to initiation of substance use among Asian American youth populations.

Cultural Influences and Help-Seeking Responses to Substance Use

There is a paucity of empirical information on help-seeking responses to substance use by Asian American youth, although there are a few studies focusing on Asian American populations as a group. The interest in understanding help-seeking responses of Asian American populations is partly related to the well-documented underutilization of treatment services by these groups (Ja & Aoki, 1998). The help-seeking responses of Asian American populations to problems of substance use are likely to be culturally embedded and influenced by their worldviews, socio-historical background, acculturation, and institutional factors (Lee, 2000; Yamashiro & Matsuoka, 1997).

Ja (1991) suggested that the topic of substance abuse brings forth a similar cultural perspective as that of mental illness. Traditional Asian values emphasize the importance of collective existence and family lineage (Chan & Leong, 1994). Consequently, cultural responses to substance abuse are heavily influenced by the emotion of shame and the fear of losing face and shaming family (Ja & Aoki, 1993). Substance users may avoid seeking external professional help for fear of shaming the family or hide their substance use from family and friends. Nemoto, Aoki, Huang, Morris, Nguyen, and Wong (1999) interviewed 92 Asian drug users in San Francisco who were not enrolled in any drug treatment program. Among the respondents, 78% reported that they had good relationships with their family members, but about 50% of them had also hidden their drug use from their family. A quote by a 27-year-old Vietnamese male vividly described his values regarding family and his fear of shaming the family.

> *My parents moved to New York with my older brother and sister. They love me, and they know I am using drugs. I will only move back when I'm off drugs. I don't want to shame my family. I don't want my parents' friends to know that they have a drug user son because it would shame my family.* (Nemoto et al., 1999, p. 833)

For family members, the negative emotion of shame usually leads to cultural responses that aim at reducing the potential loss of face. The family may engage in act of shaming, castigating, and scolding the abusers to resolve the issue (Ja, 1991). On the other hand, because of the central importance of harmonious family relationships, the family may also deny the problem and avoid dealing with the issues. A quote from a Filipino immigrant vividly described the use of denial by his family as a way to address the problem:

> *. . . We have a pretty close family. They probably know my drug use, but don't say anything. When I was younger, they asked me if I was using. I got angry and denied it, they haven't asked since.* (Nemoto et al., p. 833)

The denial of substance use often promotes codependency on drug abuse. Substance users may take advantage of the values of interdependence within the family and keep their substance dependence, which is financially supported by their family members as they still live in the home and receive money from parents (Ja & Aoki, 1993).

Because of a fear of losing face, substance users and/or their families usually attempt to resolve the problem on their own. Seeking outside professional help is commonly considered as a last resort. The fear of losing face and/or the denial of the problem, oftentimes, leads to delayed help-seeking efforts (Ja & Aoki, 1993). When they finally exhausted all their internal resources, they may seek professional help, although at that point the family usually has high expectations, little patience, and the substance user is resistant and in denial (Ja, 1991).

Besides cultural influence, the help-seeking responses of Asian American are likely to be influenced by institutional and contextual factors. Currently, the availability of a culturally appropriate and sensitive continuum of care for substance abuse treatment of Asian American populations is simply lacking, perhaps with the exception of a few major metropolitan cities such as Los Angeles, New York, or San Francisco (Asian American Recovery Services, 1996). The attempts of Asian American populations to utilize professional services are usually thwarted by cultural and/or language barriers (Ja, 1991). Asian American populations may lack knowledge of and information about appropriate helping sources. Others may face language barriers in seeking professional help (Ja & Aoki, 1993). Oftentimes, ethnic-based community and/or social services organizations are left with the nearly impossible tasks of providing services and treatment to those in need with inadequate social, financial, and professional resources.

At the cultural level, the assumptions regarding effective help may differ between the East and the West. For instance, while many therapeutic models in the West emphasize self-expression through language in the treatment process, Asian clients may simply not be socialized to use language as primary means for expressing feelings (Reynolds, 1989). The effectiveness of conventional treatment such as the Twelve Steps Program will need to be examined for its utility with the Asian American populations.

Existing knowledge regarding prevalence and pattern of substance use among Asian American youth populations is limited although it significantly informs helping professionals who are addressing substance use issues in the Asian American community. On the other hand, to effectively develop culturally appropriate and sensitive educational and intervention programs, it is imperative to examine the way Asian American youth understand and perceive substance abuse issues in the community as well as their help-seeking preferences as influenced by cultural and contextual factors.

METHODS

Sample

The study was a cross-sectional survey using a convenience sample of 87 Asian American youth respondents between age 15 and 25 with a mean age of 20.1 (S.D. 3.1). Trained bilingual interviewers visited places at which Asian American youth populations usually congregated, such as: ethnic grocery stores, ethnic churches, ESL (English as Secondary Language) classes, schools, and colleges. The interviewers conducted the survey upon consent of respondents. Ninety-six Asian American youths were approached and nine persons declined to participant in the study. The response rate was 90.6%. Participants were offered a five-dollar gift certificate as a compensation for their time. Among the 87 respondents, 31.1% self-identified ethnically as Chinese (27), 21.8% Indian (19), and 47.1% Vietnamese (43). There were slightly more male respondents than female respondents in the sample (52.9% and 47.1% respectively) (see Table 1). Among the respondents, 77% were students: 43% were in the middle/high school group (7% attending middle schools, 36% attending or had completed high school), and 57% were in the college/postgraduate group (48.8% attending or had completed college, 8.1% in postgraduate programs). Regarding their employment status, 17.2% were in full-time employment and 32.2% in part-time employment.

Significant differences were found for demographic variables of age and education across the three ethnic groups. ANOVA analyses indicated significant differences across the three ethnic groups regarding their age [$F(2,84) = 17.3$ $p < .001$]. Findings of Games-Howell tests showed that the difference was between Indian respondents and Chinese/Vietnamese respondents with respondents of Indian descent (mean: 22.9; S.D. 1.5) being older than Chinese (mean: 20.4; S.D. 3.2) and Vietnamese respondents (mean: 18.6; S.D. 2.7). In addition, findings of chi-square analyses showed that significantly more Indian respondents were in college and postgraduate programs than Chinese or Vietnamese respondents ($\chi^2 = 11.1$ $df = 2, p < .01$) (see Table 1). No significant differences were found for demographic variables of gender and employment status across the three ethnic groups.

TABLE 1. Demographic Information of the Sample (N = 87)

	%	Chinese (%)	Indian (%)	Vietnamese (%)
Gender				
Male	52.9	40.7	68.4	53.7
Female	47.1	59.3	31.6	46.3
Ethnicity		31.1	21.8	47.1
Age***				
15-18	36.8	33.3	0.0	56.1
19-21	25.3	25.9	15.88	29.3
22-25	37.9	40.7	84.2	14.6
Mean (S.D.)	20.1 (S.D. 3.1)	20.4 (S.D. 3.2)	2.9 (S.D. 1.5)	18.6 (S.D. 2.7)
$F(2,84) = 17.3$, $p < .001$				
Education**				
Middle/High school	43.0	46.2	10.5	56.1
College/Postgraduate	57.0	53.8	89.5	43.9
$\chi^2 = 11.1$ $df = 2$, $p < .01$				
Status as Student				
Full-time	73.6	70.4	52.6	85.4
Part-time	3.4	0.0	10.5	2.4
Not a student	23.0	29.6	36.8	12.2
Employment Status				
Full-time	17.2	26.9	10.5	15.0
Part-time	32.2	30.8	31.6	35.0
Not applicable	49.4	42.3	57.9	50.0

**$p < .01$ ***$p < .001$

Procedures

A 16-question survey was developed to examine perceptions of substance use problems by Asian American youth respondents. Experienced professionals working with Asian American populations and professionals who had expertise in the area of substance abuse developed the questionnaire. In addition, item construction was informed by existing literature on needs assessment of Asian populations (Lee & Law, in press; Sasao, 1991), and the survey "Assessment of Substance Dependence Treatment Needs" that was developed by the National Technical Center for Substance Abuse Needs Assessment for the purpose of conducting statewide needs assessment administered under the Center for Substance Abuse Treatment (McAuliffe et al., 1994).

Respondents were asked to rate the severity of the problem of drinking and drug use in the Asian American community. In addition, respondents' perceptions of the characteristics of Asian problem drinkers and drug users were also examined. To understand respondents' beliefs about etiology of substance abuse, the following two questions were asked: "Suppose I told you a friend of mine has a problem with drinking, what may be some possible reasons?" "Suppose I told you a friend of mine has a problem with drugs, what may be some possible reasons?" In addition, the authors were interested in examining respondents' perceptions related to substance dependency treatment as the findings will provide valuable information pertaining to the development of culturally appropriate services. Questions were asked regarding respondents' beliefs about treatment, perceived help-seeking preferences and helpful services. Respondents were asked to rate their opinions of five statements regarding beliefs about treatment along a four-point Likert-type scale from "strongly agree" to "strongly disagree." Examples of the statements are: "You really can't help people with a drug or alcohol problem until they ask for help," "Family members need and can be helped even if the addict does not want help." To understand respondents' help-seeking preferences, the following questions were asked: "If you have problems with drinking or using drugs, what would you do?" "If you have problems with drinking or using drugs, what services would be helpful?" The last four questions focused on the prevalence of substance use among respondents. In addition, demographic data regarding gender, age, ethnicity, education, and employment status were collected.

In order to outreach to non-English speaking Asian groups, the questionnaire was translated into the Asian languages of Chinese, Indian, and Vietnamese using a back translation method. In addition, the authors piloted and modified the translated version before using the questionnaire in the study.

Data Analyses

Statistical Package for Social Sciences, version 10.0.07 was used to conduct the statistical analyses. Because all items were closed-ended questions, no coding of content was required. Descriptive analyses were performed to understand the profile of the respondents and their answers to each question. Chi-square analyses and analyses of variance were used to examine the relationships among studied variables and respondents' demographic variables including ethnicity, gender, age, and education.

FINDINGS

Prevalence of Drinking and Drug Use

To examine prevalence of drinking and drug use among respondents, the interviewers asked two questions about the respondents' personal drinking and drug use pattern ("In the last 18 months, how often have you consumed alcohol?" "Have you ever used drugs for non-medical reasons?"), and two questions about substance use in their social network ("Do you personally know any Asian in the US who has a problem with drinking?" "Do you personally know any Asian in the US who has a problem with drug use?"). Respondents were in general light to moderate drinkers. Only 36% of the respondents had consumed alcohol in the past 18 months. Sixty-four percent did not consume alcohol in the past 18 months, 24.4% drank less than once a month, and 9.3% drank 1-3 days a month. Only 2.4% of respondents drank several times a week (see Table 2). Regarding their social network, 36% of the respondents personally knew Asians who had a problem with drinking (see Table 2). For those who associated with problems drinkers, they knew an average of 9.3 persons who had a problem with drinking (S.D. 4.4; range: 1-15).

No significant differences were found between respondents' prevalence of drinking and their demographic characteristics of gender and ethnicity. On the other hand, ethnicity was found to be associated with social network of drinking. Fifty percent of Vietnamese respondents reported knowing Asians who had a drinking problem, while only 22.2% of Chinese respondents and 26.3% of Indian respondents reported so ($\chi^2 = 6.4$, $df = 2$ $p < .05$). ANOVA analyses also indicated significant differences across the three ethnic groups regarding the mean size of social network [$F(2,83) = 3.2$ $p < .05$] (see Table 2). Findings of Games-Howell (GH) tests showed that the difference was between Vietnamese respondents and Chinese and Indian respondents with respondents of Chinese and Indian descent associated with more Asian problem drinkers than Vietnamese respondents.

Not surprisingly, education and age were found to be associated with prevalence of drinking. Only 13.9% of middle/high school group reported consuming alcohol in the past 18 months while 51% of the college/postgraduate group had consumed alcohol during the same time

TABLE 2. Prevalence and Social Network of Drinking and Drug Use by Ethnicity (N = 86)

	Overall (%) (n = 86)	Chinese (%) (n = 27)	Indian (%) (n = 19)	Vietnamese (%) (n = 40)
Prevalence of Drinking				
Several days a week	2.4	0.0	5.3	2.5
1-3 days a month	9.3	14.8	15.8	2.5
Less than once a month	24.4	25.9	21.1	25.0
Not at all	64.0	59.3	57.9	70.0
$\chi^2 = 5.6$ $df = 6$ $p = .47$				
Social Network of drinking*				
Yes	36.0	22.2	26.3	50.0
No	64.0	77.8	73.7	50.0
$\chi^2 = 6.4$ $df = 2$ $p < .05$				
Mean Size of Social Network*	9.3 (SD = 4.4)	10.4 (SD = 3.8)	10.5 (SD = 3.6)	8.0 (SD = 4.8)
$F(2,83) = 3.2$ $p < .05$				
Prevalence of drug use*				
Yes	2.3	0.0	10.5	0.0
No	97.7	100.0	89.5	100.0
$\chi^2 = 7.2$ $df = 2$ $p < .05$				
Social Network of drug use				
Yes	18.6	22.2	10.5	20.0
No	81.4	77.8	89.5	80.0
$\chi^2 = 1.1$ $df = 2$ $p = .58$				
Mean Size of Social Network	10.5 (SD = 3.6)	10.7 (SD = 3.6)	11.1 (S.D. = 2.9)	10.1 (SD = 3.9)
$F(2,80) = .52$ $p = .60$				

*$p < .05$

period ($\chi^2 = 12.5$, $df = 1$, $p < .001$). For those respondents age 15 to 18, only 15.6% reported consuming alcohol in the past 18 months. On the other hand, 45.5% of those respondents between age 19 to 22 and 50% age 22-25 had consumed alcohol during the same time period ($\chi^2 = 9.3$, $df = 2$, $p < .01$).

There was a relatively low prevalence of drug use among the respondents. Only 2.3% had used drugs for non-medical reasons (see Table 2). However, 18.6% of the respondents personally knew Asians who had a problem with drug use (see Table 2). Among this group, they knew an average of 10.5 persons who had a problem with drug use (S.D. 3.6; range: 1-12). No significant differences were found in respondents' prevalence and social network of drug use based on their demographic characteristics of gender, age, and education. However, ethnicity was found to be associated with prevalence of drug use. No Chinese or Vietnamese respondents reported using drug while 10.5% of Indian respondents reported using drugs for non-medical reasons (($\chi^2 = 7.2$, $df = 2$, $p < .05$).

Perceived Severity of the Problem

In order to understand respondents' perceptions of the severity of substance use problems in Asian American community, they were asked to rate the statements "Drinking is a serious problem in the Asian American community," and "Drug use is a serious problem in the Asian American community" along a four-point Likert-type scale: "strongly agree"(1), "agree" (2), "disagree" (3), and "strongly disagree"(4). Among the youth respondents, 53% agreed or strongly agreed with the statement "Drinking is a serious problem in the Asian American community." The mean score of respondents' perception of drinking as a serious problem was 2.3 (S.D. .77). Regarding drug use problems, 62.1% disagreed or strongly disagreed with the statement "Drug use is a serious problem in the Asian American community." The mean score of their perception of drug use as a serious problem was 2.6 (S.D. .82). Respondents from the three ethnic groups shared similar perceptions. The mean scores regarding drinking as a severe problem for the three ethnic groups were: 2.3 (S.D. .78) Chinese respondents, 2.5 (S.D. .77) Indian respondents, 2.2 (S.D. .77) Vietnamese respondents. The mean scores regarding drug use as a severe problem for the three ethnic groups were: 2.5 (S.D. .98) Chinese respondents, 2.6 (S.D. .90) Indian respondents, and 2.6 (S.D. .66) Vietnamese respondents. In light of these findings, respondents appeared to take a middle position in their perceptions with slightly more than half of respondents agreeing drinking was a serious problem and around two-thirds of respondents disagreeing drug use was a serious problem in the Asian American community. No significant differences were found in the respondents' perceptions based on their demographic characteristics of age, gender, ethnicity, and education.

Perceived Characteristics of Asian Americans Who Have Problems with Drinking and/or Drug Use

Respondents' perceived characteristics of Asian Americans who have problems with drinking and drug use was examined by the question: "Suppose I told you a friend of mine has a problem with drinking (drug use), what might be his/her gender, age and socioeconomic status?" A typical drinker as portrayed by our respondents is a male (92.4%), can be either an adolescent (46.2%) or an adult (51.3%), and comes from a lower class (43.4%) or middle class background (51.3%). Being a female (7.6%), an elder (2.6%) and having an upper class background (5.3%) were rarely perceived to have problems with drinking. A typical drug user is a male (92%), adolescent (77.6%), and has either a lower class (39.2%) or middle class background (48.6%). The most unlikely drinker is a woman (8%) from an upper class background (10.8%). Our respondents did not perceive the likelihood of an elder using illicit drugs (see Table 3).

No significant differences were found in respondents' perceived characteristics of an Asian drug user across ethnic groups. On the other hand, there were significant differences across ethnic groups in the perceived age ($\chi^2 = 13.4$, $df = 4$, $p < .01$) and socioeconomic status ($\chi^2 = 15.4$, $df = 4$, $p < .01$) of an Asian problem drinker. Around two-thirds of Vietnamese respondents perceived the drinker as adolescents (66.7%) while 70.4% of Chinese respondents and 66.7% of Indian respondents perceived the drinker as adults. Also, no Chinese respondents perceived elderly as likely to be drinkers while a few Indian and Vietnamese respondents perceived so. Regarding the socioeconomic status of an Asian problem drinker, 56% of Chinese and 50% of Vietnamese respondents perceived the drinker to be likely from the lower class while no Indian respondents perceived so. Instead, all Indian respondents perceived the problem drinker as having a middle class background (see Table 3). No significant differences were found between respondents' perceptions and their demographic characteristics of gender, age, and education except for respondents' perception of the socioeconomic status of Asian drug users. Over half of male respondents (52.6%) perceived a drug user to be likely from the lower class while 65.7% of female respondents perceived a drug user to be likely from the middle class (($\chi^2 = 7.3$, $df = 3$, $p < .05$).

TABLE 3. Chi-Square Results of Perceived Characteristics of Asians with Drinking or Drug Use Problems by Ethnicity

Perceived Characteristics	Overall (%)	Chinese (%)	Indian (%)	Vietnamese (%)
Drinking problems				
Gender (n = 79)		(n = 27)	(n = 14)	(n = 38)
Male	92.4	96.3	100.0	86.8
Female	7.6	3.7	0.0	13.2
$\chi^2 = 3.4$, df = 2, $p = .18$				
Age (n = 78)**		(n = 27)	(n = 15)	(n = 36)
Teenager	46.2	29.6	26.7	66.7
Adult	51.3	70.4	66.7	30.6
Elderly	2.6	0.0	6.7	2.8
$\chi^2 = 13.4$, $df = 4$, $p < .01$				
Socioeconomic status(n = 76)**		(n = 25)	(n = 13)	(n = 38)
Lower class	43.4	56.0	0.0	50
Middle class	51.3	36.0	100.0	44.7
Upper class	5.3	8.0	0.0	5.3
$\chi^2 = 15.4$, $df = 4$, $p < .01$				
Drug use problems				
Gender (n = 75)		(n = 26)	(n = 15)	(n = 34)
Male	92.0	88.5	100.0	91.2
Female	8.0	11.5	0.0	8.8
$\chi^2 = 1.8$, $df = 2$, $p = .41$				
Age (n = 76)		(n = 27)	(n = 14)	(n = 35)
Teenage	77.6	74.1	71.4	82.9
Adult	22.4	25.9	28.6	17.1
Elderly	0.0	0.0	0.0	0.0
$\chi^2 = 1.1$, $df = 2$, $p = .59$				
Socioeconomic status (n = 73)		(n = 26)	(n = 13)	(n = 34)
Lower class	39.2	26.9	23.1	54.3
Middle class	48.6	65.4	53.8	34.3
Upper class	10.8	7.7	23.1	8.6
$\chi^2 = 9.1$, $df = 4$, $p = .06$				

** $p < .01$

Beliefs About Etiology of Substance Use

To understand respondents' beliefs about etiology of substance abuse, the following two questions were asked: "Suppose I told you a friend of mine has a problem with drinking, what may be some possible reasons?" "Suppose I told you a friend of mine has a problem with drugs, what may be some possible reasons?" Respondents were asked to rank the first three choices of the following possible reasons: "social influence," "family influence (come from an alcoholic family or has family members using drugs)," "has emotional problems (e.g., stress, relational conflicts, self-esteem problems, poor coping, etc.)," and "a habit that can't be stopped." Descriptive and chi-square analyses were performed using the respondents' first choice of answer. Findings indicated that respondents shared similar beliefs regarding reasons for Asian American populations drinking or using drugs. Social influence (30.9% and 51.5%) and emotional problems (32.4% and 20.6%) were the most frequently selected first two reasons. Twenty-five percent of respondents perceived coming from an alcoholic family as the reason for a person to drink; 16.2% perceived family influence as the reason for a person to use drugs. Only 11.8% chose "a habit that can't be stopped" as the reason for Asians to have problems with drinking or drug use. No significant differences were found in the respondents' perceptions based on their demographic characteristics including ethnicity, gender, age, and education.

Attitudes Toward Treatment

Respondents were asked to rate their opinions of the following five statements regarding attitudes toward treatment along a four-point Likert-type scale from "strongly agree"(1), "agree" (2), "disagree" (3), to "strongly disagree"(4): "Formal treatment for addiction is usually not helpful," "Nothing really works for people with addiction," "People with addiction problem would be able to quit on their own if they really wanted to," "You really can't help people with a drug or alcohol problem until they ask for help," and "Family members need and can be helped even if the addict does not want help." The first two statements focused on respondents' attitudes toward the helpfulness of treatment programs. The third and the fourth statements examined respondents' perception of the issue of locus of control in relation to treatment. The fifth statement explored respondents' attitude toward treatment for family members of substance users.

The youth respondents shared similar attitudes toward treatment as no significant differences were found in the respondents' perceptions based on their demographic characteristics including ethnicity, age, gender, and education. Respondents generally showed a positive attitude toward the potential helpfulness of treatment programs. They did not agree with the statements "formal treatment for addiction is usually not helpful" (mean 2.8, S.D. 1.3) and "nothing really works for people with addiction" (mean 3.0, S.D. .9). They also believed in the usefulness of treatment programs for family members of substance users. The mean score for the statement "Family members need and can be helped even if the addict does not want help" was 2 (S.D. .7). The respondents, on the other hand, also agreed with the statements that "people with addiction problem would be able to quit on their own if they really wanted to" (mean 2.1, S.D. .8) and "you really can't help people with a drug or alcohol problem until they ask for help" (mean 2.3, S.D. 1.1). In other words, the respondents also believed in a fairly strong locus of control of the substance users to stop drinking or using drugs with or without treatment.

Perceived Help-Seeking Preferences

To examine respondents' preferred help-seeking responses to substance use problems, they were asked: "If you have problems with drinking or using drugs, what would you do?" Respondents were asked to rank three most preferred helping-seeking responses from the following choices: "do nothing," "attempt to quit on my own," "talk to supportive family members," "talk to friends," "talk to counselor/therapist," "attend Alcohol Anonymous or Narcotics Anonymous," "go to outpatient detox treatment programs," and "go to inpatient detox treatment programs." Descriptive and chi-square analyses were performed using the respondents' first choice of help-seeking preferences. The most frequently selected response was "attempt to quit on my own" (39.1%) that was followed by "talk to friends" (17.4%). Around 10% of respondents would "do nothing," "talk to supportive family members," "talk to counselor/therapist," or "attend Alcoholics Anonymous or Narcotics Anonymous." Most respondents did not view detox treatment program as a viable option. Only 2.9% would go to outpatient detox program and no respondent preferred going to inpatient detox treatment program (see Table 4).

No significant differences were found in respondents' perceptions of helping-seeking preferences based on their demographic characteristics of ethnicity, gender and age. On the other hand, Indian respondents appeared to have a different pattern of help-seeking preferences from Chinese or Vietnamese respondents. Indian respondents seemed to have a narrower range of help-seeking preferences that focused on "attempt to quit on my own" (50%) and "talk to friends" (28.6%) than Chinese or Vietnamese respondents. The presence of empty cells and the small

TABLE 4. Help-Seeking Preferences by Ethnicity (N = 69)

Help-seeking preferences	Overall (%) (N = 69)	Chinese (%) (n = 24)	Indian (%) (n = 14)	Vietnamese (%) (n = 31)
Do nothing	10.1	4.2	0.0	19.4
Attempt to quit on my own	39.1	33.3	50.0	38.7
Talk to supportive family members	10.1	8.3	7.1	12.9
Talk to friends	17.4	16.7	28.6	12.9
Talk to counselor/therapist	10.1	16.7	0.0	9.7
Attend AA or NA	10.1	16.7	14.3	3.2
Go to outpatient detox program	2.9	4.2	0.0	3.2
+ Go to inpatient detox program	0.0	0.0	0.0	0.0

$\chi^2 = 12.98$ $df = 12$, $p = .37$
+ "Go to inpatient detox program" was not included in the chi square analyses because of presence of empty cells.

sample size of Indian respondents may account for the absence of findings of significance across different ethnic groups.

Education of respondents was significantly associated with helping-seeking preferences ($\chi^2 = 14.6$, $df = 6$, $p < .05$) (see Table 5). While "attempt to quit on my own" was the first choice of help-seeking preference for respondents with middle/high school or college/post-graduate education, these two groups differed significantly in their second help-seeking preferences. For the middle/high school group, the second preferred response was "do nothing" (21.2%). None of the college/post-graduate group chose "do nothing" as a preferred response. Instead, the second preferred response for the college/post-graduate group was "talk to friends" (22.9%). Another major difference between the two groups was their attitude toward Alcoholics Anonymous or Narcotics Anonymous. "Attend Alcoholics Anonymous or Narcotics Anonymous" was the third help-seeking preference of the college/post-graduate group (17.1%) while the same response was the one of the least selected response by the middle/high school group (3.0%).

Perceived Helpful Services

The authors asked respondents "if you have problems with drinking or drug use, what kinds of services would be helpful?" Respondents were asked to rank three most helpful services from the following choices: "information about treatment and detox programs," "counseling," "support groups (e.g., AA)," and "detox programs (e.g., inpatient, outpatient, methadone detox programs)." Descriptive and chi-square

TABLE 5. Chi-Square Results of Help-Seeking Preferences by Education (N = 68)

Help-seeking preferences	Overall (%) (N = 68)	Middle/High school (%) (n = 33)	College/Postgraduate (%) (n = 35)
Do nothing	10.3	21.2	0.0
Attempt to quit on my own	39.7	45.5	34.3
Talk to supportive family members	10.3	6.1	14.3
Talk to friends	16.2	9.1	22.9
Talk to counselor/therapist	10.3	12.1	8.6
Attend AA or NA	10.3	3.0	17.1
Go to outpatient detox program	2.9	3.0	2.9
+ Go to inpatient detox program	0.0	0.0	0.0

$\chi^2 = 14.6$, $df = 6$, $p < .05$
+ "Go to inpatient detox program" was not included in the chi square analyses because of presence of empty cells

analyses were performed using the respondents' first choice of helpful services. Counseling (37.9%) was perceived to be the most helpful service, followed by "information about treatment and detox program," (25.8%), and "support groups" (21.2%). Only 15.2% of respondents perceived "detox programs" as helpful services (see Table 6).

No significant differences were found in respondents' perceptions of helpful services based on their demographic characteristics of gender, age, and education. On the other hand, ethnicity of respondents was significantly associated with their perceived helpful services ($\chi^2 = 14.2$, $df = 6$, $p < .05$) (see Table 6). The first choice of helpful services for Chinese respondents was "detox programs" (31.8%) while "detox programs" was the least selected choice among Indian and Vietnamese respondents (0% and 9.7% respectively). Indian and Vietnamese respondents perceived "counseling" as the most helpful services (61.5% and 45.2%) while "counseling" was the least selected choice of helpful services among Chinese respondents (13.6%).

DISCUSSION

The authors examined Asian American youth respondents' perceptions of substance use problems in the Asian American community, their attitude toward treatment as well as perceptions about help-seeking preferences and helpful services. In addition, prevalence and social network of drinking and drug use among youth respondents were exam-

TABLE 6. Chi-Square Results of Perceived Helpful Services by Ethnicity (N = 66)

Perceived helpful services	Overall (%) (N = 66)	Chinese (%) (n = 22)	Indian (%) (n = 13)	Vietnamese (%) (n = 31)
Information about treatment and detox programs	25.8	27.3	30.8	22.6
Counseling	37.9	13.6	61.5	45.2
Support groups (AA, NA, etc.)	21.2	27.3	7.7	22.6
Detox programs (inpatient, outpatient, methadone detox programs, etc.)	15.2	31.8	0.0	9.7

χ^2=14.2 *df*=6 *p*<.05

ined. Findings of the study provide interesting observations that have important implications for addressing substance use problems in the Asian American community.

Is Substance Abuse a Severe Problem for Asian American Youth Populations?

There is probably no simple or definite answer to the question "Is substance abuse a serious problem in the Asian American community?" Existing literature suggests a tendency of the Asian American community to minimize the severity of substance use problems. Findings of the present study, however, indicate a potential change in Asian American youth's awareness of substance use problems in their community. Findings showed a split in the respondents' opinion regarding the severity of drinking and drug use problems in the Asian American community. Respondents appeared to take a middle position with slightly more than half of respondents (53%) agreeing drinking was a serious problem and around two-thirds of respondents (62.1%) disagreeing drug use was a serious problem in the Asian American community. The split in respondents' opinion regarding the severity of substance use problems can be an indicator of increasing awareness of such problems for Asian American populations. Instead of minimizing or denying those problems, more and more Asian American youth were aware of substance use problems in the community. Still, such an awareness is more prevalent for drinking problems than for drug use problems, which is likely to carry stronger negative cultural stigma.

Findings of the present study revealed a 36% prevalence rate of drinking and 2.3% of drug use among youth respondents. Because this is not a representative sample, findings regarding prevalence of drinking and drug use of respondents cannot be generalized to other Asian American youth populations. On the other hand, such prevalence rates are comparable to rates revealed by several other major studies of Asian American youth populations that indicate a lower prevalence of drinking and drug use among Asian American youth populations as compared to other ethno-racial groups (Harachi et al., 2001 cited a 37.6% prevalence rate of drinking; Skager & Austin, 1993 cited a 3.9% prevalence rate of using illicit drugs for Chinese students). Findings of the study, however, did not indicate that Asian American youth were heavy drinkers if they did drink (Austin, 1999). Findings of relatively low prevalence rates will need to be interpreted with caution. Prevalence rates of drinking and drug use are affected by problems of self-reporting and sample-bias. Non-users might be more willing to participate in the present study than substance users, because of the attached negative cultural stigma. Respondents may under-report (or exaggerate) their frequency of drinking or using drugs. A random and representative national sample and more sophisticated reporting methods will be needed to accurately estimate the prevalence of drinking and drug use among Asian American youth populations.

Despite relatively low prevalence rates of drinking and drug use among this group of respondents, findings about the social network of drinking and drug use suggested issues that deserve attention. Although the majority of our youth respondents did not drink heavily or use drugs, more than one-third of them associated with Asian problem drinkers (36%), and about one-fifth associated with Asians who used illicit drugs (18.6%). Many studies have identified social influence and peer pressure as major factors of substance use initiation (Gillmore et al., 1990; Sasao, 1994). Respondents of the present study revealed a similar perception: "Social influence" was perceived as the most likely reason for Asians to have problems with drugs and the second most likely reason for Asians to have problems with drinking. Asian American youth populations may show lower prevalence of substance use although they do associate with other Asians who have problems with drinking or using illicit drugs. In light of these findings, preventive education for Asian American youth populations should receive adequate attention as part of the community effort to prevent substance use problems in the Asian American community. On the other hand, findings regarding social network should be interpreted with caution because the study did not collect independent information from respondents' peers and there maybe reporting bias based on respondents' answers.

Stereotypes and Myths About Substance Users

Respondents across ethnicity, gender, age, and education shared similar stereotypes of Asians who have problems with drug use or drinking problems. There was a unanimous perception that an Asian being a female, elderly, and/or having an upper class background was unlikely to be associated with substance use problems (Table 3). A typical drug user was perceived as a male adolescent from either a lower or middle class background, and a typical problem drinker as a male adolescent or adult from either a lower class or middle class background (see Table 3). While the present study did not explore underlying assumptions or values around the stereotypes, it can be postulated that those stereotypes are likely to be influenced by traditional Asian values regarding gender roles (female as submissive), respect for elders and social hierarchy.

Stereotypes and myths are usually unhelpful especially when these stereotypes are not supported by empirical evidence. In the present study, no significant differences were found in respondents' prevalence and social network of drinking and drug use based on their gender. The study by Gilmore and his associates (1990) also showed that gender and SES were not related to initiation of substance use among Asian American youth populations. The existence of community "blind spots" deserves attention. These "myths" may deter community education and intervention efforts for "model groups" such as females, elderly and upper class members. Stereotypes about problem drinkers or drug users may also make it more difficult for the "model groups" to seek help for their problems and at the same time unnecessarily create a negative, labeling effect for the identified sub-groups such as males or adolescents.

Changing Attitudes, Same Behavioral Preferences?

A major focus of the present study was respondents' attitudes toward treatment and perceptions of help-seeking preferences in response to substance use problems. The existing literature, influenced by an understanding of traditional Asian cultural values, suggested a tendency for substance users to hide the problem instead of seeking help from family members or professionals (Ja & Aoki, 1993; Neumoto et al., 1999). Findings of the present study largely supported those propositions. Findings, however, also suggested a beginning process of change in the attitude of Asian American youth toward treatment and help-seeking preferences.

Asian American youth respondents, regardless of ethnicity, age, gender, and education, showed a positive attitude toward treatment. Despite a positive attitude toward treatment, they also believed in the ability of substance users to stop using substances on their own. Findings regarding respondents' attitudes toward treatment appeared to suggest the juxtaposition of two potentially contradictory stances: "treatment is helpful" and "I can help myself even without treatment." Findings regarding respondents' help-seeking preferences for substance use problems further elucidate the dynamic process of change and continuity. The most frequently selected help-seeking preference by respondents was "attempt to quit on their own" (39.1%). Such a finding was consistent with the stance "I can help myself even without treatment." In addition, the second most frequently selected help-seeking preference by respondents was "talk to friends," which was also an attempt to utilize personal, non-professional resources (see Table 4). Despite a positive attitude toward formal treatment, few respondents preferred talking to counselor or attending support groups such as AA and NA. Detox programs were not considered as a viable treatment option (see Table 4). Findings regarding help-seeking preferences of Asian American youth respondents echoed their perceptions of helpful services. "Detox programs" was the least selected helpful service by our youth respondents as a group (see Table 6). These findings clearly indicate a gap between attitude and behavioral preferences. Findings regarding Chinese respondents' perceived helpful services and their help-seeking preferences further illustrated such a gap. The first choice of perceived helpful services for Chinese respondents was "detox programs" (31.8%) (see Table 6), although only 4.2% of Chinese youth respondents would prefer outpatient detox program, and none of them prefer inpatient detox program if they have substance use problems (see Table 4). The positive change in attitude toward treatment was not accompanied by a corresponding change in behavioral preferences.

Despite a gap between attitude and behavioral preferences and the tendency for Asian American youth respondents to utilize personal resources rather than professional help or formal treatment programs, the positive attitude toward treatment can be an indicator of increasing awareness and/or beginning acceptance of available treatment for substance use problems. In addition, among the range of available treatment options, Asian American youth respondents showed more acceptance of the less "intrusive" services such as counseling and support groups than detox programs; such observations were supported by findings regarding help-seeking preferences as well as perceived helpful services. These findings have useful implications for designing preventive and intervention efforts with Asian American youth populations.

Family Support and Substance Use Problems

Another observation is about utilization of family support for substance use problems. Despite Asian cultural values on family centrality and the well documented help-seeking patterns of Asian Americans to utilize family support, only 10.1% of youth respondents would turn to family for help if they have substance use problems (see Table 4). Such findings are congruent with the literature that suggests a tendency for Asian substance users to hide the problem (or to handle the problem on their own) instead of seeking help from family members as a result of cultural stigma and/or a fear of shaming the family (Ja & Aoki, 1993). As family support is crucial in substance users' recovery process, it is important to include parents and family members in community education and intervention efforts that target Asian American youth populations.

Contextual, Localized Knowledge as Useful Base for Community Education and Intervention Efforts

Despite the presence of many different groups of Asian people in the US and the cautions raised by many investigators regarding a simplistic view of Asian Americans as a homogeneous, undifferentiated group of people (Dawson, 1998), attempts to understand these diverse populations are often based on the ethnicity of "Asian Americans." Findings of the study revealed both similarities and differences among respondents of the three ethnic groups. On the whole, Chinese, Indian, and Vietnamese respondents shared similar perceptions regarding the severity of the problem of substance use, reasons for Asians to have substance use problems, attitude toward treatment, and help-seeking preferences. Inter-group variations were evident in respondents' perceived characteristics of problem drinkers, perceived helpful services, prevalence of drug use, and social network of drinking. It does a disservice to Asian American communities when service providers disregard inter-group differences. The localized knowledge of different groups allows community activists and service providers to implement targeted education, preventive, and treatment efforts based on localized information generated from individual communities. For instance, in the surveyed city, no Indian respondents perceived detox programs as helpful services while Chinese respondents chose "detox program" as the first helpful services (see Table 6). Similarly, more than 60% of Indian respondents viewed counseling as a helpful service while only 13% of Chinese respondents perceived so (see Table 6). Another inter-group difference focuses on the perceived characteristics of problem drinkers. Vietnamese respondents differed from Chinese and Indian respondents in their perception of Asian problem drinkers who were viewed as mostly teenagers. Indian respondents differed from Chinese and Vietnamese respondents in their perception of Asian problem drinkers who were viewed as mostly middle class members (see Table 3). With respect to prevalence and social network of substance use, more Vietnamese respondents associated with Asian problem drinkers than the other two ethnic groups. Indian respondents showed a higher prevalence rate of using drugs than Chinese or Vietnamese youth respondents (see Table 2). The present study did not examine cultural and contextual factors contributing to differential perceptions among different ethnic groups. Such localized knowledge, however, would be helpful in generating appropriate education and intervention efforts that focus on the unique needs and characteristics of each individual group.

Findings of the study support current knowledge regarding prevalence of substance use among Asian American youth populations, cultural influences on help-seeking responses, and existence of inter-group differences. Findings, however, also indicate a beginning process of change in respondents' perceptions of substance use issues in Asian American communities. Instead of minimizing the problem, there appeared to be an increasing awareness of the severity of substance use problems in the community, although such awareness was more prominent for drinking problems than drug use problems. In addition, the youth community began to show a positive attitude toward treatment, although such an attitudinal change was not yet accompanied by a change in their behavioral preferences. In addition, information on social network, perceived characteristics of substance users, and perceived help-seeking responses and helpful services generated useful implications for community education and interventions pertaining to substance use issues.

IMPLICATIONS AND CONCLUSION

The present study is a beginning effort to understand the perceptions of Asian American youth populations regarding the phenomenon of and help-seeking responses to substance use problems. Methodological limitations of the study included: the use of a non-random sampling design that limits its generalizability, reliance on respondents' self-reports of their perception that may differ from actual behaviors, and the use of a relatively small sample size that may affect the strength of findings of chi-square analyses because of the presence of empty cells or cells with expected values less than 5. On the other hand, the study provides useful information in a minimally researched area, namely, Asian American youth respondents' perceptions regarding substance use problems, their attitude toward treatment, help-seeking preferences and helpful services.

Findings regarding attitude toward treatment and perception of help-seeking preferences and helpful services have useful implications for community education and intervention efforts. Despite a positive attitude toward treatment programs, findings suggested a tendency for Asian American youth to utilize personal resources in response to substance use problems and not seek help from family or professionals. Among the small number of respondents who preferred formal treatment, there was a clear tendency to perceive counseling or support group services as helpful rather than detox programs. Such a pattern of help-seeking preferences is likely to be influenced by cultural stigma around substance use problems and seeking outside professional help for these problems. In light of these findings, preventive education for Asian American youth populations should focus on: (1) introducing the range of available treatment options especially detox programs and their relevance to substance use problems so that Asian American youths can make help-seeking choices based on an informed position; (2) educating the youth populations regarding the pros and cons of utilizing personal resources to address substance use problems (e.g., do nothing, quit on one's own); (3) providing family educational programs to help parents communicate with their children regarding issues of substance abuse as a way to enhance family ability to address substance use issues in children; and most important of all, (4) assisting parents and youth to openly discuss cultural stigma around substance use problems as a way to initiate beneficial community dialogue around the issue.

The agency that initiated this study has utilized various strategies in its community educational efforts. A primary task was to develop culturally appropriate curriculum and educational materials regarding substance use issues for Asian youth and adults as there is a lack of these much needed, but rarely available, materials. For instance, the agency developed a booklet "Keeping Your Kids Drug Free" that was translated into 5 Asian languages including Chinese, Korean, Japanese, Laotian, and Vietnamese for dissemination (Asian American Community Services, 2002). In addition, the agency implemented community education using a wide range of activities such as workshops, presentations, art contests, and booth displays at prominent places that Asians gather. Because of cultural stigma around substance use issues, many Asian Americans are not yet ready to openly discuss substance use problems. Consequently, staff employed more flexible ways to engage Asian American youth and their parents. For example, drug and alcohol education was presented in relation to issues that carry less stigmatization. These issues include but are not limited to parenting, cross-cultural adjustment, self-assertiveness, women's health, self-esteem, and leadership training. Utilizing community networks also plays an important role in community education efforts. Activities were conducted in collaboration with public schools, ethnic churches, ethnic language schools, and English as a Secondary Language (ESL) classes. Strategies for implementing culturally appropriate and sensitive community education are almost endless, but constantly demand flexibility, creativity, and responsiveness on the part of service providers.

Findings of the study also have implications for designing and implementing treatment for Asian American youth populations who have substance use problems. First, there should be a comprehensive system of care including a range of services for Asian American youth populations. Such a system of care should focus on counseling and support group services as the gate keeping services as there is more acceptance of these services among Asian American youth populations. Second, treatment should utilize the cultural strengths of self-reliance in the recovery process. Third, in view of the tendency for Asian American youth populations to utilize private, personal resources in response to substance use problems, issues of confidentiality should be addressed early on in the treatment process.

Besides ethnicity, differential perceptions of Asian American youth respondents regarding substance use problems were also observed along age and educational differences that were more developmental than cultural in nature. Still, these observed differences have useful implications for preventive educational efforts. Respondents of the college/postgraduate group had a higher prevalence of drinking than the middle/high school group (51% vs. 13.9%). Such a pattern was expected since the older youth have increased accessibility to alcohol and were legally allowed to purchase alcohol. Despite lower prevalence of drinking among respondents of the middle/high school group, they seemed to have limited options and were less willing to utilize external resources and formal treatment when they had substance use problems. In fact, more than one-fifth of middle/high school respondents chose "doing nothing" and almost half chose "attempt to quit on my own" if they had problems with drinking and drug use. They rarely preferred seeking help from family members (6.1%) or using professional help other than talking to counselors (see Table 5). While it was not possible to account for the differences in help-seeking preferences between the younger and older youth groups, which can be a result of maturity or information accessibility, there is a clear need to implement targeted educational efforts to middle and high school Asian American youth regarding available treatment options as well as enlisting family support in the process.

In sum, findings of the study bring forth issues that have useful implications for future research as well as preventive and treatment efforts. In terms of research direction, future investigators will need to develop knowledge regarding: (1) prevalence and social network of substance use among Asian American youth population across ethnic groups; (2) the use of behavior-specific questions to explore actual help-seeking behaviors to address substance use problems among Asian American youth populations; (3) a more refined understanding of social, cultural, institutional, and contextual barriers for Asian American youth populations in seeking professional help, (4) protective and risk factors in family that affect substance use initiation and help-seeking responses, and (5) the process of cultural change and continuity that influences youth's perceptions of and responses to substance use problems. Regarding research design, future studies will need to use representative and random samples, a larger sample for more precise and refined statistical analysis, and multiple reporting sources in examining social network of substance use. Implications for community education and intervention efforts include: (1) educate the youth community regarding available treatment options and their relevance to substance use problems with a special focus on detox programs, (2) challenge and dissipate the community "myths" about substance users, (3) develop culturally sensitive treatment procedures that would normalize the act of seeking professional help, reduce feelings of shame, ensure confidentiality; and utilize cultural strengths of self-reliance in the recovery process, and (4) design and implement culturally appropriate and sensitive education and intervention efforts based on localized knowledge of unique characteristics of local Asian communities instead of reference to a broad, generalized understanding of an undifferentiated group of Asian Americans.

REFERENCES

Asian American Community Services. (2002). *Keeping your kids drug free*. Columbus, OH: Asian American Community Services.

Asian American Recovery Services. (1996). *An Asian outreach intervention model* (Report submitted to SAMHSA's Center for Substance Abuse and Treatment). San Francisco, CA: Author.

Austin, G. A. (1999). Current evidence on substance abuse among Asian American youth. In *Current evidence on substance abuse among Asian American youth*. (DHHS Publication No. SMA 98-3193, pp. 169-219).

Bachman, J. C., Wallace, J. M., Jr., O'Malley, P. M., Johnston, L. D., Kurth, C. L., & Neighbors, H. W. (1991). Racial/ethnic differences in smoking, drinking, and illicit drug use among American high school seniors, 1976-1989. *American Journal of Public Health, 81*, 372-377.

Barnes, G. M., & Welte, J. W. (1986). Patterns and predictors of alcohol use among 7-12 grade students in New York State. *Journal of Studies on Alcohol, 47*, 53-62.

Barnes, G. M., Welte, J. W., & Dintcheff, B. A. (1993). Decline in alcohol use among 7-12 grade students in New York State, 1983-1990. *Alcoholism: Clinical and Experimental Research, 17*, 797-801.

Chan, S., & Leong, C. W. (1994). Chinese families in transition: Cultural conflicts and adjustment problems. *Journal of Social Distress and the Homeless, 3*, 263-281.

Chi, I., Lubben, J. E., & Kitano, H. H. L. (1988). Heavy drinking among young adult Asian males. *International Social Work, 31*, 219-229.

Chi, I., Lubben, J. E., & Kitano, H. H. L. (1989). Differences in drinking behavior among three Asian-American groups. *Journal of Studies on Alcohol, 50*, 15-23.

Dawson, D. A. (1998). Beyond Black, White and Hispanic: Race, ethnic origin and drinking patterns in the United States. *Journal of Substance Abuse, 10*, 321-339.

Gerstein, R. G., & Harwood, H. J. (1990). *Treating drug problems (Vol. 1)*. Washington, DC: National Academy Press.

Gilmore, M. R., Catalano, R. F., Morrison, D. M., Wells, E. A., Iritani, B., & Hawkins, J. D. (1990). Racial differences in acceptability and availability of drugs and early initiation of substance use. *American Journal of Drug and Alcohol Abuse, 16*, 185-206.

Harachi, T. W., Catalano, R. F., Kim, S., & Choi, Y. (2001). Etiology and prevention of substance use among Asian American youth. *Prevention Science, 2*, 57-65.

Ja, D. (1991). *Substance abuse treatment and the Asian American community: Issues and implication*. Paper presented at Office for Treatment Improvement Consultation, Honolulu, Hawaii, April 21, 1991.

Ja, D., & Aoki, B. (1993). Substance abuse treatment: Cultural barriers in the Asian-American community. *Journal of Psychoactive Drugs, 25*, 61-71.

Ja, D., & Aoki, B. (1998). Cultural barriers in the Asian-American community. In P. B. Organista, K. M. Chun, & G. Marin (Eds.), *Reading in ethnic psychology* (pp. 386-401). New York: Routledge.

Lee, M. Y. (2000). Understanding Chinese battered women in North America: A Review of the Literature and Practice Implications. *Journal of Ethnic and Cultural Diversity in Social Work* (previous *Journal of Multicultural Social Work*), *8*, 215-241.

Lee, M. Y., & Law, P. F. M. (in press). Perception of Sexual Violence Against Women in Asian American Communities. *Journal of Ethnic and Cultural Diversity in Social Work*.

McAuliffe, W. E. et al. (1994). *Assessment of substance dependence treatment needs: A telephone survey manual and questionnaire, Revised edition*. Cambridge, MA: National Technical Center for Substance Abuse Needs Assessment.

Neumoto, T., Aoki, B., Huang, K., Morris, A., Nguyen, H., & Wong, W. (1999). Drug use behaviors among drug users in San Francisco. *Addictive Behaviors, 24*, 823-838.

Reynolds, D. K. (1989). *Flowing bridges, quiet waters: Japanese psychotherapies, Morita and Naikan*. Albany: State University of New York Press.

Sasao, T. (1991). *Statewide Asian drug service needs assessment: A multimethod approach*. Sacramento, CA: California Department of Alcohol and Drug Abuse.

Sasao, T. (1994). *Patterns and correlates of alcohol, tobacco and other (ATOD) use among high school students in the San Gabriel Valley, California* (Technical Report). Rosemead, CA: Asian Pacific Family Center.

Sasao, T. (1999). Identifying at-risk Asian American adolescents in multiethnic schools: Implications for substance abuse prevention interventions and program evaluation. In *Identifying at-risk Asian American adolescents in multiethnic schools: Implications for substance abuse prevention interventions and program evaluation* (DHHS Publication No. SMA 98-3193, pp. 143-167).

Skager, R., & Austin, G. (1993). *Fourth biennial statewide survey of drug and alcohol use among California students in grades 7, 9, and 11: Winter 1991-1992: Report to the attorney general*. Sacramento, CA: Office of the Attorney General, California Department of Justice.

Sue, D. (1987). Use and abuse of alcohol by Asian Americans. *Journal of Psychoactive Drugs, 19*, 57-66.

U.S. Census Bureau. (2000). *Census 2000 Summary File 1 (SF1) 100 Percent Data*. [WWW Document]. Retrieved May 2, 2002 from factfinder.census.gov/servlet/QTTable?ds-mae DEC 2000 SF1 U&gp id = p 1000 US&gr name = DEC 2000SF1 U DT.

U.S. Department of Commerce. (1998). *Statistical abstract of the United States, 1998: The national data book (118th Ed.)*. Springfield, VA: National Technical Information Services.

Yamashiro, G., & Matsuoka, J. K. (1997). Help-seeking among Asian and Pacific Americans: A multiperspective analysis. *Social Work, 42*, 176-186.

Zane, N., Park, S., & Aoki, B. (1999). The development of culturally valid measures for assessing prevention impact in Asian American communities. In *The development of culturally valid measures for assessing prevention impact in Asian American communities* (DHHS Publication No. SMA 98-3193, pp. 61-89).

Ties That Protect: An Ecological Perspective on Latino/a Urban Pre-Adolescent Drug Use

Flavio Francisco Marsiglia
Bart W. Miles
Patricia Dustman
Stephen Sills

SUMMARY. An ecological risk and resiliency framework was applied to explore how social contexts, especially the role of families and schools, are affecting Latino/a pre-adolescent substance use in the urban Southwest. A mixed research design, using both quantitative and qualitative methodologies, guided the study. Quantitative data were collected through surveys administered as part of a school-based prevention intervention experiment (N = 2,125). Individual interviews conducted with a randomly selected number of matched students (N = 60) provided the

---

Flavio Francisco Marsiglia, PhD, is Associate Professor and Director and Patricia Dustman, EdD, is Associate Director, Southwest Interdisciplinary Research Consortium (SIRC), School of Social Work, Arizona State University. Bart W. Miles is Social Work PhD Candidate and Stephen Sills is Sociology PhD Candidate, Arizona State University.

The research presented in this article is part of the Drug Resistance Strategies grant, funded under award number R01 DA05629-07 of the National Institutes of Health/National Institute on Drug Abuse.

[Haworth co-indexing entry note]: "Ties That Protect: An Ecological Perspective on Latino/a Urban Pre-Adolescent Drug Use." Marsiglia et al. Co-published simultaneously in *Journal of Ethnic & Cultural Diversity in Social Work* (The Haworth Social Work Practice Press, an imprint of The Haworth Press, Inc.) Vol. 11, No. 3/4, 2002, pp. 191-220; and: *Social Work with Multicultural Youth* (ed: Diane de Anda) The Haworth Social Work Practice Press, an imprint of The Haworth Press, Inc., 2002, pp. 191-220. Single or multiple copies of this article are available for a fee from The Haworth Document Delivery Service [1-800-HAWORTH, 9:00 a.m. - 5:00 p.m. (EST). E-mail address: docdelivery@haworthpress.com].

http://www.haworthpress.com/store/product.asp?sku=J051

10.1300/J051v11n03_03

qualitative data. The main theme emerging throughout both data sets was a strong resilience against drug use of the participating 7th grade urban youth. The vast majority of students did not use hard drugs, and agreed that alcohol use was inappropriate at their age. A high degree of attachment and strong ties to their parents and their school environment emerged as a shared protective factor. Recommendations include social work interventions that support the resiliency characteristics of urban Latino/a youth in different social contexts such as communities, schools, and families. Limitations of the study are reviewed and suggestions for future research are offered.

KEYWORDS. Resiliency, drug use, family, Latinos/as, Hispanics

INTRODUCTION

The purpose of this research is to advance our understanding of the protective and risk factors that shield Latino and other pre-adolescents from drug use. National survey data show that drug use has increased significantly among adolescents over the past decades (Botvin et al., 2000a). It has been estimated that 13.9 million American youth 12 and older use illicit drugs, with a 2.4% increase between 1996 and 1997 (SAMHSA, 1998). Commonly, these increases in drug use are associated with risk factors located within a risk and protective factors continuum (Smokowski et al., 1999; NIDA, 1999). These factors can have a risk or a protective effect at different times and in different contexts. Home and school have been identified as key contexts influencing adolescents' substance use (Bauman & Phongsaun, 1999; Ellickson & Morton, 1999; Luekefeld et al., 1998; McWhirter et al., 1998).

In urban settings with high concentrations of ethnic minorities, there is a tendency to describe the social contexts of home and school as strained and faltering, therefore, increasing at-risk factors of youth (Adams, 1999). Risk factors present at home and school have been specifically associated with substance abuse among Latino youth (Botvin et al., 2000b; Cabrera Strait, 1999; Chalk & Phillips, 1996). The influence of family, on the other hand, has been identified as a powerful protective factor against substance use (Herman et al., 1997; Howard, 1996;

Swaim et al., 1998), as has investment in school and good academic performance (Seydlita & Jenkins, 1998; McWhirter et al., 1998; Swaim et al., 1998) and involvement in after-school and religious activities (Mahoney & Stattin, 2000; Johanson et al., 1996). In addition, biculturalism and ethnic pride have been identified as strengthening the resiliency of Latino adolescents against drug abuse (Belgrave et al., 1997; Marsiglia et al., 2001; Marsiglia & Holleran, 1999; Kulis et al., 2000). Connectedness to home and school is hypothesized here to be a key protective factor against drug use (Seligman & Csikszentmihalyi, 2000).

The assumption is that despite the strains experienced by homes, schools, and communities, these social contexts play a protective role in preventing or reducing delinquent behavior through attachment and control (McWhirter et al., 1998; Seydlita & Jenkins, 1998; Smokowski et al., 1999). In other words, the purpose of this research is to explore how selected social contexts protect children against the stressors they encounter in their daily lives and keep them healthy (Newcomb & Bentler, 1988). The central question guiding this study is "What resiliency role do the social contexts of home and school play in the ability of Latino/a urban pre-adolescents in the Southwest to refuse drug offers?" This question will be explored from an ecological risk and resiliency perspective.

THEORETICAL APPROACH

The emphasis on families, schools, and communities follows an eco-systems perspective, which is fundamental to social work practice. The Ecological Risk and Resiliency Approach (Bogenschneider, 1996) will be followed because it takes into account the relationship between the individual and her/his social context, addressing both the risk and protective factors influencing behavioral outcomes. Researchers using this approach argue that greater attention should be paid to basic social conditions. Studies, they argue, need to contextualize individually based risk factors by examining what puts people at risk. Social factors such as ethnicity and culture are relevant to disease prevention and treatment because they influence access to important resources, including social support, and impact multiple disease outcomes, including drug abuse. Although membership in particular ethnic or geographic communities is not in itself a risk factor, it may influence access to both prevention resources and effective service delivery systems.

Bronfenbrenner's (1986) ecological risk and resiliency approach is used to examine the complex issues associated with the ability to resist drugs among Latino/a and other youth in the urban Southwest–a borderland population of mostly Mexican American heritage with strong cultural and language ties to Mexico and to Mexican American culture in the U.S. This ecosystem perspective considers structural factors that prove critical when differentiating drug use patterns, particularly within and between ethnic and racial groupings (Brunswick, 1999).

Resiliency is measured by the degree to which people (or communities) are productive and healthy despite hardships, traumas, and obstacles in their environmental (Bogenschneider, 1996). Personal attributes are important determinants of resiliency, but cultural factors are also important as they can amplify risks and resiliencies in the environment. The ecological risk and resiliency approach will be specifically applied to the study of a sample of Latino/a and other youth ability to refuse drugs.

LITERATURE REVIEW

Drug Use Among Latino Youth

Latinos/as are a heterogeneous umbrella group, and, as such, present many differences in terms of etiology of use, frequency of use, and drugs of choice (Cervantes et al., 1990/91). Because this study was conducted in the Southwest, the attention is focused on Mexicans and Mexican Americans. The Mexican American population has higher rates of heavy drinking and alcohol related problems than many other Latino subgroups (Cervantes et al., 1990/91). Mexican American women have higher rates of both abstinence and frequent heavy drinking than other Latinas, and the prevalence of alcoholism is higher among U.S.-born Mexican American women than among Mexican women immigrants (Aguirre-Molina & Caetano, 1994; Caetano, 1988). Mexican American adolescents with strong Mexican cultural identification are less likely than those with weaker ethnic identification to be regular users of tobacco, and more likely to believe that tobacco use is harmful (Casas et al., 1998). This pattern reflects several factors, including varying degrees of adherence to traditional Mexican substance use norms. Mexican culture holds strong social norms against drinking and drug abuse by women (Canino, 1994; Van Wilkinson, 1989); but tolerates heavy drinking for men, especially in rural areas (DeWalt, 1979; Madsen & Madsen, 1979).

Family Context as a Protective Factor

Perhaps the most important protective factor arising from Mexican American culture is *familism*, a cultural orientation in which the family of origin is of primary importance, even after marriage (Suarez-Orozco & Suarez-Orozco, 1995). Mexican and Mexican American families tend to have stronger family pride, family closeness, respect for parents, mutual obligation, trust and cohesion than non-Hispanic White families (Chandler et al., 1999, Olson et al., 1983). Traditional Mexican norms such as parental monitoring and involvement with children, and the tendency of married couples to settle close to parents and other family members, also act protectively as they provide children with more attention by a greater number of caring adults and situate children in more cohesive communities (Chandler et al., 1999; Denner, 2001; Gonzales, 1993).

On the other hand, migration can dislocate families and seriously limit their ability to rely upon relatives, compadres (ritualistic relatives), neighbors, and friends (Patterson & Marsiglia, 2000). The protective aspects of culture can also be weakened by acculturation and acculturation stress, resulting in vulnerability to drug use (Barnes, 1979; Beauvais, 1998; Bonnheim & Korman, 1985). Acculturation stress can weaken adolescents' connections with traditional support systems such as family. Recent immigrants who do not yet have the skills (such as language use) necessary to navigate the host society have a difficult time developing replacement sources of support in the new culture (Rogler, Cortes, & Malgady, 1991).

Despite the challenges associated with migration and acculturation, family context remains a vital factor associated with adolescent substance use (Resnick, 2000). Family strength (often called cohesiveness) and family sanctions against substance use are associated with youth resiliency against drug use (Howard, 1996; Swaim et al., 1998). On the other hand, family factors that promote adolescent substance use include perception of family use, actual family use, family discord, family separation, lack of family guidance, and absence of a father (Duncan et al., 1995; Friedman et al., 2000; Iannotti, 1996; Nurco et al., 1998; Smokowski, 1999). Many treatment and prevention strategies acknowledge the role of the family in substance use and abuse and include them in their interventions (Vega & Gil, 1998). However, the role of the family varies among groups, emerging as a diverse issue with differing impact on families–especially with regard to ethnic and racial differentials (Vega & Gil, 1998).

School Context as a Protective Factor

The role of schools in urban communities has been covered extensively in the literature (Agnew, 1999; Botvin, 2000; Resnick, 2000; Ripple & Luthar, 2000). Youth who drop out of school have higher rates of delinquency, drug use, theft, and violent crimes (Guagliardo et al., 1998; Obot & Anthony, 1999; Swaim et al., 1998). Communities that report high delinquency rates also record high truancy rates, low student educational performance, and low socioeconomic status (Farrington, 1992).

Schools and teachers provide physical care, ensure safety, develop social skills, reinforce pro-social behavior, and exercise control (Chazan, 1992). Since the 1930s, emphasis has been placed on the role of schools in curbing delinquent behaviors such as drug use (Everett, 1933). In general, student behaviors and attitudes reflect the degree of adjustment to the school environment. Positive school adjustment functions as a protective factor against drug using peer affiliation (Swaim et al., 1998). Recently the role of teachers in schools also has been linked to resiliency factors in adolescent drug use research (Smokowski, 1999). Understanding the way in which the described social contexts operate to shield Latino youth from drugs is vital in aiding youth, families, school personnel, and social work practitioners with their prevention efforts against the increase of substance use among adolescents.

METHODS

A mixed method research design guided the implementation of this study. Both quantitative and qualitative data were gathered and analyzed. Quantitative data were collected through the administration of surveys as part of a school-based intervention research project. This article reports only the quantitative data collected through a pretest survey administered at all schools (control and experimental) before a drug prevention experiment took place. The ethnographic or qualitative data were collected through recorded face-to-face interviews conducted by graduate students trained in ethnographic methods.

Sample

All 45 middle schools within a large size Southwestern city were recruited for the study, and 35 schools from 9 different school districts agreed to participate. Within these schools, every 7th grader was selected as a participant in the study. The 35 schools produced samples ranging in size from 56 to 725 students; their proportion of Mexican, Mexican-American, other Latino, and multi-ethnic Latino origin students ranged from 21.2% to 98.6%.

The total sample consisted of 6,035 students. Most of them (n = 3,318) were Mexican or Mexican American students, followed by 1,141 students of other Latino or multi-ethnic Latino origin (e.g., Mexican and White, Mexican and American Indian), 1,049 European American students, and 527 African American students. According to student responses, 74.3% qualified for a free school lunch and 8.0% qualified for reduced priced lunches. The 7th graders averaged 12.53 years of age (*SD* = .65 years; overall range of 9 to 18 years), with little age variability among the racial/ethnic groups.

The results reported in this article utilized a sub-sample of the total sample. Only student surveys from eight schools randomly selected to have an ethnographer were used in the analysis. There were 2,125 completed surveys in those eight schools and sixty of those students completing the survey were successfully matched with those interviewed by the ethnographers assigned to their school. Table 1 summarizes demographic data on the 2,125 student sub-sample and the sixty matched interviewees.

Survey Data

The surveys (each up to 82-items) utilized a three-form design (Graham, Hofer, & MacKinnon, 1996; Graham, Hofer, & Piccinin, 1994; Graham, Taylor, & Cumsille, 2001) using limited combinations of items to reduce the number of items each individual student received in his/her survey, while maximizing the total number of items available for later analysis. Students responded to demographic items (9 items); recent alcohol, cigarette, and marijuana use (6 items); anti-drug personal norms (3 items); descriptive norms (2 items); and anti-drug use intentions (3 items). The remainder of the 23 relevant items were distributed across three groups (A, B, and C) with each student receiving all questions from two of the three groups (i.e., A and B, B and C, or C and A). All of the main survey based scales of interest to this study ap-

TABLE 1. Demographic Overview

	Non-Inter-viewed Students		Interviewees			Non-Interviewed Students		Interviewees	
Gender	Percent	N	Percent	N	Free/Reduced Lunch	Percent	N	Percent	N
Male	52.6	1052	38.3	23	Free lunch	82.3	1719	62.1	36
Female	47.4	949	61.7	37	Reduced lunch	6.8	143	13.8	8
Total	100.0	2001	100.0	60	Neither reduced nor free	10.8	226	24.1	14
					Total	100.0	2088	100.0	58
Ethnicity	Percent	N	Percent	N	Home Language	Percent	N	Percent	N
Other Hispanic	3.5	73	3.4	2	English only	28.0	593	40.0	24
American Indian	3.7	77	10.3	6	Mostly English	10.1	214	13.3	8
Other Multi-Ethnic	4.0	83	13.8	8	Both English and Spanish, about equal	32.9	698	23.3	14
African-American	5.3	110	1.7	1	Mostly Spanish	10.2	217	6.7	4
Mexican Multi-Ethnic	11.0	226	8.6	5	Spanish only	16.9	358	13.3	8
Non-Hispanic White	11.1	228	12.1	7	Other language	1.9	40	3.3	2
Mexican/Chicano	61.3	1263	50.0	29	Total	100.0	2120	100.0	60
Total	100.0	2060	100.0	58					
Academic Goals	Percent	N	Percent	N	Self-Reported Grades	Percent	N	Percent	N
4 years of college	52.0	1100	59.3	35	Mostly A's	9.1	192	13.6	8
2 years of college	22.5	476	28.8	17	A's and B's	33.0	696	45.8	27
Trade/vocational school	2.6	55	3.4	2	Mostly B's	9.0	190	3.4	2
High school	19.7	417	6.8	4	B's and C's	27.6	583	22.0	13
8th grade	3.3	69	1.7	1	Mostly C's	5.8	122	3.4	2
Total	100.0	2117	100.0	59	C's and D's	10.7	226	6.8	4
					Mostly D's	1.2	26	1.7	1
					D's and F's	3.0	64	3.4	2
					Mostly F's	0.6	12	0.0	0
					Total	100.0	2111	100.0	59

pear acceptably to highly reliable, including recent substance use (α = .89), parent injunctive norms (α = .73), friend injunctive norms (α = .82), personal norms (α = .84), self-efficacy (α = .78), personal intentions (α = .84), and substance use expectancies (α = .77).

University trained proctors administered the 45-minute survey, (one form containing both English and Spanish versions) during regular school hours in science, health, or homeroom classes, with the students in a few schools assembled together for survey administration. Table 1 presents a basic demographic profile of the students who were interviewed and all their school peers in the eight selected schools that completed the survey.

Ethnographic Data

Narratives were gathered using structured questions designed to explore the students' forms of understanding situational and temporal contexts. The narratives, in addition to serving as mirrors of reality, represented the actual mode of thinking used in the students' everyday life (Widdershoven, 1993). The interviewers utilized a semi-structured interview guide, which focused on youth culture and how youth respond to substance use situations. Multiple interviewers at the eight schools utilized the same interview guide to elicit narration by the interviewees. The narratives shared by the adolescents provide an insiders' perspective into the protective and risk factors present in their homes, schools, and neighborhoods, and the impact of these factors on drug use. Because the ethnographers had prior experience in the schools, a pre-established contextual knowledge and rapport existed. Twenty interviewees were randomly selected from each of the eight schools. Some of the key questions used in the interviews were: "Can you tell me a story about drugs in your life, in your friends' lives, in your family or in your neighborhood? If you needed some help getting out of a situation that involved drugs, alcohol, or cigarettes, who would you go to? How would your friends have acted in that situation? Who do you hang out with at school? Are they the same people you hang out with when you're not at school?"

Of the original pool of 160 students, interviews were conducted with a total of 141. From the 141 interviews, 60 were successfully matched with the survey data using the students' initials and birth dates. Using hermeneutical analysis techniques, emergent themes were drawn from the interviews and coded using NUD*IST software, version 4.0. The emergent themes form the foundation of the qualitative findings.

Mixed Method Procedures

The two sources of data were used to inform and complement each other. The survey data provided insight into the phenomenon through aggregate data or the "what," while the ethnographic data aimed at providing meaning or the "why" and "how." All the survey respondents were selected from the eight schools from which interviewees were drawn (N = 2,125). Interview responses then were matched to individual surveys, resulting in 60 clear matches. General descriptive statistics of the interviewed population were compared to those of the non-interviewed school population. T-tests were conducted to compare the mean scores of survey respondents that were interviewed with the responses of the rest of the survey respondents who were not interviewed by the ethnographers. In order to protect the anonymity of the participants, only gender and age information will be provided when referring to a particular student; no names will be used.

FINDINGS

Descriptive Statistics

When descriptive statistics were compared, distinctions emerged between the 60 matched cases of students who completed both the written survey and the in-person interview, and the 2,065 students who simply answered the survey but were not interviewed. Those interviewed were found to be disproportionately female, English speakers, and with above average grades. Because the selection process for the intensive interviews required an additional signed parental consent form to be returned to the school, the authors surmise that female students, and students with better attendance records, were more likely to comply, and that their parents would be more likely to allow their children to participate and return the required extra consent forms. Additionally, when ethnicity and socioeconomic status were considered, as measured by the proxy of free or reduced lunch eligibility, those interviewed were less likely to be Mexican/Chicano (though more likely to be American Indian or Non-Hispanics Multi-ethnic) and less likely to receive either free or reduced lunch subsidies. Finally, there were differences in the long-term academic aspirations of those interviewed; they were more likely to indicate post-secondary education plans than the general population of the schools from which they were drawn. As our results show, the interview subjects also differed based on the attachment, commitment, and involvement with their families and schools. The survey respondents and the smaller number of interviewees provide a glimpse into the risk and resiliency spectrum present within the overall sample. The narratives, in particular, are a rich exemplar of how the students' home, school and neighborhood contexts were supporting their resiliency.

t-tests were used to determine whether the mean values of core drug use related variables were significantly different between those who were interviewed and the other students in their schools. The interviewees presented fewer risk factors and more protective factors than the non-interviewed sub sample (see Table 2).

Drug use profiles for all respondents showed that the majority of students–both those interviewed and those not interviewed–reported no use of alcohol, cigarettes or marijuana in the recent past, and they agreed that alcohol use was inappropriate at their age. While both groups of students showed low levels of drug use in the aggregate, differences between the interviewees and non-interviewees were, however, statistically significant in many instances. Importantly, in all measures of last 30-day use of alcohol, marijuana, and cigarettes, and lifetime use of alcohol and marijuana, interviewees were found to use significantly less than other non-interviewed survey respondents. This difference may be due to the need for an additional parental consent for the interview participants. This distinction in drug use resiliency is also apparent in the ethnographic interviews.

Although the interviews were conducted with a relatively low at-risk group, the transcripts provide valuable insights into the experiences and understandings of the participating youth. The following section will focus on data gathered from the 60 students completing the written survey and the intensive interview. The results were organized around overarching themes emerging from the survey and ethnographic data sets.

Resiliency Themes Emerging in Families, Schools, and Neighborhoods

The Family Context

Survey results reported by the students who were also interviewed by ethnographers highlight the importance of family as a protective factor and the themes of resiliency emerging from the narratives about family life support. Both sources of data support the premise that social bonding and resilience resulted from attachment, commitment, and involvement with family. In examining these survey findings, it is important to remember that students received at random three somewhat different forms of the questionnaire containing the pertinent family survey items. Only about two-thirds of the 60 student interviewees answered each of

TABLE 2. T-Tests of Mean Differences on Drug Use Related Survey Items, Comparing Interviewees and Non-Interviewees

	Students Not-Interviewed			Interviewees				
Core Variables	N	Mean	Std. Error of Mean	N	Mean	Std. Error of Mean	t-statistic	sig.
# Drinks in entire life	2049	3.234	0.052	59	2.915	0.240	−1.696	*
# Cigarettes in entire life	2054	2.314	0.045	60	2.167	0.233	−0.783	
# Marijuana "hits" in entire life	2043	1.726	0.034	59	1.373	0.145	−3.190	***
Used smokeless tobacco ever (Yes = 1; No = 0)	2052	1.063	0.006	60	1.100	0.052	0.813	
Used crack, LSD, downers, etc., ever (Yes = 1; No = 0)	2054	1.078	0.007	60	1.083	0.043	0.151	
Used uppers (speed) ever (Yes = 1; No = 0)	2053	1.061	0.007	60	1.083	0.049	0.525	
Used inhalants ever (Yes = 1; No = 0)	2047	1.244	0.012	59	1.169	0.049	−2.010	*
# Alcohol drinks last 30 days	2049	1.861	0.037	60	1.617	0.168	−1.865	*
Frequency used alcohol last 30 days	2044	1.433	0.022	60	1.267	0.082	−2.755	***
# Cigarettes last 30 days	2051	1.349	0.023	59	1.153	0.079	−3.482	***
Frequency used cigarettes in last 30 days	2052	1.246	0.017	59	1.068	0.048	−5.905	***
# Marijuana "hits" in last 30 days	2043	1.581	0.034	59	1.237	0.119	−4.019	***
Frequency used marijuana in last 30 days	2041	1.350	0.022	59	1.186	0.092	−2.349	**
Drinking at your age OK	2047	3.292	0.019	59	3.288	0.114	−0.042	
Smoking at your age OK	2046	3.380	0.018	59	3.458	0.103	0.910	
Marijuana at your age OK	2045	3.373	0.020	58	3.569	0.099	2.498	**
Likelihood of accepting future alcohol offer	2040	1.784	0.018	59	1.644	0.099	−1.738	*
Likelihood of accepting future cigarette offer	2040	1.620	0.016	59	1.559	0.088	−0.846	
Likelihood of accepting future marijuana offer	2026	1.630	0.019	59	1.390	0.087	−3.544	***
Estimation of # of other students who tried drugs once	2030	1.275	0.014	59	2.373	0.128	9.669	***
Estimation of # of regular drug users in your school	2024	2.081	0.022	58	2.931	0.115	9.116	***
Estimation of regular participation in drug use by classmates	1987	2.506	0.050	58	2.672	0.304	0.657	

*** $\alpha = 0.005$
** $\alpha = 0.01$
* $\alpha = 0.05$

the family items. Their responses express a high degree of attachment and connectedness to their parents, complemented by strong parental authority and control (see Table 3).

Most of the interviewee respondents who answered the relevant family items (84%) identified themselves as being "close" or "very close" to their parents and feeling that their parents were proud of them most of the time (50%). The survey results demonstrated that parents, especially mothers, played a strong role in educating these students about drugs. Seventy-three percent (73%) indicated that their parents have taught them the most about the consequences of using drugs. Parental

TABLE 3. Attachment and Parental Authority as Reported by Interviewees on Written Survey[1]

Attachment/Connectedness					
	A little close	Neutral	Close	Very close	
Closeness to parents (N = 40)	3 (8%)	7 (18%)	13 (33%)	17 (43%)	
	Strongly Disagree	Disagree	Agree	Strongly Agree	
Feel I belong in this school (N = 29)	1 (3%)	3 (10%)	10 (34%)	15 (52%)	
	No one	Media	School	Friends	DadMom
Who taught R about drugs (N = 33)	4 (12%)	1 (3%)	3 (9%)	1 (3%)	24 (73%)
	Never	Almost never	Sometimes	Often	Most of the time
Freq. parents proud of you (N = 36)	0	4 (11%)	8 (22%)	6 (17%)	18 (50%)
Parental Authority					
	All of the time	Sometimes	Never		
Parents allow R to drink at parties (N = 40)	1(3%)	9 (23%)	30 (75%)		
	Never	Almost never	Sometimes	Often	Most of the time
Freq. parents question where R goes (N = 35)	0	0	2 (6%)	4 (11%)	29 (83%)
	Never	Almost never	Sometimes	Often	Most of the time
Freq. parents set time R comes home (N = 39)	0	2 (5%)	9 (23%)	11 (35%)	17 (44%)
	Never	Almost never	Sometimes	Often	Most of the time
Freq. parents forbid activities (N = 31)	1 (3%)	13 (42%)	7 (23%)	4 (12%)	6 (14%)
	Never	Almost never	Sometimes	Often	Most of the time
Freq. parent allows R to go out (N = 30)	3 (10%)	4 (13%)	15 (50%)	3 (10%)	5 (17%)
	Not angry at all	A little angry	Pretty angry	Very angry	
Parent's reaction if R had alcohol (N = 36)	1 (3%)	1 (3%)	4 (11%)	30 (83%)	
	Not angry at all	A little angry	Pretty angry	Very angry	
Parent's reaction if R smoked cigarettes (N = 35)	2 (6%)	2 (6%)	3 (9%)	28 (79%)	
	Not angry at all	A little angry	Pretty angry	Very angry	
Parent's reaction if R smoked marijuana (N = 36)	0	4 (11%)	4 (11%)	28 (80%)	

*Note all percentages are rounded to the nearest whole percent

1. Because of the multiple form structure of the survey questionnaire, one-third or more of the interviewees were not asked each of these questions

authority was demonstrated by the fact that the majority (74%) of respondents' parents never allowed them to drink at parties, reinforced boundaries by questioning them about where they were going (83%), and set time limits (72%). On the other hand, most interviewee respondents (77%) indicated that their parents allowed them to go out and less than half of them were regularly forbidden to do certain activities (49%). Finally, respondents overwhelmingly believed that their parents would be very angry if they were to drink alcohol (83%), smoke cigarettes (79%), or use marijuana (78%).

The survey results present the interviewee respondents as youth closely connected with their parents, with whom they appear to share a sense of trust and maintain good communication. The ethnographic data confirm and further explain the survey results. The majority of youth who were interviewed identified a strong influence of social control and few reports of strain in the immediate family. The strongest influence of social control was parental influence on drug use, including the connectedness with mothers as the most commonly reported bond. Three main resiliency themes emerged from the ethnographic data within the realm of family context; they were: (1) Parental control, (2) Parental support, and (3) Shared time.

1. Parental control. Parental control was identified in many forms, such as parents setting boundaries and parents reinforcing expected behaviors. An example of these practices is found in the following comment.

> I'd probably go to my parents, and they'd probably be mad at me. But, kinda like, in a way they'll be mad at you, but then they'll kinda be happy that you told them so they can help you out. That's a parenting thing that a parent will understand. But my friends, I don't know. I guess they'd help me if I had helped them. Hopefully, but. . . . To get help, like to get real help, I'd have to go to my parents 'cause I know they'll still love me then. They care about me. (Male, age 13)

In general, setting boundaries was described as parents getting upset, setting clear rules, being disappointed, or punishing unacceptable behavior. When was asked if he would go along with friends who were doing something he did not approve, a 14 year old male replied, "No. Because I wouldn't want to do that . . . They [my parents] would tell me not to do bad things." A 13 year old female responded to the same question by saying, "No. Because my Mom will get mad. Because they don't like for me to do bad stuff." Parental positive reinforcement of prosocial behavior was described frequently as praise as well as more affective responses of "being happy" or "being glad." The youth more often identified positive reinforcement than they did boundary setting.

2. *Parental support*. The theme of parental support emerged out of the written surveys and the students' narratives describing their help seeking behaviors. For example, parents were the most common response to the survey question about whom you would go to if you had a problem with drugs. In their narratives as in their survey responses (see Table 3), parents were mentioned as the first source of help and advice.

> I think, my Mom. Because I can tell her anything and she just goes along with it, and she helps me, and all that. (Female, age 13)

> My parents. They would probably talk to me about it; my friends; that they might be like. . . . How did they do it? (Female, age 14)

Other interviewees explicitly chose their parents over other adults in their lives. They talked about trust, using phrases like "they care about me." Both adolescent females and males offered the following observations about their parents as being available and trustworthy,

> [I'd talk] with a teacher that comes here for that, or if not, maybe I would tell my parents or someone I trust. Mmm, I think it's better with my parents because they know what they're going do better than the teachers, but I trust my parents more, to . . . to talk to them. (Female, age 14)

> Well, first, I think I'd go to my parents 'cause, you know, they're always. . . . They're always defending me and, you know, they've taught me everything so far, so I'd pretty much go to my parents. Yeah, 'cause, you know. . . they would help me. (Female, age 13)

> I'd go to my Mom and my Dad because most of the time they're really always. . . . All the time, they're really always there for me. So, I would just go and I'll tell them what's going on and they'll pray about it and then . . . Like, pretty soon they'll have the answer to what's right or what's wrong. (Male, age 14)

Although the students mentioned their parents as their primary source of advice, their stories mostly involved their mothers. For example,

> I'd have to say my Mom 'cause if my Dad. . . . I know he'll yell and scream at me. Like, "You done this. You never told me." Blah, blah, blah. And like make it all bad. And, "Your body's gonna be all different" and "You're gonna get all new friends." But my Mom, I don't think she'll tell my Dad. It's like . . . If anything really bad happens to me, she'll try to see if she can help. With my Mom. . . . I can talk to her when I want to talk to her. And, like, you know, she's a woman and so it's like easier to talk to her. 'Cause my Dad. . . . Some of my friends, they live with their Dad 'cause their Mom got divorced, and I think it's pretty hard to talk . . . I mean, if it's a man, you know? (Female, age 13)

Both adolescent males and females seem to rely mostly on their mothers for help and advice, however, other family members were mentioned as sources of support and help and as role models. Such was the case below. When asked whom would he go to for help, the student replied:

> Probably my brother 'cause he would like back me up. Yeah. He's 18 and he would help me, like, to read the situation and would probably tell me how it's very important to talk to him, and [ask me] why are you doing that and . . . (Male, age 14)

As this quote illustrates, older siblings were sometimes described by the interviewees as performing parental roles. There was a complete absence of any reliance on professional or institutionalized forms of help.

3. *Shared time*. The majority of the students identified their out of school socialization as taking place within the family's sphere of influence. Mothers were once more identified as the main person with whom they shared unstructured time outside of the school. One female respondent gave an example of this practice by saying: "I stay home. I help my Mom at home." Another added,

> Most of the time on weekends, I don't hang out with them [friends]. Only like when we go somewhere together. But, most of the weekend I spend time with my Mom or something to do with family. (Female, age 13)

Commonly, after-school socialization included family members such as cousins and siblings: "just my sister and me hang around when we are not in school" (Female, age 14). Sharing time with non-family members is heavily scrutinized as illustrated by the following vignette.

> 'Cause, my parents . . . they are so protective of me. They don't want me to go to my friend's house because they might . . . Like my friend. . . . Me and my best friend Lisa, we went to the mall and my Mom didn't know that we're best friends yet, and then she wouldn't let me go to the mall with her Dad because she wasn't sure he wouldn't try kidnaping me. And so, I think. . . . She's really protective of me. (Female, age 13)

The rest of the students participating in the ethnographic component of the study appear to be enjoying a close and rewarding relationship with their parents especially their mothers. Their parents are available to them, provide the support students feel they need and at the same time communicate clear messages in terms of what is and what is not permissible.

The School Context

The school context also proved to be important in social support and bonding. Most survey respondents (87%) expressed a strong sense of belonging to school (see Table 3). Teachers were identified as key players in supporting a sense of belonging and social bonding. However, drug offers and drug use frequently occurred in school. Next to parents, the teacher was the person a youth most likely would seek out if they had a problem with drugs.

> I would go to a teacher or to an adult because you don't know what they are going to do to you. They can hold you and take you for treatment. (Male, age 14)

Teachers were identified as a good alternative to parents, especially for students coming from very strict homes.

> I'd be scared to death to go to my family, so I wouldn't go to them [parents] first. I'd probably like ask one of my teachers for help. Like, "I don't . . . I want to stop, but I can't . . ." And if they could help me, then I might go to my family. I have a pretty good relationship with all of my teachers. (Female, age 13)

The respondents also reported several examples of teachers' use of modeling and discipline–how a teacher handled drugs in the classroom.

> Last week a group of boys were using drugs and I told a teacher that they were using it, and they got them and they were looking for the drugs, and they couldn't find it. And a boy threw it into a trash and the teacher found it. And I was glad because I thought they were going to do something to me. [And later] I remember when we were gonna make cookies at life skills class, and the kids–I don't know what happened or anything–but the teacher opened one of them, and they caught him, and they were putting marijuana in the cookies. (Female, age 14)

Yet, the youth maintained school norms, illustrated by instances in which several youth reported drugs or drug use to school officials. Those instances were followed by positive reinforcement by authority figures. Many of the respondents stated that there was drug use in school, but only a few identified offers. Several youth reported drug use by peers to a school authority. Below is an illustration of these practices supported by a positive social structure despite the presence of drugs.

> Last year I had this friend that had brought weed, and he gave it away so we could take care of it. He had gotten caught, and they sent him to the office. We talked to my teacher and the principal. That was about it. Yes. We threw it away and later on we thought there would be more, like the people that hang out with them. We got it and put it into this paper. So we went to the teacher, and she took us to the principal. They suspended him. (Female, 14 years old)

Youth identified school personnel next to the police as the adults they would go to if they had a problem with drugs. When asked whom he would go to for help one 13 year old male responded, "To the police . . . the teacher or the principal." When asked the same question, another male student replied, "The counselors from school, because I don't know them, and I prefer to speak with someone I don't know, because if I spoke with someone I did know, I would feel ashamed." Several youth identified the counselor or principal, but more often they named their teacher. Counselors and principals were mentioned as more anonymous sources of help. As stated above, going to the family and in some cases the teacher (seen in a familial light) would bring "shame" to the family name. This type of helping seeking behavior seems to be an unintended consequence of "familismo." Strong identification with family and family honor may prevent some youth from asking for help out of respect to the family.

Although the school experienced both the presence of drugs, and drug offers, the risks were minimized by the social support of the school structure and the social bonding and modeling by the adults within the school. The school context allowed learning opportunities for youth to address drug issues within a strong pro-social supportive environment while, at the same time, providing institutional reinforcement for pro-social behaviors.

The After-School Context

The school was described by the interviewees as a social context nurturing resiliency. By contrast, the after-school context lacked positive social structures and relied solely on the strong social support of the family system. There was a significant absence of opportunity for social bonding outside of the students' families. Most of the participants reported that they did not play outside or have friends in their neighborhood, and only one youth identified going to community center activities. The great majority of the youth did not have after-school peer socialization opportunities and, in many cases, did not have permission to leave the house once home from school. These responses illustrated that strong parental control focused on protectiveness and safety concerns. For example:

> I can't go out on school days. I go out on Saturdays and Sundays because that is when my Mom lets me go out on my bike. I go around here. She doesn't let me go anywhere else. Every time I ask her, she wants me to tell her the address and everything. If something comes up, she goes and picks me up. (Male, 13 years old)

Other respondents described similar situations: "At home I'm, like totally over protected. Can't really go anywhere. So, I just hang out with my next-door neighbor" (Male, 14 year old). "No . . . No, I do not have friends outside of school. I do not play outside of school. Because no, they do not let me go out a lot. I never leaves my home" (Female, 14 years old). "My parents don't let me. They are afraid. I stay at home. I do my chores like clean and mop and I also do my homework" (Female, 13 years old).

Other youth identified two separate peer groups for leisure time. In most instances, the reason was due to proximity of homes and the protectiveness/safety issue. "I have different friends in my neighborhood. I just hang around with them and I go outside and play kick ball and stuff" (Female, 14 years old). When asked why she had different friends she responded:

> I live kind of far from them. Like some of them live in trailers and I live over here. Like on 1st Avenue. . . And that is why, because my dad won't let me go anywhere. Well they don't let me go on the streets because my dad says that's bad. That it's bad because I could do something like smoke or something can happen to me. Like people, you know how there is bad people around? They can grab me and rape me. Bad stuff can happen on the street.

When asked why his peer and school group was the same, the respondent replied, "Cause they live close to me, they are just school friends." A 14 year old female respondent reported that, for her, it is easier to have just one big group of friends.

> Because it's just easier. I mean, it's easier if you have like one group of friends than if you have like one here, then at home, you have a group, and then, you know, what you have here and everything. So, if you just have one big group, it's much easier.

Although some students said they go out with the same groups and had after-school socialization opportunities, a factor even for these youth was the role of family in outside-of-school socialization. Students specifically noted that out-of-school time with friends was limited. For example: "When I am at home, I usually don't hang out with all of them. At school I hang out with most of them, not at home. At home I usually hang out with my sister or my cousins, my family. We play mostly at school, but sometimes at our houses" (Male, 13 years old).

The lack of involvement with community centers and city parks was almost universal. Only one youth mentioned going to community centers after school. This student said that he went to the YMCA. However, many youth noted that they did not play outside or have friends in the neighborhood. Only a few youth mentioned that they went to the park to play. One of the reasons for that may be the presence of gangs. A 14 year old male student gave one instance: "I used to hang out with gang members. . . . Every time I go to the park, I see them over there writing their signs and saying stuff." One of the main reasons that the students reported minimal or no peer relationships outside of school was due to safety concerns and the protective nature of their parents. These reactions resulted from the strain produced in the neighborhood. In fact, a few youth reported that their families moved out of neighborhoods, providing examples of parental social control. A student provided an example:

> Well in our neighborhood, we want to move out of our neighborhood because there are a lot of people that go there to buy drugs in the apartments that we live in. My dad is trying to find a house for us to move into because our current neighborhood is very dangerous and there is a lot of gunfire there. I hardly ever leave my house. Or I run if I am going to a friend's house or I am taken. That is why they want to move because they say it's very dangerous for us. (Female, 13 years old)

Home and school appear to be perceived by parents and students as connected and relatively safe. After school activities are not available to them or are not accessible. Unstructured time outside of the home is not part of the experience of this group of students.

Risks Factors Present in Families, Schools, and Neighborhoods

Students, at times, encountered family environments where there was drug use or where they were using. One student described such an experience: "Uh, my Mom. . . . My Mom did drugs and my Step-Dad did drugs. I'm not sure about my Step-Dad. My Mom's doing them now" (Male, 14 years old). The risk factors present in neighborhoods and the impact of those factors on the substance use of a family also were apparent in the following perspective:

> In my neighborhood they do a lot of drugs and things happen. In my family too . . . My grandma's son, he does a lot of drugs too. My sister too. My sister tried to get me into it, and I didn't really like it. My brother too and that same day I got into it and after two days, I got out of it. I felt very bad and I told my grandma. When I do things I tell my grandma, because I tell her everything. I told her, "you know grandma I did something bad and I wasn't supposed to do it; it was the wrong thing, I know it can mess up my mind and I can't do things in school like think or nothing." I told her. Now my

> family doesn't do that no more. In the neighborhood, people go by, and go to that house where they sell drugs. (Female, 13 years old)

This response touches on many of the aspects of family influences, both risk and resiliency. But for this respondent, it was the parental figure of her grandmother that changed her actions to pro-social behaviors.

Most commonly, families were described as playing a role at ameliorating the risk of drug use. Once students or their families become engaged in risk behaviors, the boundaries between the different social contexts become more diffused. A student offered an example of the crossing over effects of risk and resiliency when the interviewer asked about any personal experiences with drugs.

> A long time ago, before I started going to church, I used to do a lot of drugs. And, I wasn't really like going to school a lot. I would like to stay home and do like really bad stuff. Like do drugs and stuff. (Male, 14 years old)

He mentioned that he had not attended school when he was involved with drugs. The absence of the school attachment was a contributing factor to his drug use. When questioned about his mother's response, he continued,

> I would get in a lot of trouble. And, I would always tell her that I really didn't care about anything, and she would tell me that, "You better start caring 'cause one of these days, you might get caught and go to jail." And I kept on telling her, "So?" and "I don't care." and "Just leave me alone. I'm gonna go out and go to my friends." And she would try to keep me in the house so I wouldn't go out and do anything wrong anymore.

This respondent also described how important his step-father was to his sense of parental support, and explained how he would seek both his mother's and step-father's advice if he were in trouble.

> Most of the time, they are there for me. When I do right, they'll be proud of me. But, when I do wrong, I know I did wrong so I like. . . . I just stay in the room for a couple . . . for a while and just think about what I did and then I'll go in and apologize to them because I know they'll feel bad. But then, my Step-dad, he used to. . . . He

> goes to church. And he talked to me, and I started going to church, and he got married to my Mom, and just because, now that he got to me, I stopped doing that stuff. Now, I go to church and everything. I go to my Mom and my Dad because most of the time they're really always . . . All the time, they're really always there for me. So, I would just go and I'll tell them what's going on and . . . And they'll pray about it and then . . . like, pretty soon they'll have the answer to what's right or what's wrong.

This quote also highlights the role of after-school involvement with a community institution. The role of the church as a source of social support is clearly apparent in this narrative. The threat of jail was not identified as a deterrent, yet the investment of a family member, his step-dad, and involvement with his church steered the youth away from drugs.

DISCUSSION

These findings confirm other research identifying family bonding and school commitment as sources of resiliency for Latino youth (Cabrera Strait, 1999; Marsiglia & Holleran, 1999; Robertson et al., 1998: Swaim et al., 1998). The neighborhoods of the large Southwestern city where the study took place are characterized by a demographic explosion, with a growing Latino population, high poverty rates, high mobility rates, and high drug use rates. Yet youth are still resistant to substance use offers. Thus, the common belief that high poverty and minority concentrations increase the likelihood of substance use does not fit in this case. This study defies these commonly held notions, which are often utilized to perpetuate myths and stereotypes of minority and impoverished populations.

The after school context presented the surprising finding that a majority of the interviewed youth did not socialize with their same school peer group after school, or they did not have a peer group after school. Often the youth said that this was due to the dangers of their neighborhood context, such as gangs. Moreover, only one youth mentioned involvement in after school institutions such as community centers, boy/girl scouts, and church groups. Involvement in structured activities is a key component in drug use prevention (Mahoney & Stattin, 2000), yet this is absent in the interviews with these youth.

The presence and strength of families in these youths' lives emerged as the cornerstone of their resiliency (Akers & Lee, 1999). The family provides the youth with advice, direction, modeling, and support when it comes to drug use and other deviant behaviors. The family represents the foundation of resiliency in the lives of this predominately Latino/a youth sample. The school functioned as a protective institution in the resiliency of these youth. The school provided structured support, discipline, and modeling of pro-social behaviors for these youth.

The strong ties to school and family protected these youth and counterbalanced the risks present in their neighborhoods. The school, and particularly the families, provided a social bond and support that was fundamental to the resilience of these youth. The presence of opportunity and risks in this urban setting was countered by the commitment of these youth to family and school. The schools and families reciprocated this commitment in their support and reinforcement of the youth's pro-social behaviors.

Limitations

The participants were mostly pre-adolescents, at a developmental stage where experimentation with drugs increases rapidly. The protective effects of family and school may or may not continue as these youths grow older and more detached from family and teachers. Because both the survey and ethnographic data sets used in this analysis are cross-sectional, the study lacks longitudinal and developmental comparisons. Follow-up interviews and follow-up surveys may capture the developmental changes, and the students' adjustments to them. Resiliency may continue as documented or may begin to switch to peer groups. These changes need to be understood and anticipated to effectively support them.

In some key respects, the matched group of 60 interviewees was not completely representative of the larger group of 2,125 students surveyed at the eight schools. The interviewees were more resilient and less at-risk than their classmates. Although they were originally randomly selected, the additional parental permission slips made the sub-sample less representative and the matching to completed surveys reduced their numbers further in some analyses reported here. Students with poor attendance records (and probably higher drug use) were less likely to be included among the interviewees. To be included they needed to be at school during both data gathering activities and have actively participated in obtaining their parents' signed permission. These facts limit the generalizability of the mixed-method findings. The ethnographic data cannot be generalized to the larger sample or other middle school students. In future studies, innovative approaches may need to be developed to more effectively reach the at-risk student population at the same time that human subject procedures are observed.

Implications

The implication for social work practice is that the emphasis on the family is fundamental in interventions targeting Latino/a youth. Additionally the implication of inclusion of family in clinical work with Latino/a youth regarding substance use/abuse is essential. Future social work research in this area should focus on the strengths present within minority families and communities rather than emphasizing the negative stereotypes. Addressing the issue of minority youth substance abuse in an urban context requires a unification of cultural competency, strengths based practice, and global ethnographic questions (Dewees, 2001).

On the macro level, the placement of institutional support for the Latino/a families is essential to enhancing youth resiliency. Another vital element is the impact of schools in creating attachment and commitment with the youth. Schools influence youth investment in academics, with a majority of the youth in this study seeing college in their future. The school on a mezzo level serves to create social bonds that resist the strains of the urban context and lack of community activities. The school is a vital link between the community and the family system and has tremendous potential for intervention strategies. The call for social work is to develop and enhance this linkage through expanding social work practices within school settings.

The absence of after-school opportunity is a profound finding, and rather disturbing. The lack of this macro support structure is a key element that should not be overlooked or ignored by social workers. This finding begs the question, why are there no after school opportunities in these communities of need? Critical evaluation of this finding needs to address where in the city are the after school resources, why are they there, and why are they not in these communities? The revelation from these questions may call for social workers to advocate change in the allocation of resources by local governments. If, in fact, the neighborhoods have after school services, the question will change to why do Latino students not use them? Issues of access and equity may need to be addressed.

The recommendations offered as a result of this analysis highlight several possibilities for social workers to strengthen the social bond that already exists between the students and their families and schools, and to create and increase the community bonding opportunities that were absent in these findings. For example one major recommendation that stems from this research is that prevention programs should target families, schools and communities as partners in the intervention strategies. The role of community organizers and school social workers would be indispensable in the development of such programs.

A key role social workers can play is the role of cultural mediator (Marsiglia & Holleran, 1999). As such, social workers will provide services that nurture and maintain the protective effects of family and culture of origin as youth go through the acculturation process. Lowering the negative consequences of acculturation stress on the youth and assisting them in maintaining their protective ties to family and culture of origin could have great prevention impact on youth.

A possible concrete step in that direction would be to create Family Centers in schools–welcoming places where families could access resources, support and educational groups, information and referral services, activities for youth and families, and family assistance programs. Such collaborative efforts also should target and reinforce youth attachment and family commitment to schools and communities. The lack of after school activities leaves a need for social workers to advocate for the development of after school programs and community centers in these neighborhoods. These recommendations emphasize ways to strengthen the resilient social bond with both school and family that was found in the study, and to increase the community bonding that was absent in the findings. These would enhance the web of protective factors already present within families and schools, as well as adding an important strand of community bonding.

REFERENCES

Adams, G. (1999). Introduction: At-Risk adolescents. *Journal of Adolescent Research, 14*(1), 7-9.

Agnew, R. (1999). A general strain theory of community differences in crime rates. *Journal of Research in Crime and Delinquency*, 36(2), 123-155.

Aguirre-Molina, M. & Caetano, R. (1994). Alcohol Use and Related Issues. In: Molina, C. & Aguirre-Molina, M. (Eds.), *Latino Health in the US: A Growing Challenge* (pp. 393-424). American Public Health Association: Washington, D.C.

Akers, R. & Lee, G. (1999). Age, social learning, and social bonding in adolescent substance use. *Deviant Behavior: An Interdisciplinary Journal*, 19, 1-25.

Barnes, G. E. (1979). Solvent abuse: A review. *International Journal of the Addictions*, 14, 1-26.

Bauman, A. & Phongsavan, P. (1999). Epidemiology of substance use in adolescence; prevalence, trends and policy implications. *Drug and Alcohol Dependence*, 55, 187-207.

Beauvais, F. (1998). Cultural identification and substance use in North America–An annotated bibliography. *Substance Use and Misuse*, 33, 6, 1315-1336.

Belgrave, F., Townsend, T., Cherry, V., & Cunningham, D. (1997). The influence of Afrocentric worldview and demographic variables on drug knowledge, attitudes, and use among African American youth. *Journal of Community Psychology*, 25(5), 421-433.

Bogenschneider, K. (1996). An ecological risk/protective theory for building prevention programs, policies, and community capacity to support youth. *Family Relations*, 45, 127-138.

Bonnheim, M.L. & Korman, M. (1985). Family interaction and acculturation in Mexican-American inhalant users. *Journal of Psychoactive Drugs*, 17(1), 25-33.

Botvin, G. (2000). Preventing drug abuse in schools: Social and competence enhancement approaches targeting individual level etiologic factors. *Addictive Behaviors*, 25(6), 887-897.

Botvin, G., Griffin, K., Diaz, T. & Ifill-Williams, M. (2000b). Drug abuse prevention among minority adolescents: Posttest and one year follow up of a school-based preventive intervention. *Prevention Science*, 2(1), 1-13.

Botvin, G., Griffin, K., Diaz, T., Scheier, L., Williams, C. & Epstein, J. (2000a). Preventing illicit drug use in adolescents: Long-term follow-up data from a randomized control trial of a school population. *Addictive Behaviors*, 25 (5), 769-774.

Bronfenbrenner, U. (1986). Ecology of the family as context for human development: Research perspectives. *Developmental Psychology*, 22, 723-742.

Brunswick, A. (1999). Structural strain: An ecological paradigm for studying African American drug use. In M. De La Rosa, B. Segal & R. Lopez (Eds.). *Conducting drug abuse research with minority populations: Advances and issues* (pp. 3-19). New York, NY: The Haworth Press, Inc.

Cabrera Strait, Saki. (1999). Drug use among Hispanic youth: Examining common and unique contributing factors. *Hispanic Journal of Behavioral Sciences*, 21(1), 89-104.

Caetano, R. (1988). Alcohol use among Hispanic groups in the United States. *American Journal of Drug and Alcohol Abuse*, 14(3), 293-308.

Canino, G. (1994). Alcohol use and misuse among Hispanic women: Selected factors, processes, and studies. *International Journal of the Addictions*, 29(9), 1083-1100.

Casas, J.M., Bimbela, A., Corral, C.V., Yanez, I., Swaim, R.C., Wayman, J.C., & Bates, S. (1998). Cigarette and Smokeless Tobacco Use among Migrant and Non-immigrant Mexican American Youth. *Hispanic Journal of Behavioral Sciences*, 20, 102-121.

Cervantes, R.C., Gilbert, M.J., DeSnyder, N.S., & Padilla, A.M. (1990/91). Psychosocial and cognitive correlates of alcohol use in younger adult immigrant and U.S.-born Hispanics. *International Journal of the Addictions*, 25, 687-708.

Chalk, R. & Phillips, D. (1996). *Youth development and neighborhood influences: Challenges and opportunities* (Workshop Summary). Washington, D.C.: The National Academy of Sciences.

Chandler, C.R., Tsai, T.M., & Wharton, R. (1999). Twenty years after: Replicating a study of Anglo- and Mexican-American cultural values. *The Social Science Journal*, 36(2), 353-367.

Chazan, M. (1992). The home and the school. In J. Coleman (Ed.). *The school years: Current issues in the socialization of young people* (2nd ed). (pp. 164-195). New York, NY: Routledge.

Coleman, J. (1992). Current issues in adolescent process. In J. Coleman (Ed.). *The school years: Current issues in the socialization of young people* (2nd ed.). (pp. 164-195). New York, NY: Routledge.

Denner, J., Kirby, D., Coyle, K., & Brindis, C. (2001). The protective role of social capital and cultural norms in Latino communities: A study of adolescent births. *Hispanic Journal of Behavioral Sciences*, 2001, 23(1), 3-21.

DeWalt, B.R. (1979). Drinking behavior, economic status and adaptive strategies of modernization in a highland Mexican community. *American Ethnologist*, 6, 510-530.

Dewees, M. (2001). Building cultural competence for work with diverse families: Strategies from the privileged side. *Journal of Ethnic & Cultural Diversity in Social Work*, 9, 33-51.

Duncan, S., Duncan, T., Biglan, A. & Ary, D. (1998). Contributions of social context to the development of adolescent substance use: A multivariate latent growth modeling approach. *Drug and Alcohol Dependence*, 50, 57-71.

Duncan, T., Tildesley, E., Duncan, S. & Hops, H. (1995). The consistency of family and peer influences on the development of substance use in adolescence. *Addictions*, 90, 1647-1660.

Ellickson, P. & Morton, S. (1999). Identifying adolescents at risk for hard drug use: Racial/Ethnic variations. *Journal of Adolescent Health*, 25, 382-395.

Everett, E. (1933). An approach to the problem of juvenile delinquency through casework in the school. *Journal of Educational Sociology*, 6(8), 491-499.

Farrington, D. (1992). Juvenile delinquency. In J. Coleman (Ed.). *The school years: Current issues in the socialization of young people* (2nd ed.) (pp. 123-163). New York, NY: Routledge.

Friedman, A. & Glassman, K. (2000). Family risk factors versus peer risk factors for drug abuse: A longitudinal study of African American urban community sample. *Journal of Substance Abuse Treatment*, 18, 267-275.

Gonzales, Phillip B. (1993). Historical Poverty, Restructuring Effects, and Integrative Ties: Mexican American Neighborhoods in a Peripheral Sunbelt Economy. In Joan Moore and Raquel Pinderhughes, editors. *In the Barrios: Latinos and the Underclass Debate*. New York: Russell Sage Foundation.

Graham, J.W., Hofer, S.M., & MacKinnon, D.P. (1996). Maximizing the usefulness of data obtained with planned missing value patterns: An application of maximum likelihood procedures. *Multivariate Behavioral Research*, 31, 197-218.

Graham, J.W., Hofer, S.M., & Piccinin, A.M. (1994). Analysis with missing data in drug prevention research. In L.M. Collins & L.A. Seitz (Eds.), *Advances in Data Analysis for Prevention Intervention Research* (pp. 13-63), NIDA Research Monograph 142, Washington, D.C.: National Institute on Drug Abuse.

Graham, J.W., Taylor, B.J., & Cumsille, P.E. (2001). Planned missing data designs in analysis of change. In L. Collins & A. Sayer (Eds.), *New methods for the analysis of change*, (pp. 335-353). Washington, DC: American Psychological Association.

Guagliardo, M., Huang, Z., Hicks, J. & D'Angelo, L. (1998). Increased drug use for old-for-grade and dropout urban adolescents. *American Journal of Prevention Medicince*, 15(1), 42-48.

Herman, M., Dornbusch, S., Herron, M. & Herting, J. (1997). The influence of family regulation, connection, and psychological autonomy on six measures of adolescent functioning. *Journal of Adolescent Research*, 12(1), 34-67.

Howard, D. (1996). Searching for resilience among African American youth exposed to community violence: Theoretical issues. *Journal of Adolescent Health*, 18, 254-262.

Iannotti, R., Bush, P. & Weinfur, K. (1996). Perception of friends' use of alcohol, cigarettes, and marijuana among urban schoolchildren: A longitudinal analysis. *Addictive Behaviors*, 21(5), 615-632.

Johanson, C., Duffy, F. & Anthony, J. (1996). Association between drug use and behavioral repertoire in urban youths. *Addictions*, 91(4), 523-534.

Kulis, S., Marsiglia, F. & Hecht, M. (2001). Gender labels and gender identity as predictors of drug use among ethnically diverse middle school students. *Journal of Research on Adolescence*, 11(1), 21-48.

Luekefeld, C., Logan, T., Clayton, R., Martin, C., Zimmerman, R., Cattarello, A., Milich, R. & Lynam, D. (1998). Adolescent drug use, delinquency, and other behaviors. In T. Gullotta, G. Adams & R. Montemayor (Eds.). *Delinquent violent youth: Theory and intervention* (98-128). Thousand Oaks, CA: Sage Publishers.

Madsen, W. & Madsen, C. (1979). The cultural structure of Mexican drinking behavior. In: Marshall, M. (ed.) *Beliefs, Behaviors, and Alcoholic Beverages* (pp. 38-54). Ann Arbor. MI: University of Michigan Press.

Mahoney, J. & Stattin, H. (2000). Leisure activities and adolescent antisocial behavior: The role of structure and social context. *Journal of Adolescence*, 23, 113-127.

Marsiglia, F.F., Kulis, S., & Hecht, M.E. (2001). Ethnic labels and ethnic identity as predictors of drug use among middle school students in the Southwest. *Journal of Research on Adolescence*, 11 (1), 21-48.

Marsiglia, F. F. & Holleran, L. (1999). I've learned so much from my mother: Narratives from a group of Chicana high school students. *Social Work in Education*, 21(4), 220-237.

McWhirter, J., McWhirter, B., McWhirter, A. & McWhirter, E. (1998). *At-risk youth: A comprehensive response* (2nd ed.). Pacific Grove, CA: Brooks/Cole.

Newcomb, M.D. & Bentler, P.M. (1988). *The consequences of adolescent drug use: Impact on the lives of young adults*. Newbury Park, CA: Sage.

NIDA. (1999). *Preventing Drug Use Among Children and Adolescents: A Research-Based Guide*. Washington D. C.: National Institute of Health.

Nurco, D., Kinlock, T., O'Grady, K. & Hanlon, T. (1998). Differential contributions of family and peer factors to the etiology of narcotic addiction. *Drug and Alcohol Dependence*, 51, 229-237.

Obot, I., & Anthony, J. (1999). Association of school dropout with recent and past injecting drug use among African American adults. *Journal of Addictive Behaviors*, 24(5), 701-705.

Olson, D.H., McCubbin, H., Barnes, H.I., Larsen, A.S., Muxen, M.J., & Wilson, M.A. (1983). *Families*. Beverly Hills, CA: Sage.

Patterson, S. & Marsiglia, F.F. (2000). "Mi casa es su casa": A beginning exploration of Mexican Americans' natural helping. *Families in Society*, 81,1, 22-31.

Resnick, M. (2000.) Resilience and protective factors in the lives of adolescents. *Journal of Adolescent Health*, 27, 1-2.

Ripple, C. & Luthar, S. (2000). Academic risk among inner city adolescents: The role of personal attributes. *Journal of School Psychology*, 38(3), 277-298.

Rogler, L.H., Cortes, D.E., & Malgady, R.G. (1991). Acculturation and mental health status among Hispanics: Convergence and new directions for research. *American Psychologist*, 46, 585-597.

Robertson, L., Harding, M., & Morrison, G. (1998). A comparison of risk and resilience indicators among Latino/a students; Differences between students identified as at-risk, learning disabled, speech impaired and not at-risk. *Education and Treatment of Children*, 21, (3), 333-353.

SAMHSA. (1998). *Annual national drug survey results released: Overall drug use is level, but youth drug use increase persists*. Washington D.C.: SAMHSA Press Office.

Seydlitz, R. & Jenkins, P. (1998). The influence of families, friends, schools, and communities on delinquent behaviors. In T. Gullotta, G. Adams & R. Montemayor (Eds.). *Delinquent violent youth: Theory and interventions* (53-97). Thousand Oaks, CA: Sage Publishers.

Seligman, W. & Csikszentmihalyi, M. (2000). Positive psychology: An introduction. *American Psychologist*, 55(1), 5-15.

Smokowski, P., Reynolds, A. & Bezruczko, N. (1999). Resilience and protective factors in adolescence: An autobiographical perspective from disadvantaged youth. *Journal of School Psychology*, 37(4), 425-448.

Suarez-Orozco, C. & Suarez-Orozco, M. (1995). *Transformations: Immigration, Family Life, and Achievement Motivation Among Latino Adolescents*. Stanford, CA: Stanford University Press.

Swaim, R., Bates, S. & Chavez, E. (1998). Structural equation socialization model of substance use of Mexican-American and White non-Hispanic school dropouts. *Journal of Adolescent Health*, 23, 128-138.

Van Wilkinson, W. (1989). The influence of lifestyles on the patterns and practices of alcohol use among south Texas Mexican Americans. *Hispanic Journal Behavioral Science*, 11(4), 354-65.

Vega, W. & Gil, A. (1998). Different worlds. In W. Vega & A. Gil (Eds.). *Drug use and ethnicity in early adolescence* (pp. 1-12). New York, NY: Plenum Press.

Widdershoven, G. (1993). The story of life: Hermeneutic perspectives on the relationship between narrative and life history. In A. Liebling & R. Josselson (Eds.). *The narrative study of lives: Volume 1* (pp. 1-20). Newbury Park, CA: Sage Publications.

Reproductive Attitudes and Behavior Among Latina Adolescents

Jillian Jimenez
Marilyn K. Potts
Daniel R. Jimenez

SUMMARY. This study examines the relationship between acculturation and sexual activity, contraceptive use and attitudes toward self. The sample consisted of 290 Latinas participating in a statewide adolescent pregnancy prevention program funded by the California Department of Health Services. Respondents were divided into three groups for purposes of analysis: those born outside the United States, those born in the United States who spoke primarily Spanish in the home, and those born in the United States who spoke primarily English in the home. Results indicated that less acculturated adolescents were less likely to engage in sexual activity. Place of birth was the most important predictor of differences in reproductive attitudes and behavior; language spoken in the home was not a predictor of sexual activity. There were no significant differences in contraceptive use among the sexually active respondents

Jillian Jimenez, PhD, and Marilyn K. Potts, PhD, are Professors of Social Work, Department of Social Work, California State University, Long Beach. Daniel R. Jimenez, PhD, is Lecturer, Department of Social Work, California State University Long Beach.

The authors wish to thank the California State Department of Health Services for allowing them to use these data.

[Haworth co-indexing entry note]: "Reproductive Attitudes and Behavior Among Latina Adolescents." Jimenez, Jillian, Marilyn K. Potts, and Daniel R. Jimenez. Co-published simultaneously in *Journal of Ethnic & Cultural Diversity in Social Work* (The Haworth Social Work Practice Press, an imprint of The Haworth Press, Inc.) Vol. 11, No. 3/4, 2002, pp. 221-249; and: *Social Work with Multicultural Youth* (ed: Diane de Anda) The Haworth Social Work Practice Press, an imprint of The Haworth Press, Inc., 2002, pp. 221-249. Single or multiple copies of this article are available for a fee from The Haworth Document Delivery Service [1-800-HAWORTH, 9:00 a.m. - 5:00 p.m. (EST). E-mail address: docdelivery@haworthpress.com].

http://www.haworthpress.com/store/product.asp?sku=J051

10.1300/J051v11n03_04

in the three groups. Respondents born outside of the United States had more negatives attitudes toward self on one measure; respondents born in the United States who spoke primarily Spanish in the home were more likely to plan to attend college, and to delay sexual activity because their parents would be upset, than the other groups. The authors suggest factors that may explain these differences in attitudes and behavior among the three groups.

KEYWORDS. Latina, acculturation, sexual activity, contraception

INTRODUCTION

Latina adolescents have the highest birthrate of any identified ethnic group in the United States. The rate of pregnancy among Latina adolescents in the United States doubled from 1987 to 1997 (Henshaw, 1997). The main increase occurred from 1990 to 1995, when the rate was 163 per 1,000; rates declined slightly after that (Ventura et al., 2000). In 1999, 1 in 11 Latinas age 15 to 19 gave birth (Curtin & Martin, 2000). Mexican-origin adolescents had the highest birth rate of all ethnic groups in 1997 (National Campaign to Prevent Teen Pregnancy [NCPTP], 1999).

Sexual activity is far less easy to measure than birth rate; the best and latest estimates, drawn from a nationally representative sample in 1995, are that more than half (52%) of unmarried Latina adolescents (age 13 to 19) had ever had sex; 48% reported having sex in the last 12 months before the survey. Among those Latinas who were 15 to 17 years old, 49% had had sex (Ventura, 2000). Another study found that of those Latina adolescents who reported having sex in the last three months, 74% had used contraception the last time they had sex (Abma et al., 1997). In 1999, less than half (43%) of Latina high school students surveyed reported condom use at their last sexual experience (Kann et al., 2000). Thus, a high percentage of Latina adolescents who do engage in sexual activity are not protected from Sexually Transmitted Infections (STIs).

Abma et al. (1997) found that among those adolescents who became pregnant, more (54%) Latinas than those from other groups reported that their pregnancies were intended; only one-third of non-Latino White and one-fourth of African American adolescents reported their pregnancies as intended (Abma et al., 1997). Adolescent pregnancy, intended or not, has serious consequences for both mother and child. Latinas who become pregnant in high school are one-fourth as likely to complete school as those who do not (Ahn, 1994). Moreover, the likelihood of poverty and child abuse increases substantially for children of adolescent mothers (Haveman, Wolfe, & Wilson, 1997; Lee & George, 1999).

AIDS rates are higher among Latino youth than among non-Latino White youth, but not higher than among African American youth (CDC, 2000). Because of poor health care access and lack of information about AIDS, Latinos are likely to be diagnosed with HIV later than other groups and more likely to die of the disease (Bishop-Townsend, 1996). Sexually active Latinas are seriously at risk for HIV and other STIs. Latina adolescents are more likely to become infected than young Latino men (Townsend, 1996).

Latino children and adolescents are more likely to be uninsured and have less access to health care than African American or non-Latino White children and adolescents (Zambrana & Logie, 2000). In California, poor Latino immigrant families are often medically uninsured (Shinkman, 1997). Due in part to the large group of uninsured immigrants, Latinas in California have lower levels of early prenatal care than African American, non-Latino White, and Asian American women (Baezconde-Garbanti & Portillo, 1999). As a consequence of the limitations of the health care system, access to reproductive health care by Latinas in California is more limited than it is for other groups. This fact affects the availability of contraception, the prevalence and treatment of STIs, and other reproductive health issues facing Latina adolescents.

PURPOSE

The purpose of this study was to compare reproductive attitudes and behavior of Latina adolescents who were (a) born outside the United States (b) born in this country and spoke Spanish at home and (c) born in this country and spoke English at home. As in previous research with Latino populations (Driscoll et al., 2001), both place of birth and language spoken in the home were used as measures of acculturation. The study compared attitudes toward self, educational goals, future aspirations, and religiosity among Latina adolescents according to their levels of acculturation. In addition, the predictors of sexual activity and contraceptive use in this sample of Latina adolescents were examined.

The findings are based on secondary data analysis of survey data gathered under the auspices of the California Department of Health Services in 1997 and 1998 through the Community Challenge Grant Program. This program was designed to reduce adolescent and unwed pregnancies and build life skills in high-risk groups. Adolescent girls who participated in the program were administered questionnaires upon entering an after-school program designed to influence attitudes and behavior related to sexuality and pregnancy.

LITERATURE REVIEW

Acculturation and Reproductive Behavior Among Latinas

Much of the research on Latina adolescents' reproductive attitudes and behavior has focused on Mexican American adolescents. Within this population, traditional Mexican values are likely to influence both immigrant adolescents and those born in the United States, since acculturation is a process taking place over time. Marin (1992) described acculturation as a three-stage process, which involved learning factual information from the new culture; accepting core skills (such as language); and integrating attitudes, values, and beliefs from the dominant culture. Kaplan and Marks (1990) defined acculturation as a process of change in beliefs, attitudes, and values that occurs when two cultural groups interact over a period of time. Sabogal and Perez-Stabel (1995) described acculturation as the process of modifying attitudes, cultural norms, and behaviors as a result of interaction with another culture.

Perez and Padilla (2000), in a study of 203 Latino adolescents representing three generations, found that acculturation occurred in a linear manner, with the third generation exhibiting the most dominant American cultural orientation. The authors concluded that the amount of time spent in the host culture is the most important variable influencing acculturation.

Among Latino adolescents, acculturation is likely to be inversely related to traditional Mexican cultural values that stress familism and traditional roles for women (Falicov, 1984) over individual sexual fulfillment and decision-making. In Mexico, gender roles are formed around traditional concepts of *machismo* (masculinity) and *marianismo* (femininity). The latter includes the valorizing of virginity, chastity, and obedience to males (Pavich, 1986). Padilla and Baird (1991) in their study of Mexican American adolescents (n = 84) found that most Mexican American adolescents continue to hold these traditional attitudes toward gender roles, especially the importance of virginity for girls and the relationship between sex and love. Furthermore, Flores et al. (1998) examined antecedents of sexual behavior among Mexican American adolescents (n = 37) and found that traditional cultural values (as opposed to mainstream American values) influenced Mexican American female adolescents' preference for partners with strong family orientations. The authors suggested that this value is consonant with familismo, the traditional Mexican American cultural value emphasizing the importance of the family. Both male and female adolescents believed that loving the person is a salient reason to have sex; the authors noted that the connection of love and sex reflects traditional Mexican American cultural values.

Felix-Ortiz and Newcomb (1994) developed a multidimensional measure of cultural identity for Latino and Latina adolescents (n = 130) that included language, values, and behavior. Interestingly, the authors found that while behavior and language did discriminate between cultural identity groups (bicultural, Latino-identified, and American-identified), the values/attitudes measures did not, suggesting that traditional values may be held by more acculturated generations of adolescents. On the other hand, the importance of language as a measure of acculturation was upheld by the results of this study.

Several studies have looked at acculturation and sexual risk behaviors in Latino adolescents. One study found that acculturation was strongly associated with sexual activity among Latina adolescents and young women; foreign born Latinas or less acculturated Latinas were less sexually active than U.S.-born or more acculturated Latinas (n = 711), but they were also less likely to use contraceptives (Ford & Norris, 1993). On the other hand, Brindis et al. (1995) found that foreign-born Latino high school students (n = 1,789) were more likely to be sexually active, but, similar to Ford and Norris's study, less likely to use contraceptive than were native born Latino students. Less acculturated Latinas, therefore, may be more at risk for pregnancies and STIs. Another study found that levels of acculturation impact gender differences among Latino adolescents (n = 497); that is, the percentage engaging in sex was higher for less acculturated male adolescents than for less acculturated female adolescents. As level of acculturation increased, these differences diminished (Upchurch et al., 2001). Aneshensel et al. (1990), using a large (n = 1,023) random sample, surveyed the ethnic differences in reproductive behavior among non Hispanic White and Mexican American female adolescents. The authors found that Mexico born Mexican American adolescents had the lowest rate of early sexual intercourse, but the highest rate of early births, because they were most likely to become pregnant if sexually active and most likely to give birth if pregnant. United States born Mexican American adolescents were intermediate between the Mexico born adolescents and the non Hispanic White adolescents; the latter group was the most likely to be sexually active, but the least likely to become pregnant and the most likely to elect abortion. More positive attitudes toward their pregnancy and better birth outcomes have been found among less acculturated Latina adolescents than among their more acculturated counterparts (Frisbie et al., 1998); however, more acculturated Latina adolescents had more positive attitudes toward sexuality than their counterparts (Flores et al., 1998).

Explanations for some of these differences were offered by Wood and Price (1997), who argued that the social scripts of machismo and marianismo, which tolerate male sexual promiscuity, along with Catholicism, which prohibits contraception, contribute to high risk sexual behavior among more traditional Latinos. Moreover, according to Wood and Price's review of the research, less acculturated Latino males have more sexual partners than more acculturated Latino males and are, therefore, more likely to put their partners at risk.

In seeking to determine which risk factors are implicated in adolescent sexual activity, one study comparing Latinos, African Americans, and European American adolescents found that low religiosity predicted sexual activity for Latinos, but not for Latina youth (Perkins et al., 1998). Physical abuse and sexual abuse predicted sexual activity for adolescent girls of all ethnicities as did time alone, alcohol use, and low-grade point average. Low grade point average was a predictor for all ethnic groups studied, as was time home alone and alcohol use. Plotnik's (1992) research also suggests that adolescents with higher educational expectations are less likely to be sexually active and more likely to use contraception. Similarly, adolescents with expectations of working in a professional occupation were found to be less likely to have a child than those without such expectations (Sugland, Manlove, & Romano, 1997). The latter study found this relationship to hold across ethnic and social class groups.

Liebowitz, Castellano, and Cuellar (1999) studied 413 Mexican American adolescents in Texas who were 11 to 14 years of age in order to predict the absence of sexual activity. The best predictors were child's religiosity, child's educational goals, and child's perception of the congruency of parent-child sexual values. These findings are somewhat contradictory to those of Perkins et al. (1998), who found that low religiosity did not predict sexual activity in Latina adolescents. Strong religious beliefs have been positively associated with traditional values and inversely associated with contraceptive use and sexual behavior among Latina teenage girls in earlier research (Brindis, 1992; Holden, Nelson, Velasquez, & Ritchie, 1993), suggesting that religiosity would serve to reduce sexual behavior as well as contraceptive use.

Findings regarding sources of information about sexuality and contraception for Latina adolescents are somewhat contradictory. One study indicated that these adolescents tend to seek advice from their mothers, aunts, sisters, and friends (Rew, 1997), whereas another study found that Latina adolescents receive little information about birth control from their parents (Baumeister, Flores, & Marin, 1995).

Compared with African Americans and European Americans, both adult and adolescent Mexican Americans are less likely to have discussed contraception with others (Padilla & Baird, 1991; Stroup-Benham & Trevino, 1991; Catania et al., 1992). Padilla and Baird (1991) found that Mexican-American adolescents have limited knowledge of contraceptive effectiveness. One study found that sexually active Latino adolescents who characterized their mothers as responsive in discussing sexuality were more likely to talk to their partners about contraception and more likely to use condoms (Whitaker, Miller, May, & Levin, 1999). Another study found that Latinas who perceive their mothers as disapproving of adolescent sexual activity, and whose mother have rules about dating and are in favor of their daughters waiting until marriage to have sex, were less likely to engage in advanced sexual behaviors (Hovell et al., 1994). However, although they may disapprove of sexual activity, if an adolescent becomes pregnant, Latino parents are more likely to encourage motherhood as the primary role for their daughters, according to earlier research (Dore & Dumois, 1990). Belief in traditional gender roles may encourage families to accept motherhood as the final stage in an adolescent girl's development, thus de-emphasizing school and career (Driscoll, 2001).

Factors Related to Sexual Activity and Contraceptive Use

Latino adolescents are less likely to use condoms than non-Latino White or African American adolescents (Abma et al., 1997; Ford, Sohn, & Lepkowski, 2001). Some studies have suggested that Mexican American females are not able to insist that their partners use a condom (Flores, 1992; Gomez & Martin, 1996). Sneed (2001) examined the reasons 618 Latino adolescents did or did not use condoms at first intercourse. The most common reasons cited for not using condoms were "don't know" (26%), "not available" (26%), and "didn't think of it" (24%). Males were significantly more likely to report using condoms for protection at first intercourse than were females.

One explanation of the low condom use among Latinos is suggested by a study of the effect of ethnicity among over 1,000 college students in which Latinos and Asians were found to be slightly more conservative sexually than the other groups (Baldwin & Whiteley, 1992). The implications of conservative attitudes toward sexuality were reported in another study of 1,600 Latino men and women (Marin & Gomez, 1996, cited in Marble, 1996). These authors noted that conservative gender role beliefs are strongly related to sexual coercion by male partners and lack of condom use.

Research on the reproductive behavior of adult Latinos suggests that adolescents may be at an increased risk for HIV. In a study of 226 HIV positive Latino men and women receiving services at an outpatient clinic, Marks and Cantero (1998) found that as acculturation increased, men and women were increasingly likely to have engaged in unsafe sex, usually with their intimate lovers, in the most recent sexual encounter since testing seropositive. On the other hand, in a study of the general population of Latinos, Marin and Flores (1994) found that more acculturated Latinas were more likely to use condoms with secondary partners than were less acculturated Latinas. Marks and Cantero explained this difference by pointing out that their respondents were seropositive and, therefore, had less reason to protect themselves with their intimate partners than respondents who were presumably seronegative who chose to have sex with secondary partners.

Studies of Latino adult attitudes toward condom use have important implications for Latino adolescents, since their attitudes are likely to have been influenced by Latino adults. In a study of 513 Latina and 184 non-Latino White women, Gomez and Marin (1996) found that non-Latino White women had better knowledge about HIV, more sexual comfort, more self-efficacy in using condoms, and more sexual power than did Latina women. Soler, Qaudagno, and Sly (2000) studied low income African American, Latina, and non-Latino White women in Miami from 1994 to 1995 (n = 393) and found that African American women and Latinas reported more consistent condom use than non-Latino White women, although Latina women scored lowest on condom-related self-efficacy and were less comfortable talking about condom use with their partners. The authors suggested that Latina women utilized indirect methods of assuring condom use so "as to remain within the constraints imposed by machismo" (p. 8). Marin et al. (1998) found that less acculturated Latino adults (male and female) reported less self-efficacy in discussing condom use with their partners, largely because they felt it was not respectful for men to discuss sex with women. These studies suggest that cultural factors are strongly implicated in attitudes toward contraceptive use in adult Latinos; these same factors are likely to be important to attitudes among Latina adolescents and vary by level of acculturation in this group.

Summary

The relationship between acculturation and sexual activity among Latina adolescents is not clear. Some studies have indicated that contraceptive use is related to acculturation in Latinas (Marin & Flores, 1994; Marin et al., 1998; Gomez & Marin, as cited in Marble, 1996); another study found that Latinas were more likely to use condoms than non-Latino White women (Soler, Qaudagno & Sly, 2000). Flores et al. (1998) found that more acculturated Latinas had more positive attitudes toward sexuality. The research on the relationship between religiosity and sexual behavior among Latina adolescents is contradictory. Research thus far has found a negative association between strong educational goals, future professional aspirations, and adolescent sexuality and a positive relationship between these goals and using contraception and not becoming pregnant.

Much is still unknown about the relationship between acculturation and reproductive attitudes and behavior and about the specific factors linked to reproductive behavior. This study examined the relationship between acculturation and reproductive attitudes and behavior in Latina adolescents. Additionally, the study looked at the association between acculturation and attitudes toward self, educational goals, future aspirations and religiosity.

METHODS

Sample

The sample consisted of 290 Latinas participating in a statewide adolescent pregnancy prevention program (Community Challenge Grant

Program: Funding Local Solutions to Reduce Teen and Unwed Pregnancies and Fatherlessness) funded by the California Department of Health Services. This program targeted adolescents at risk of pregnancy and was implemented through grants to nearly 1,000 lead agencies throughout the state. Recruitment took place through schools, clinics, health fairs, and community organizations. The present analyses utilize existing data from three sites in the Los Angeles area: Montebello Unified School District, White Memorial Medical Center, and YMCA Harbor Area. All who attended the first meeting of a voluntary educational program aimed at reducing adolescent pregnancy were asked to participate in the study and nearly all agreed to do so. It should be recognized that the existing data set used for these analyses did not contain information regarding country of origin. However, these three sites are located in predominately Mexican American neighborhoods; thus, the sample is presumed to be predominately Mexican American.

Data Collection

The present analyses are based on data from self-administered pre-tests completed by participants prior to the first session of the adolescent pregnancy prevention program. Consent was obtained from research participants and their parents/guardians.

Instrument

The self-administered pre-test consisted of 30 questions. Of relevance to the present analyses, participants were first asked to provide demographic data (e.g., age, ethnicity, born within or outside the United States, and primary language spoken in home). The remaining items employed a four-point scale. Respondents were instructed to mark one of the following response options: YES!, yes, no, or NO!. Items concerned reasons for waiting to have sex (e.g., my mother or father would be upset, I am afraid of STDs, and I am afraid of a pregnancy) and attitudes toward sex (e.g., it's OK for a teenage boy/girl to have sex with someone he/she likes but doesn't know well, I want to marry a virgin, and it is a good idea to try sex before marriage). Additional items concerned future aspirations (e.g., I have a good idea of where I am headed in the future, I feel that I can change the future by what I do today, and I don't spend time planning for the future because planning doesn't work for me) and views of oneself (e.g., I wish I had more to be proud of, someone in my family loves and supports me, and I know how to overcome problems in my life). Future plans were also addressed (e.g., finish high school, get job training, and attend college).

Finally, participants were asked a series of questions about their sexual activity and contraceptive use. Questions included whether they had ever had sex, whether they had ever been pregnant, and the method of contraception used during both their first and last sexual experiences.

Data Analysis

Responses from the four-point scales were collapsed into two categories (yes vs. no). This was done for two reasons: (a) to minimize the likelihood of small cell sizes given the small numbers of respondents in many categories and (b) because it has been reported that less acculturated Latinos tend to prefer a dichotomous response format and may tend to ignore the range of the scale continuum (Land & Hudson, 1997). A three-category variable reflecting level of acculturation was created: (a) immigrant, (b) born in the United States and Spanish spoken in the home, and (c) born in the United States and English spoken in the home. Chi-square was used for all bivariate analyses. Logistic regression was used to assess the effects of level of acculturation on sexual activity and contraceptive use, controlling for other factors in the model, because the dependent variables were dichotomous. These factors were selected based on their significant associations with acculturation in the bivariate analyses. Hierarchical procedures were used: Block 1 included country of origin and language spoken in the home; Block 2 added age; Block 3 added attitudes toward sexuality and reasons for waiting to have sex; Block 4 added attitudes toward self and educational goals. Zero-order correlations were used to ascertain the degree of mutlicollinearity between all independent variables.

FINDINGS

Demographic Characteristics

The 290 respondents were divided fairly equally between those who were 14 to 15 (n = 165; 56.9%) and 16 to 19 (n = 125; 43.1%) years old. The mean age was 15.39 (sd = 1.07). A large majority (n = 231; 80.2%) had been born in the United States, although about two-thirds (n = 161; 62.5%) reported Spanish as the primary language spoken in the home.

Sexual Activity and Contraceptive Practices

About one-third (n = 88; 32.6%) reported that they had had sex previously. Of those, most (n = 53; 61.6%) had experienced their first sexual encounter at 14 to 15 years of age (mean = 13.85, sd = 1.86). Few of those who had had sex (n = 13; 14.8%) had ever been pregnant. Of those who had ever been pregnant, the mean number of pregnancies was 1.14 (sd = 0.36).

Of the 88 who reported ever having had sex, the primary method of contraception during their first sexual experience was a condom (n = 49; 61.2%). Only 2 (2.5%) had used birth control pills during this first experience. Over one-third (n = 29; 36.2%) reported no contraceptive use. In contrast, during their last sexual experience, a slight majority (n = 41; 53.2%) reported using birth control pills, while only 3 (3.9%) reported using a condom. Again, over one-third (n = 31; 40.3%) admitted to no contraceptive use. The mean number of partners within the last six months was 1.36 (sd = 1.01) and the mean number of sexual experiences within the last six months was 8.90 (sd = 14.33).

Sexual Activity and Contraceptive Use by Country of Origin and Language Used in Home

Differences in sexual activity were apparent by level of acculturation (see Table 1). Those who were born outside of the United States (and assumed to be the least acculturated) were significantly more likely than those in the remaining groups to report not being sexually active. A large majority (n = 49; 83.1%) of those in the immigrant group reported no prior sexual activity, compared to a much smaller majority of those in the non-immigrant groups. In contrast, those who were born in the United States and spoke English in the home (and assumed to be the most acculturated) showed the highest proportion of being sexually active (n = 32; 41.0%). There was no significant difference across groups in terms of their contraceptive use. Of those who were sexually active, a slight or substantial majority of respondents in all three groups reported using contraceptives. This ranged from 18 (54.5%) of those who were born in the United States and spoke English in the home to 8 (80.0%) of those who were born outside of the United States.

Attitudes Toward Sexuality and Reasons for Waiting to Have Sex by Country of Origin and Language Used in Home

Differences by acculturation level were apparent for only one of the six attitudes toward sexuality (see Table 2). Those who were born in the

TABLE 1. Sexual Activity and Contraceptive Use, by Country of Origin and Language Used in Home (N = 290)

	Born Elsewhere		Born in US and Spanish in Home		Born in US and English in Home	
	(n = 59)		(n = 153)		(n = 78)	
	f	%	f	%	f	%
Not Sexually Active	49	83.1	107	69.9	46	59.0
Sexually Active	10	16.9	46	30.1	32	41.0
$X^2 = 9.22, p \leq .01$						
	(n = 10)		(n = 45)		(n = 33)	
Contraceptive Use[1]	8	80.0	31	68.9	18	54.5
No Contraceptive Use	2	20.0	14	31.1	15	45.5
$X^2 = 2.86$, ns						

[1]Of those who were sexually active (n = 88). Contraceptive use pertains to last time had sex.

United States and spoke English in the home were most likely to agree that their parents would want them to use protection if they had sex. They were followed closely by those who were born in the United States and spoke Spanish in the home. Immigrants were least likely to endorse this view.

Differences by acculturation level were noted for three of the eight reasons for waiting to have sex (see Table 2). Those who were born in the United States and spoke Spanish in the home were most likely to (a) believe that their parents would be upset if they had sex and (b) be afraid of STDs. In contrast, respondents who were born outside of the United States were more likely than those in the non-immigrant groups to endorse waiting until marriage as a reason for refraining from having sex.

Attitudes Toward Self by Country of Origin and Language Used in Home

Only one of eight items concerning attitudes toward self differed by acculturation level. Respondents who were born outside of the United States were more likely than non-immigrants to agree with the item, "I wish I had more to be proud of" (see Table 3).

TABLE 2. Attitudes Toward Sexuality and Reasons for Waiting to Have Sex, by Country of Origin and Language Used in Home (N = 290)[1]

	Born Elsewhere		Born in US and Spanish in Home		Born in US and English in Home	
	(n = 59)		(n = 153)		(n = 78)	
	f	%	f	%	f	%
Attitudes						
OK for teenage boy to have sex with someone he likes						
Yes	7	12.3	14	9.3	10	13.0
No	50	87.7	137	90.7	67	87.0
	$X^2 = 0.87$, ns					
OK for teenage girl to have sex with someone she likes						
Yes	2	3.4	13	8.7	11	14.5
No	57	96.6	137	91.3	65	85.5
	$X^2 = 5.00$, ns					
Want to marry a virgin						
Yes	35	62.5	91	62.8	48	63.2
No	21	37.5	54	37.2	28	36.8
	$X^2 = 0.01$, ns					
Good idea to try sex before marriage						
Yes	7	12.1	37	25.3	22	28.9
No	51	87.9	109	74.7	54	71.1
	$X^2 = 5.73$, ns					
Parents think only married people should have babies						
Yes	39	66.1	110	72.8	54	70.1
No	20	33.9	41	27.2	23	29.9
	$X^2 = 0.95$, ns					
Parents would want me to use protection if I had sex						
Yes	45	84.9	134	91.2	70	97.2
No	8	15.1	13	8.8	2	2.8
	$X^2 = 6.04$, $p \leq .05$					

	Born Elsewhere		Born in US and Spanish in Home		Born in the US and English in Home	
	(n = 59)		(n = 153)		(n = 78)	
	f	%	f	%	f	%
OK to have baby while in high school						
Yes	4	7.1	11	7.4	5	6.6
No	52	92.9	137	92.6	71	93.4
	$X^2 = 0.06$, ns					
Reasons for Waiting						
Parents would be upset						
Yes	45	80.4	135	92.5	63	84.0
No	11	19.6	11	7.5	12	16.0
	$X^2 = 6.84$, $p < .05$					
Afraid of STDs						
Yes	46	85.2	140	96.6	70	92.1
No	8	14.8	5	3.4	6	7.9
	$X^2 = 8.06$, $p < .05$					
Afraid of pregnancy						
Yes	45	83.3	127	88.8	60	78.9
No	9	16.7	16	11.2	16	21.1
	$X^2 = 3.93$, ns					
Haven't met right person						
Yes	34	60.7	92	61.7	39	51.3
No	22	39.3	57	38.3	37	48.7
	$X^2 = 2.26$, ns					
Waiting until marriage						
Yes	40	72.7	86	61.9	33	44.0
No	15	27.3	53	38.1	42	56.0
	$X^2 = 11.74$, $p < .01$					
Not old enough						
Yes	39	70.9	88	63.3	40	51.9
No	16	29.1	51	36.7	37	48.1
	$x^2 = 5.22$, ns					
Would feel guilty						
Yes	35	63.6	78	56.9	39	50.6
No	20	36.4	59	43.1	38	49.4
	$X^2 = 2.22$, ns					
Best friend would be upset						
Yes	15	28.3	54	39.1	22	29.3
No	38	71.7	84	60.9	53	70.7
	$X^2 = 3.10$, ns					

[1]Most variables contained missing data.

TABLE 3. Attitudes Toward Self, by Country of Origin and Language Used in Home (N = 290)[1]

	Born Elsewhere		Born in US and Spanish in Home		Born in US and English in Home	
	(n = 59)		(n = 153)		(n = 78)	
	f	%	f	%	f	%
Wish I had more to be proud of						
Yes	48	85.7	98	65.3	54	70.1
No	8	14.3	52	34.7	23	29.9
	$X^2 = 8.19$, $p \leq .05$					
Someone in family loves and supports me						
Yes	52	96.6	145	95.4	74	94.9
No	2	3.4	7	4.6	4	5.1
	$X^2 = 0.22$, ns					
Know how to overcome problems in my life						
Yes	46	82.1	117	80.1	61	78.2
No	10	17.9	29	19.9	17	21.8
	$X^2 = 0.32$, ns					
Do things as well as most people my age						
Yes	44	81.5	125	84.5	58	77.3
No	10	18.5	23	15.5	17	22.7
	$X^2 = 1.72$, ns					
Have something to offer my community						
Yes	29	54.7	73	48.3	28	37.8
No	24	45.3	78	51.7	46	62.2
	$X^2 = 3.87$, ns					
Like my body and the way I look						
Yes	30	54.5	100	68.0	43	57.3
No	25	45.5	47	32.0	32	42.7
	$x^2 = 4.25$, ns					
At times, think I am no good at all						
Yes	29	51.8	90	60.4	52	69.3
No	27	48.2	59	39.6	23	30.7
	$X^2 = 4.21$, ns					
Wish other people would respect me more						
Yes	38	70.4	106	72.5	56	75.7
No	16	29.6	40	27.4	18	24.3
	$X^2 = 0.47$, ns					

[1]Most variables contained missing data.

Educational Goals and Future Aspirations by Country of Origin and Language Used in Home

While most respondents in all three groups reported that they planned to finish high school, there was a significant difference in terms of their intentions to attend college (see Table 4). Those who were born in the United States and spoke Spanish in the home were most likely to indicate college aspirations, followed closely by those who were born in the United States and spoke English in the home. No differences were noted with respect to plans to obtain job training or in beliefs regarding one's ability to determine one's future.

Importance of Religion by Country of Origin and Language Used in Home

The importance of religion did not differ by acculturation ($X^2 = 0.13$, df = 2, ns). Respondents in all three groups tended to state that religion was important to them: 70.7% for immigrants, 71.2% for respondents born in the United States who spoke English in the home, and 68.9% for respondents born in the United States who spoke Spanish in the home.

Logistic Regression: Predictors of Sexual Activity

For the logistic regression analyses shown in Table 5, sexual activity was the dependent variable. Those who were sexually active were coded 1; thus, negative betas and odds ratios lower than 1.00 indicate that these respondents were less likely to be sexually active. Dummy variables (coded yes = 1 and no = 0) were used for all independent variables excluding age (which was continuous). Table 5 depicts the results for the final model only.

Block 1 of the logistic regression model included only acculturation. Notably, respondents who were born in the United States were over 3 times more likely than immigrants to be sexually active (odds ratio = 3.33). However, language spoken in the home did not affect sexual activity. The variables in this block predicted only 4% of the variance in sexual activity.

The addition of age in block 2 revealed that older respondents were significantly more likely than younger respondents to be sexually active, with an odds ratio of 1.88. R^2 for the overall model was .13, indicating a small increase over block 1 in the proportion of variance accounted for.

TABLE 4. Educational Goals and Future Aspirations, by Country of Origin and Language Used in Home (N = 290)[1]

	Born Elsewhere		Born in US and Spanish in Home		Born in US and English in Home	
	(n = 59)		(n = 153)		(n = 78)	
	f	%	f	%	f	%
Plan to finish high school						
Yes	48	81.4	125	81.7	67	85.9
No	11	18.6	28	18.3	11	14.1
	$X^2 = 0.74$, ns					
Plan to get job training						
Yes	27	45.8	80	52.6	37	47.4
No	32	54.2	72	47.4	41	52.6
	$X^2 = 1.05$, ns					
Plan to attend college						
Yes	30	50.8	109	71.2	52	66.7
No	29	49.2	44	28.8	26	33.3
	$X^2 = 7.91$, $p \leq .05$					
Have good idea of where headed in future						
Yes	52	91.2	123	80.9	61	79.2
No	5	8.8	29	19.1	16	20.8
	$X^2 = 3.85$, ns					
Feel can change future by what do today						
Yes	41	78.8	126	86.3	59	81.9
No	11	21.2	20	13.7	13	18.1
	$X^2 = 1.78$, ns					
Don't spend time planning for future; planning doesn't work						
Yes	19	35.8	58	40.0	30	42.3
No	34	64.2	87	60.0	41	57.7
	$X^2 = 0.53$, ns					

[1]Most variables contained missing data.

TABLE 5. Logistic Regression: Predictors of Sexual Activity (N = 290)[1]

Independent Variable	*B*	SE	Odds Ratio	p
Block 1 (Acculturation Variables)				
Born in United States	1.20	.53	3.33	.02
English in home	.10	.38	1.11	.79
Model $X^2 = 8.04$ df = 2, $p = .02$, $R^2 = .04$				
Block 2 (Demographic Variable)				
Age	.63	.17	1.88	< .001
Block $X^2 = 16.46$, df = 1, $p < .001$				
Model $X^2 = 24.50$, df = 3, $p < .001$, $R^2 = .13$				
Block 3 (Attitudes Toward Sexuality and Reasons for Waiting)				
Parents would want me to use protection if I had sex	−1.05	.61	.35	.08
Parents would be upset	− .97	.50	.38	.05
Afraid of STDs	− .65	.60	.52	.28
Waiting until marriage	−2.44	.38	.09	<.001
Block $X^2 = 63.42$, df = 4, $p < .001$				
Model $X^2 = 87.92$, df = 7, $p < .001$, $R^2 = .42$				
Block 4 (Attitudes Toward Self and Educational Goals)				
Wish I had more to be proud of	.21	.40	.23	.61
Plan to attend college	−.37	.36	.69	.30
Block $X^2 = 1.37$, df = 2, $p = .50$				
Model $X^2 = 89.29$, df = 9, $p < .001$, $R^2 = .43$				

[1]Results depicted for final model.

After controlling for other variables in the model, respondents' belief that their parents would want them to use protection, as well as their fear of STDs, no longer predicted sexual activity. However, their perception that their parents would be upset if they had sex, as well as their endorsement of waiting until marriage as a reason for refraining from having sex, remained significant predictors of not being sexually active. The addition of these factors in block 3 increased the proportion of variance accounted for to 42%. This substantial increase suggests that such perceptions are more important predictors of sexual activity than acculturation per se, although immigrant status remained significant.

Finally, attitudes toward self and educational goals no longer predicted sexual activity. The addition of these factors in block 4 increased the proportion of variance accounted for by only 1%.

Logistic Regression: Predictors of Contraceptive Use

Table 6 shows the results of the logistic regression analyses with contraceptive use as the dependent variable. Only those who were sexually active were included in these analyses. Those who used contraceptives were coded 1; thus, negative betas and odds ratios lower than 1.00 indicate that these respondents were less likely to report contraceptive use. Independent variables were coded as described above. Table 6 depicts the results for the final model only.

TABLE 6. Logistic Regression: Predictors of Contraceptive Use Among Those Sexually Active (N = 88)[1]

Independent Variable	*B*	SE	Odds Ratio	p
Block 1 (Acculturation Variables)				
Born in United States	−1.94	1.27	.14	.13
English in home	.04	.60	1.04	.95
Model X^2 = 1.06 df = 2, p = .59, R^2 = .02				
Block 2 (Demographic Variable)				
Age	.04	.27	1.04	.87
Block X^2 = 0.15, df = 1, p = .70				
Model X^2 = 1.21, df = 3, p = .75, R^2 = .02				
Block 3 (Attitudes Toward Sexuality and Reasons for Waiting)				
Parents would want me to use protection if I had sex	1.65	1.05	5.22	.11
Parents would be upset	1.02	.70	2.77	.15
Afraid of STDs	2.96	1.23	19.29	.02
Waiting until marriage	1.09	.84	2.96	.20
Block X^2 = 12.88, df = 4, p = .01				
Model X^2 = 14.09, df = 7, p = .05, R^2 = .23				
Block 4 (Attitudes Toward Self and Educational Goals)				
Wish I had more to be proud of	−.27	.69	.76	.69
Plan to attend college	1.32	.57	3.75	.02
Block X^2 = 5.81, df = 2, p = .06				
Model X^2 = 19.90, df = 9, p = .02, R^2 = .31				

[1]Results depicted for final model.

Neither immigrant status nor country of origin predicted contraceptive use and only 2% of the variance in contraceptive use was predicted by these variables. The addition of age in block 2 showed that age was not a significant predictor and did not add to the predictive power of the model.

Of the attitudinal factors added in block 3, only fear of STDs was a significant predictor of contraceptive use. Notably, those who endorsed this item were over 19 times more likely than other respondents to report the use of contraceptives (odds ratio = 19.29). The addition of these factors increased the proportion of variance accounted for appreciably (to 23%).

The addition of attitudes toward self and educational goals in block 4 showed that endorsement of the item, "I wish I had more to be proud of," had no effect on contraceptive use. In contrast, those who stated that they planned to attend college were nearly 4 times more likely than other respondents to report the use of contraceptives (odds ratio = 3.75). The proportion of variance accounted for by the final model was 31%.

DISCUSSION

Respondents in this study were 290 Latina adolescents between 14 and 19 years of age. While the majority of the respondents were born in the United States, two-thirds reported speaking Spanish in the home. Over two-thirds of the respondents reported never having engaged in sexual intercourse. Of those who were sexually active, over half reported using contraception at their last sexual experience.

Limitations

Several limitations should be noted. First, the results are not generalizable to the population of Latina adolescents. The sample was non-random, consisting of voluntary participants in three adolescent pregnancy prevention programs located in Los Angeles County. Motivational factors, in particular, may have differed from those of the general population. Second, although the three sites are located in predominately Mexican American neighborhoods, the existing dataset utilized contained no information about country of origin beyond whether participants were born within or outside the United States. Clearly, various Latina subgroups may differ from each other in important ways. Third, these data were gathered by means of self-administered questionnaires. Others (Land & Hudson, 1997) have maintained that face-to-face interviews are preferable to other methods of data collection among Latinos. Furthermore, there is some evidence that Latinos are more likely than other ethnic groups to refrain from using the full continuum of response categories (Land & Hudson, 1997). Our decision to collapse responses into two categories may have helped mitigate this problem, but a response set bias may have affected the results nonetheless. Finally, the use of generation status and language use are imperfect indicators of acculturation. Although these indicators are the two most commonly used, and are closely related to more elaborate measures, acculturation is more appropriately viewed as a multidimensional process that includes change in a variety of dimensions (Samaniego & Gonzales, 1999). The authors' inferences regarding the relationship between acculturation and reproductive attitudes and behavior should be interpreted with this in mind.

Acculturation and Reproductive Attitudes and Behavior

Respondents were divided into three groups for purposes of analysis: those born outside the United States, those born in the United States who spoke primarily Spanish at home, and those born in the United States who spoke primarily English in the home. Of these groups, those born outside the United States were significantly less likely to be sexually active than the other groups. Being born in this country, regardless of language spoken at home, was associated with more sexual activity among the Latinas in this study. This result is consistent with those of Flores et al. (1998), who found that more acculturated Latinas had more positive attitudes toward sexuality than did less acculturated Latinas, and with those of Ford and Norris (1993) who found that less acculturated urban Latina adolescents were less sexually active than U.S.-born urban adolescents. These results contradict those of Brindis et al. (1995), who found that foreign-born adolescents were more likely to engage in sexual activity than U.S.-born adolescents.

Interestingly, among those respondents who were sexually active, no differences were found for contraceptive use between the two groups, contrary to the findings of Ford and Norris (1993) that less acculturated Latinas were less likely to use contraceptives. In this study over one-third of the sexually active respondents did not use contraception at last sexual experience. Previous research has indicated that Latina adolescents were less likely to use contraceptives than those from other groups (Abma et al., 1997; Ford, Sohn, & Lepkowski, 2001); others have imputed this difference to more conservative gender roles held by Latinos (Marin & Gomez, 1996, cited in Marble, 1996).

In the bivariate analysis, those respondents who were born outside the United States were less likely to agree that their parents would want them to use protection if they had sex. These respondents were also more likely to agree that they wanted to wait until marriage to engage in sexual activity. One explanation for this finding is that respondents born outside of the United States were less likely to have discussed the possibility of sexual activity with their parents, thereby reducing the chances that their parents had discussed contraception with them. Their desire to delay sexual activity until marriage was stronger than that of adolescents born in the United States, whether speaking Spanish or English in the home. Traditional Latino culture discourages the sexual activity of adolescent girls, who are supported in sexual abstinence by the cultural value of marianismo (Pavich, 1986). As a corollary to these more traditional attitudes toward sexual activity, those respondents born outside the United States were less likely to cite their fear of STIs as a reason for waiting to have sex. They may have been less aware of STIs than respondents in the other two groups, or they may have viewed STIs as a less important reason to delay sexual activity than their desire to wait until marriage.

Respondents who were born in the United States and spoke primarily Spanish in the home were more likely than the other two groups to endorse the statement that their parents would be upset as their reason for delaying sexual activity. These adolescents may have felt more pressure to complete their schooling and fulfill their parents' expectations than the other two groups. Similarly, when looking at educational goals and future aspirations, respondents in this group were more likely to say they planned to attend college than the other two groups. This response also may have been shaped by parental expectations. While respondents born in the United States were likely to be more acculturated than respondents born outside the United States, the fact that their parents spoke Spanish in the home suggests that their parents may have immigrated to this country. Research suggests that first generation immigrants have higher expectations for their children than other groups (Bulcroft & Carmody, 1996; Tschann, 1999).

Acculturation and Attitudes Toward Self

Attitudes towards self did not vary among the three groups of respondents with one exception. Respondents born outside the United States were more likely to "wish that they had more to be proud of" than did either group of respondents born in the United States. First generation immigrant adolescents may be struggling with the conflict between traditional parental values and peer expectations. Insofar as traditional Latino culture emphasizes adolescent dependency and resistance to peer pressure, as Tschann (1999) argued, immigrant Latina adolescents might find peer expectations in the United States a source of conflict and personal devaluation.

Religion and Attitudes Toward Sexuality

In this study there was no difference in sexual activity or contraceptive use between those who viewed religion as important and those who did not. This result is inconsistent with that of Liebowitz et al. (1999), who found that religiosity was one of the predictors of the absence of sexual activity in a sample of Latino and Latina adolescents in Texas. On the other hand, Perkins et al. (1998) studied adolescent girls and found that religiosity did not predict sexual activity in Latinas. Earlier research had found that strong religious beliefs were inversely associated with sexual activity and contraceptive use (Brindis, 1992; Holden et al., 1993). There may be a gender effect that exists in the relationship of religion to reproductive activity: This relationship may be stronger for males.

Predictors of Sexual Activity and Contraceptive Use

In the regression analysis, place of birth remained the most powerful predictor of sexual activity, even after controlling for the attitudinal factors discussed above; that is, those born outside the United States were less likely to engage in sexual activity than those born in the United States, regardless of language spoken at home. Other, somewhat less powerful predictors of sexual activity were age (the older, the more sexually active), and two reasons for delaying sexual activity: parents would be upset and desire to wait until marriage. For contraceptive use among those sexually active, only fear of STIs and planning to attend college were predictors. Findings from this study suggest that less acculturated adolescents are less likely to engage in sexual activity. Place of birth was a more powerful predictor of differences in reproductive attitudes and behavior than was language spoken at home, suggesting that adolescents born outside the United States are more traditional in these respects than adolescents whose families spoke Spanish at home, but who were born in the United States. In this study, language spoken at home was not an important predictor of sexual activity; only place of birth was powerfully linked to adolescent sexual activity among Latinas. Latina adolescents who are born in the United States are at higher risk of engaging in sexual activity than those who are born elsewhere.

Implications

Pregnancy prevention programs should target Latina adolescents born in the United States. Inasmuch as fear of STIs and desire to attend college were associated with contraceptive use, pregnancy prevention programs should include these dimensions in their education and counseling efforts. Social workers and other allied professionals working with Latina adolescents should recognize that acculturation is a risk factor for sexual activity and ultimately for adolescent pregnancy. While cultural attitudes and beliefs that encourage Latinas born outside the United States to delay sexual activity are not likely to be recreated by pregnancy prevention programs, there are other factors, such as fear of STIs and desire to attend college that can be emphasized to empower Latina adolescents to delay sexual activity and to use contraception when they are sexually active. Counseling efforts and program design should incorporate these factors.

REFERENCES

Abma, J.C., Chandra, A., Mosher, W.D., Peterson, L. & Piccinino, L. (1997). Fertility, family planning and women's health: New Data from the 1995 National Survey of Family Growth. *Vital Health Statistics*, 23 (19).

Ahn, N. (1994). Teenage childbearing and high school completion: Accounting for individual heterogeneity. *Family Planning Perspectives*, 26(1),17-21.

Aneshensel, C., Becerra, R., Fielder, E., & Schuler, R. (1990). Onset of Fertility-Related Events during Adolescents: A Prospective comparison of Mexican American and non-Hispanic White females. *American Journal of Public Health*, 80 (8), 959-963.

Baezconde-Garbanti, L. & Portillo, C. (1999). Disparities in Health Indicators for Latinas in California. *Hispanic Journal of Behavioral Sciences*, 21 (3), 302-330.

Baumeister, J., Flores, E. & Marin, B. (1995). Sex information given to Latina adolescents by parents. *Health Education Research*, 10, 233-239.

Baldwin, J. & Whiteley, S. (1992). The effect of ethnic group on sexual activities related to contraception and STDS. *Journal of Sex Research*, 29 (2), 189-208.

Bulcroft, R. & Carmody, D. (1996). Patterns of parental independence giving to adolescents: Variations by race, age, and gender of child. *Journal of Marriage and the Family*, 58 (4), 866-884.

Bishop-Townsend, V. (1996). STDs: Screening, Therapy and long-term implications for the adolescent patient. *International Journal of Fertility and Menopausal Studies*, 41 (2), 109-114.

Brindis, C. (1992). Adolescent pregnancy prevention for Hispanic youth. *Journal of School Health*, 62, 345-351.

Brindis, C.D., Wolfe, A.L., McCarter, V., Ball, S., & Starbuck-Morales, S. (1995). The association between immigrant status and risk-behavior patterns in Latino adolescents. *Journal of Adolescent Health*, 17 (2) 99-105.

Catania, J.A., Coates, T.J., Kegeles, S., Fullilove, M.T., Peterson, J., & Jarin, B. (1992). Condom use in the multi-ethnic neighborhood of San Francisco. *American Journal of Public Health*, 98, 284-287.

Centers for Disease Control. (2000). Youth risk behavior surveillance–United States, 1999. *MMWR*, 49 (05), 1-96.

Cuellar, I. & Roberts, R. (1997). Relations of depression, acculturation, and socioeconomic status in a Latino sample. *Hispanic Journal of Behavioral Sciences*, 19 (2), 230-239.

Curtin, S.C. & Martin, J.A. (2000). Births: Preliminary data for 1999. *National Vital Statistics Report*, 48 (14). Hyattsville, MD: National Center for Health Statistics.

Dore, M.M. & Dumois, A.O. (1990). Cultural differences in the meaning of adolescent pregnancy. *Families in Society*, 7 (2), 93-101.

Driscoll, A., Biggs, M.A., Brindis, C., & Yankah, E. (2001). Adolescent Latino reproductive health: A review of the literature. *Hispanic Journal of Behavioral Sciences*, 23 (3), 255-326.

Esparza, D.V. & Esperat, C.R. (1996). The effects of childhood sexual abuse on minority adolescent mothers. *Journal of Obstetric, Gynecologic and Neonatal Nursing*, 25, 321-328.

Falicov, C.J. (1984). Mexican families. In M. McGoldrick, J.K. Pearce, & G. Giordano (Eds.) *Ethnicity and Family Therapy* (pp. 134-163), New York: Guilford.

Felix, Ortiz, M. & Newcomb, M. (1994). A multidimensional measure of cultural identity for Latino and Latina adolescents. *Hispanic Journal of Behavioral Sciences*, 16 (2), 99-108.

Flores, E., Eyre, S. & Millstein, S. (1998). Sociocultural beliefs related to sex among Mexican American adolescents. *Hispanic Journal of Behavioral Sciences*, 20, 60-81.

Ford, K. & Norris, A.E. (1993). Urban Hispanic adolescents and young adults: Relation of acculturation to sexual behavior. *Journal of Sex Research*, 30, 316-323.

Ford, K., Sohn, W., & Lepkowski, J. (2001). *Family Planning Perspectives*, 33 (3), 100-106.

Frisbie, W.P. (1994). Birth weight and infant mortality in the Mexican origin and Anglo populations. *Social Science Quarterly*, 75 (4), 881-895.

Gibson, M. (1998). Promoting academic success among immigrant students: Is acculturation the issue? *Educational Policy*, 12 (6), 615-634.

Gomez, C. & Martin, B. (1996). Gender, culture, and power: Barriers to HIV-prevention strategies for women. *Journal of Sex Research*, 33 (4), 355-363.

Allan Guttmacher Institute. (1994a). *Sex and America's teenagers*. New York: Author.

Allan Guttmacher Institute. (1994b). *Teenage reproductive health in the United States*. New York: Author.

Haverman, R., Wolfe, B., & Wilson, K. (1997). Childhood poverty and adolescent schooling and fertility outcomes: Reduced-form and structural estimates. In G.J. Duncan & J. Brooks-Gunn (Eds.), *Consequences of growing up poor* (pp. 419-464). New York: Russell Sage Foundations.

Henshaw, S.K. (1997). *U.S. teenage pregnancy statistics*. New York: The Alan Guttmacher Institute.

Holden, G.W., Nelson, P.B., Velasquez, J., & Ritchie, K.L. (1993). Cognitive, psychosocial and reported sexual behavior differences between pregnant and non pregnant adolescents. *Adolescence*, 28, 557-570.

Hovell, M., Sipan, C., Blumber, E., Atkins, C., Hofstetter, C.R., & Kreitner, S. (1994). Family influences on Latino and Anglo adolescents' sexual behavior. *Journal of Marriage and the Family*, 56, 973-986.

Hurtado, M. & Gauvain, M. (1997). Acculturation and planning for college youth of Mexican Descent. *Hispanic Journal of Behavioral Sciences*, 19 (4), 506-517.

Kahn, L., Kinchen, S.A., Williams, B.I., Ross, J.G., Lowry, R., Gunbaum, J.A., & Kolbe, I.J. (2000). Youth risk behavior surveillance–United States, 1999. *MMWR*, 49 (05), 1-96.

Kaplan, M.S. & Mark, G. (1990). Adverse effects of accuturation: Psychological distress among Mexican American young adults. *Social Science and Medicine*, 31, 1313-1319.

Land, H. & Hudson, S. Methodological considerations in surveying Latina AIDS caregivers: Issues in sampling and measurement. *Social Work Research*, 21 (4), 233-257.

Lee, B.J. & George, R.M. (1999). Poverty, early childbearing, and child matreatment: A multinomial analysis. *Children and Youth Services Review*, 21 (9/10), 755-780.

Liebowitz, S.W., Castellano, D.C. & Cuellar, I. (1999). Factors that predict sexual behaviors among young Mexican American adolescents: An exploratory study. *Hispanic Journal of Behavioral Sciences*, 21 (4), 470-479.

Marin, G. (1992). Issues in the measurement of acculturation among Hispanics. In K.F. Geisinger (Ed.), *Psychological testing of Hispanics* (pp. 235-251). Washington, DC: American Psychological Association.

Marin, B.V. & Flores, E. (1994). Acculturation, sexual behavior, and alcohol use among Latinas. *International Journal of the Addictions*, 29, 1101-1114.

Marin, B. & Gomez, C. (1996). Latino gender roles impede condom use. Paper presented at the 11th International Conference on AIDS, Vancouver, British Columbia. Cited in Marble, M. (1996). *Women's Health Weekly*, 7/29/96, p. 2.

Marin, B., Tschann, J., Gomez, C., & Gregorich, S. (1998). Self-efficacy to use condoms in unmarried Latino adults. *American Journal of Community Psychology*, 26 (1), 53-69.

Marks, G. & Cantero, P.J. (1998). Is acculturation associated with sexual risk behaviors? An investigation of HIV-positive Latino men and women. *AIDS Care*, 10 (3), 283-296.

Miranda, A. & Matheny, K.B. (2000). Socio-psychological predictors of acculturative stress among Latino adults. *Journal of Mental Health Counseling*, 22 (4), 306-318.

Miranda, A. & Umhoefer, D. (1998). Depression and social interest differences between Latinos in dissimilar acculturation stages. *Journal of Mental Health Counseling*, 20 (2), 159-172.

National Campaign to Prevent Teen Pregnancy. (1999). *Fact Sheet: Teen pregnancy and childbearing among Latinos in the United States.* Washington, D.C.: Author.

National Center for Educational Statistics. (1994). Digest of Education statistics. (DHHS Publication No. NCES 94-115). Washington, DC: U.S. Government Printing Office.

Padilla, A. & Baird, T. (1991). Mexican American adolescent sexuality and sexual knowledge: An exploratory study. *Hispanic Journal of Behavioral Sciences*, 13, 95-105.

Pavich, E.G. (1986). A Chicana perspective on Mexican culture and sexuality. *Journal of Social Work and Human Sexuality*, 4, 47-65.

Perez, W. & Padilla, A.M. (2000). Cultural orientation across three generations of Hispanic adolescents. *Hispanic Journal of Behavioral Sciences*, 22(3), 390-398.

Perkins, D. & Luster, T. (1998). An ecological, risk-factor examination of adolescents' sexual activity in three ethnic groups. *Journal of Marriage and the Family*, 60 (3), 660-674.

Plotnick, R.D. (1992). The effects of attitudes on teenage premarital pregnancy and its resolution. *American Sociological Review*, 57 (6), 800-811.

Rew, L. (1997). Health-related, help-seeking behaviors in female Mexican American adolescents. *Journal of the Society of Pediatric Nursing*, 2, 156-162.

Sabogal, F., Perez-Stable, E., & Eliseo, J. (1995). Gender, ethnic and acculturation differences in Hispanic and non-Hispanic White adults. *Hispanic Journal of Behavioral Sciences*, 17, 139-159.

Samaniego, R. & Gonzales, N. (1999). Multiple mediators of the effects of acculturation status on delinquency for Mexican American adolescents. *American Journal of Community Psychology*, 27 (2), 189-209.

Shinkman, R. (1997). Studies: California Latinos Behind in Access to Health Care. *Modern Healthcare*, 27 (50), 25.

Soler, H., Quadagno, D., & Sly, D. (2000). Relationship dynamics, ethnicity and condom use among low-income women. *Family Planning Perspectives*, 32 (2), 82-90.

Sneed, C.D. (2001). 'Don't know' and 'Didn't think of it': Condom use at first intercourse by Latino adolescents. *AIDS Care*, 13 (3), 303-309.

Stroup-Benthan, C. & Trevino, F. (1991). Reproductive characteristics of Mexican American, mainland Puerto Rican, and Cuban American women. *JAMA*, 265, 222-226.

Sugland, B.W., Manlove, J.M. & Romano, A.D. (1997). Perceptions of opportunity and adolescent fertility: Operationalizing across race/ethnicity and social class. Paper presented at the annual meeting of the Population Association of America. Washington, DC.

Tschann, J. (1999). Assessing interparental conflict: Reports of parents and adolescents in European American and Mexican American families. *Journal of Marriage and the Family*, 61 (2), 269-284.

Upchurch, D., Aneschensel, C. Mudgal, J., & McNeely, C. (2001). Sociocultural contexts of time to first sex among Hispanic adolescents. *Journal of Marriage and the Family*, 63 (4), 1158-1170.

Ventura, J., Mosher, W.D., Curtin, S.C., Abma, J.C., & Henshaw, S. (2000). Trends in pregnancy and pregnancy rates by outcome: Estimates for the United States, 1976-96. *Vital Health Statistics*, 21 (56): United States Department of Health and Human Services: Hyattsville, MD. 1-23.

Whitaker, D.J., Miller, K.S., May, D.C., & Levin, M.L. (1999).Teenage partners communication about sex and condom use: The importance of parent-teenager discussions. *Family Planning Perspectives*, 31 (3), 117-121.

Wood, M.L. & Price, P. (1997). Machismo and marianismo: Implications for HIV/AIDS risk reduction and education. *American Journal of Health Studies*. 13 (1), 44-53.

Zambrana, R. & Logie, L.A. (2000). Latino Child Health: Need for Inclusion in the U.S. National Discourse. *American Journal of Public Health*, 90 (12), 1827-1834.

The GIG: An Innovative Intervention to Prevent Adolescent Pregnancy and Sexually Transmitted Infection in a Latino Community

Diane de Anda

SUMMARY. The GIG[1] is an innovative community based intervention which offers education regarding pregnancy and sexually transmitted infection (STI) risks and prevention in the context of a social event that is open to the adolescent community. This intensive, six hour intervention features live and recorded music, celebrities from local radio stations, raffles and prizes, and a number of educational activities providing instruction regarding pregnancy and STI risks and prevention. A total of 609 Latino adolescents completed matched pre and posttest measures. The increase in the total mean score from pretest to posttest was found to be statistically significant, as were the separate analyses for items related to pregnancy and those related to STIs. Information regarding specific attitudes and areas of knowledge are provided. Important intervention components related to the research literature are discussed along with areas of success, especially with regard to risk factors, and those in need of further attention in future intervention events. Recommendations for reinforcing

Diane de Anda, PhD, is Associate Professor, Department of Social Welfare, School of Public Policy and Social Research, University of California, Los Angeles.

[Haworth co-indexing entry note]: "The GIG: An Innovative Intervention to Prevent Adolescent Pregnancy and Sexually Transmitted Infection in a Latino Community." de Anda, Diane. Co-published simultaneously in *Journal of Ethnic & Cultural Diversity in Social Work* (The Haworth Social Work Practice Press, an imprint of The Haworth Press, Inc.) Vol. 11, No. 3/4, 2002, pp. 251-277; and: *Social Work with Multicultural Youth* (ed: Diane de Anda) The Haworth Social Work Practice Press, an imprint of The Haworth Press, Inc., 2002, pp. 251-277. Single or multiple copies of this article are available for a fee from The Haworth Document Delivery Service [1-800-HAWORTH, 9:00 a.m. - 5:00 p.m. (EST). E-mail address: docdelivery@haworthpress.com].

http://www.haworthpress.com/store/product.asp?sku=J051

10.1300/J051v11n03_05

and enhancing the GIG messages are presented along with implications of the findings for social work and health care professionals responsible for designing interventions for at-risk youth.

KEYWORDS. Adolescent pregnancy, sexually transmitted infections, Latino adolescents, intervention, prevention

INTRODUCTION

Adolescent sexual behavior has become a social concern because of the potential for related health risks. Although emotional/psychological risks of early sexual experiences have been recognized, the major focus of policymakers, service professionals, and the public has been with regard to pregnancy and sexually transmitted infections (STI), including HIV/AIDS. The rates for pregnancy and childbirth among adolescents as well as for sexually transmitted infections have been carefully monitored and adolescent populations at particular risk identified. Latino adolescents are one such population at risk.

The adolescent pregnancy rates climbed steadily from 95.1 per 1000 for 15 to 19 year olds and 62.4 per 1000 for 15 to 17 year olds in 1972 to an all time high of 117.1 (in 1990) and 74.4 (in 1989), respectively. The first half of the 1990s saw a slow decline followed by a more rapid decrease to below the 1972 rate by 1997: 93.0 for 15 to 19 year olds and 57.7 for 15 to 17 year olds (Alan Guttmacher Institute, 1999a). However, while the pregnancy rate between 1990 and 1996 dropped 20% for African American adolescents and 16% for White adolescents, the pregnancy rate for Hispanic/Latino adolescents increased between 1990 and 1992 and by 1996 decreased by only 6% (Alan Guttmacher Institute, 1999b). Moreover, the birth rate for Hispanic/Latino adolescents (149.3) is the highest among all adolescent populations. The rate for non-Hispanic Black adolescents is slightly lower (141.0) even though their pregnancy rate is higher, because non-Hispanic Black adolescents have higher abortion rates than their Hispanic/Latino cohorts (Health, United States, 2000).

Latino youth are at particular risk for HIV/AIDS infection: "In 1996-1998, non-Hispanic black and Hispanic adolescents in every age group had higher rates of AIDS than non-Hispanic white adolescents"

(Health, United States, 2000, p. 72). Although the AIDS rates are relatively low in this age group, the extremely high rates of young adults in their twenties indicate that, given the long incubation period, the rate of HIV infection is very high in the adolescent population (Health, United States, 2000). In addition to HIV/AIDS, the rate of sexually transmitted infections is estimated to be one in four in the sexually active youth population (Centers for Disease Control and Prevention, 2002).

Moreover, national survey data indicate that Latino youth also demonstrate risk factors with regard to pregnancy and sexually transmitted infection. Only about half (55.2%) of Latino adolescents (43% of females) reported using a condom at last sexual intercourse; less than 8% (7.8%) used birth control pills; 16.6% (23.0% males) had four or more sexual partners, and 22.5% used alcohol or drugs at last intercourse. In addition, 14.2% had their first experience of sexual intercourse prior to age 13. (It is important to note that Hispanic/Latino youth also had the highest percentage of abstinent youth, 32.7% versus 25.3% for African American and 27.0% for White youth.) (Youth Risk Surveillance, 1999).

The risk factors among the Latino youth population are important to address, because of the growth of the Latino population over the last decade and the projected growth over the next few decades. The Latino population as a whole increased to 12.5% of the nation's population, becoming the largest minority population in the United States (Census 2000). Furthermore, the Latino population is younger than other population groups, so that Latino youth comprised 17% of the youth population in 2000 and is projected to rise to 24% by 2025 (Driscoll, Biggs, Brindis, & Yankah, 2001). With 54.1% of Latino high school youth reporting that they have had sexual intercourse, and 36.3% in the past three months, this represents a substantial youth group at risk.

Given the above risks, it is critical that prevention efforts that have demonstrated effectiveness be directed at Latino youth populations. However, although a myriad of interventions have been developed over the last two decades, there is significant debate regarding their effectiveness and conflicting interpretations of the empirical research findings (see Literature Review). Nevertheless, there is concurrence that programs which have demonstrated the greatest success are those which are composed of multiple, diverse components, include peer educators and role models, and are culturally relevant to the target group (DiCenso, Gutatt & Griffith, 2002; Kirby, 2002; Kim, Stanton, Dickersin & Galbraith, 1997). The GIG intervention evaluated in this article is one component of a pregnancy and STI prevention program, includes youth leaders in the conducting of the intervention, and has been uniquely tailored to the youth culture of the participants.

PURPOSE

The aim of the GIG intervention is to impact both knowledge and attitudes. In terms of knowledge, the objectives include increasing accurate understanding of: (1) means of transmission and increased risks for transmission of sexually transmitted infections; (2) diagnosis and the visibility/nonvisibility of symptoms of sexually transmitted infections; (3) treatability/curability of specific sexually transmitted infections; (4) adequate and inadequate methods for protection against pregnancy and STI transmission (e.g., abstinence, withdrawal). Attitude change includes recognition of (1) the loss of future opportunities attendant to adolescent parenthood; (2) shared responsibility with regard to protection from pregnancy and STIs; (3) coercion in a sexual relationship; and (4) the impact of substance use on the ability to practice safe and responsible sex.

LITERATURE REVIEW

Overview

Concern over the rates of adolescent pregnancy and sexually transmitted infections has stimulated the creation of numerous intervention programs aimed at prevention and reduction of contributing risk factors. Hubbard, Giese and Rainey (1998) and Thomas (2000) trace the history of these programs, designating four "generations" in their evolution as the outcomes of the preceding generation of interventions failed to confirm their effectiveness. The first generation focused on increasing knowledge regarding the risks and negative consequences of adolescent pregnancy. Second generation interventions added values clarification, communication, and decision making skills as important factors. Third generation interventions adopted an abstinence only approach, generally abstinence until marriage and often to the exclusion of information regarding other methods of protection and contraception. The fourth and current generation interventions combine the above approaches to achieve a more comprehensive approach, are theory based, and have been subjected to more rigorous evaluation than those in previous generations.

The above categorization of current interventions, however, may not be totally accurate in that prevention efforts appear extremely diverse in content, focus, and approach, and run the gamut from abstinence only interventions (funded in particular by the Office of Pregnancy and Parenting under the Adolescent Family Life Act of 1981), to programs aimed at increasing condom use to prevent STIs (especially HIV/AIDS), and comprehensive programs that offer multiple options and generally employ skill-building approaches to intervention.

In a recent conference presentation to the staff of agencies with prevention programs funded by the state of California, Claire Brindis (2002), the state evaluator, identified the five types of programs which comprise these state funded interventions: (1) abstinence only, (2) youth development, (3) comprehensive family life education, (4) youth development and abstinence, (5) youth development and comprehensive family life education. She further indicated that empirical findings attest to the greater effectiveness of the last approach.

Coyle et al.'s (2001, 1999) longitudinal, randomized controlled study of nearly 4000 (n = 3869) youth in Texas and California demonstrated the effectiveness of a comprehensive, multi-component intervention in increasing behaviors which provide protection with regard to pregnancy and STIs. In his review of 73 intervention research studies, Kirby (2002) also concluded that comprehensive, multiple component interventions which address both sexual and non-sexual antecedents tended to be more effective. He qualified this position, however, with the caution that not all youth are in need of a comprehensive intervention, and that the appropriate intervention should be based on an assessment of the factors related to the adolescent's sexual risk-taking behavior. Moreover, Kirby identified two other types of intervention programs which have demonstrated positive outcomes: clinic protocols and service learning programs. His conclusion regarding both of these types of interventions, however, was based on a small number of studies. For example, his appraisal of clinic protocols was based on positive results regarding increased use of contraception and condoms in four out of six studies and reduction of pregnancy rates (while in the program) in three out of four studies evaluating youth service (to the community) programs.

In direct contrast, Thomas' (2000) review of abstinence based programs led him to conclude that there was a lack of "measurable success" (p. 16), particularly with regard to behavior change. Among the nine intervention programs evaluated, the few behavioral changes that were achieved were not sustained at long term follow-up or, in the case of Postponing Sexual Involvement (Howard, 1992; Howard & Mc Cabe, 1990), upon replication (Kirby, Korpi, Barth, & Cagampang, 1995). The programs fared better with respect to knowledge and attitude changes; however, methodological weaknesses (e.g., lack of representative sampling) did not allow for generalization and bring the findings into question.

Kirby's (2002) assessment of programs is somewhat different. First he warns that generalization and conclusions about effectiveness are difficult, because of the heterogeneity of these interventions in content, message, methods employed, duration, etc. Moreover, only three evaluations of abstinence programs met the criteria for inclusion in his analysis, and two of these had significant methodological problems. Despite the fact that none of the three studies had any significant impact on behavior, he cautions that the lack of studies with methodological rigor allows no conclusions to be drawn or generalized to all abstinence only programs.

Impact by Outcome Measure

Knowledge and Attitudes

The success of intervention programs has varied, often depending upon the types of outcome measures. Interventions with outcomes focused on changing knowledge and attitudes have reported the greatest success in achieving their objectives. Kim's (1997) "quantitative review" of 34 studies measuring gains in knowledge found 88% (n = 30) reported statistically significant gains in knowledge with the improvement rate favoring the randomized controlled (13/14) versus the non-randomized controlled studies (17/20).

Coyle et al.'s (2001, 1999) study (described previously) found not only significant differences in knowledge gains between the intervention and the control group at posttest, but sustained differences at the 7, 19, and 31 month follow-up.

On the other hand, Aaron et al.'s (2000) evaluation of a randomized controlled sample of 582 middle school students found differences in knowledge gains only after "booster sessions" the year subsequent (grade 8) to the initial intervention (7th grade).

Intent

Those few programs that have measured intent (e.g., to use protection, to reduce specific sexual risk behaviors, etc.) as an outcome variable have had mixed results. For example, Kim's (1999) analysis found a 60% improvement rate in intent in 10 (out of 40) studies that utilized that variable, and these were primarily non-randomized control studies.

Levy et al.'s (1995) evaluation of a school based AIDS prevention program on middle school children who became sexually active between seventh and eighth grade (n = 312) found mixed and ambiguous effects on intent, with no difference between experimentals and controls in the intention to have sex or use condoms in the next 12 months, but greater intention to use condoms with foam among the intervention group. The lack of difference in condom use without foam may be explained by a ceiling effect, since 97% of both the experimental and control group indicated intent to use a condom.

In contrast, Jemmott, Jemmott, and Fong (1992) found that among the 157 African American males participating in their study, a greater number of experimental versus control subjects reported "weaker intentions to engage in risky sexual behavior in the next three months" (p. 375).

Behavior

Interventions evaluated in terms of their impact on behavior related to pregnancy or STI risk and prevention have demonstrated considerably less effectiveness, with differences depending upon the specific behaviors measured.

Initiation of sex. Abstinence or delaying of initiation of sexual intercourse was, for the most part, not achieved. For example, Kim et al.'s (1997) review found only six studies which measured abstinence, and of these only two found significant differences between experimentals and controls (one randomized and one non-randomized controlled study). Similarly, Kirby's (2002) review identified two interventions that delayed the onset of sexual intercourse, the Children's Aid Society CARRERA Program, a collection of long-term intensive programs, and a program combining a health education curriculum and service learning component. It is noteworthy with regard to the latter that the researchers (O'Donnell et al., 1999, 2001) indicated that the curriculum alone was not successful in delaying initiation of sex in their sample of 2029 adolescents.

Hubbard et al.'s (1998) replication study found significant differences in initiating sex between experimentals (intervention participants) and controls; however, the difference is questionably meaningful in that the number of adolescents available for the analysis (those who were sexually inexperienced at last measure) diminished considerably from his initial n of 212 to an n of 69 for the experimental group and an n of 56 for the control group. As a result, the difference in the number of youth who initiated sex since the last measure, although statistically significant, amounted to only 5 students (E = 19, C = 24).

Finally, DiCenso et al.'s (2002) meta-analysis of 13 studies with females (n = 9642) and 11 studies with males (n = 7418) that included initiation of sexual intercourse as an outcome variable found no difference in delay of sexual intercourse between intervention participants and controls.

Condom Use and Contraception. DiCenso et al. (2002) also demonstrated the ineffectiveness of a number of studies (females' n = 799; males' n = 1262) with regard to improvement in the use of birth control (at last intercourse). Kim et al.'s (1997) analyses reported mixed results: significant improvement in condom use among 100% (7 of 7) of the non-randomized controlled studies examined and among 50% (4 of 8) of the randomized controlled studies. (It is important to note that non-random assignment has been associated with inflation of differences between experimental and control group subjects.)

In contrast, Kirby's (2002) analysis found condom and contraceptive use to have improved significantly in four studies of clinic protocol interventions and three community based interventions with methodologically sound evaluations, including randomization, large samples, and long term follow-up data. Kirby reported the results of one of these latter studies, Coyle et al. (1999), at 7 month follow-up. In a subsequent study, Coyle et al. (2001) found an increased use of condoms and contraception among intervention participants versus controls at 31 month follow-up.

Sexual Risk Behavior. A few studies have examined the effects of interventions on sexual risk behavior, such as multiple sexual partners. Kim et al. (2001) found a 73% decrease in the number of sexual partners in 7 of the 11 studies employing it as an outcome variable, 3 out of 5 randomized controlled and 4 out of 6 non-randomized controlled studies. Coyle et al. (1999, 2001) found no significant differences between experimentals and controls at 7 and 31 month follow up (n = 1371).

Thomas's (2000) review of abstinence programs identified only one program measuring this outcome, and no significant differences were found at posttest. Finally, Levy et al. (1995), in their study of 312 middle school students, found the intervention did not differentially reduce the number of sexual partners between intervention and control groups.

Pregnancy and STI. Oddly enough, although the ultimate aim of the intervention programs reported herein is the prevention of adolescent pregnancy, pregnancy rates have been examined as an outcome variable in relatively few studies. None of the 40 studies in Kim et al.'s (2002) meta-analysis measured pregnancy rates. In his review of abstinence programs, Thomas (2000) found only one program which examined pregnancy rates as an outcome; Postponing Sexual Involvement reported a 33% lower rate of pregnancy in the intervention group in their study with non-random assignment.

Even in studies whose aim is to prevent and reduce STIs in the adolescent population, the outcome variables are risk factors related to STIs (multiple sexual partners, unprotected sexual intercourse, etc.) rather than the STI rate itself. None of the major reviews and meta-analyses cited above identified research with STI rates as an outcome variable. This may be the case because the intervention settings do not lend themselves to any type of laboratory verification, and there may be both constraints on requesting that information of minors and questions regarding the validity of self-report data. However, a survey research study by Millstein and Moscicki (1995) of 571 sexually active female adolescents (13-19 years of age) found that "risky sexual behavior showed a significant association with STD status (Chi-square [change] 18.9, $df = 1,472$, $\beta = .26$, $p \leq .0001$) with more risky behavior associated with positive STD results" (p. 87).

Multiple Behaviors. A few studies show improvement in multiple areas. For example, Jemmott et al. (1992), in their randomized controlled study of 157 African American male adolescents, found that those who had received a 5 hour intensive HIV/AIDS prevention intervention scored significantly higher at posttest than controls in knowledge and had less favorable attitudes towards and stronger intention against engaging in sexual risk behaviors. At the three month follow-up, significant differences were maintained with regard to knowledge and intentions, and the intervention group reported a significantly lower incidence of engaging in sexual risk behaviors.

Coyle et al. (2001) found improvement in 7 out of 15 psychosocial variables (e.g., knowledge, attitudes, self-efficacy, perceived risk, intention) as well as condom and contraceptive use. Hubbard's (1998) replication study reported lower frequencies of initiation of sex, greater use of prevention, and higher frequency of communication with parents about birth control and STI/HIV protection. However, reduction in the sample size by nearly 50% for some of the analyses raises some questions regarding the findings.

Conclusions

The literature on pregnancy and STI prevention interventions offers no definitive answers regarding specific best practice models that impact all relevant areas: knowledge, attitude, intent, and behavior. Even evaluations presented by reviews and meta-analyses of the literature have not been congruent in their examination and assessment of the extant body of research. Kirby (2002) presents a number of positive findings and concludes on an optimistic note: "In sum, it is very encouraging that there are now four different and somewhat complementary types of programs for adolescents with rather strong evidence that they effectively reduce either unprotected sex that place youth at risk of pregnancy or STD/HIV, or that they reduce actual pregnancy" (p. 56).

Thomas (2000), focusing solely on abstinence interventions, provides a strong criticism of the literature, particularly its methodological limitations: "Up to the present time, no evaluated program with an exclusive abstinence message has been evaluated in such a way as to show a significantly positive impact on behavior; some have shown a desirable effect on attitude" (p. 16).

Kim et al.'s (2001) meta-analysis of 40 AIDS risk reduction programs concludes that interventions appear to impact knowledge and behavior related to condom use, but not abstinence. They indicate that the lack of "published articles of sufficient rigor" (p. 211) weakens the evidence for intervention effect with regard to attitude and intention.

Finally, DiCenso et al.'s (2002) review and meta-analysis of randomized controlled studies intended to reduce adolescent pregnancy presents the harshest evaluation:

> The results of our systematic review show that primary prevention strategies do not delay the initiation of sexual intercourse or improve the use of birth control among young men and women. Meta-analyses showed no reduction in pregnancies among young women, but data from five studies, four of which evaluated abstinence programmes and one of which evaluated a school based programme, show that interventions may increase pregnancies in partners of male participants. (p. 6)

All of the above concur that the intervention research literature is extremely heterogeneous, rife with methodological limitations, and in need of further research with more methodological rigor before certain conclusions regarding prevention efforts can be reached. Despite their differing perspectives, there is also agreement regarding a number of characteristics that appear to be associated with more successful interventions: (1) The intervention is theory-based. (Most often, social cognitive theory is cited.) (2) Peers are used as educators and role models. (3) The intervention includes skills training (e.g., negotiation, communication, and refusal skills) in addition to information aimed at knowledge and attitude change. (4) The intervention involves the community and is culturally relevant. (5) The intervention is of sufficient duration to reinforce the content.

THE INTERVENTION

The GIG is an innovative community based intervention which offers education regarding pregnancy and sexually transmitted infection (STI) risks and prevention in the context of a social event that is open to the adolescent community. This intervention is the community outreach component of a larger, primarily school-based multiple intervention program funded by the state and conducted by a large community social service agency with the cooperation of the school and assistance of a limited number of the school staff. Each GIG event, which is scheduled from 6:00 p.m. to midnight on a Friday or Saturday, takes place in an off-campus, city facility, features a disc jockey, celebrities from the local radio stations, live and recorded music, raffles and prizes, and a number of activities providing instruction regarding pregnancy and STI risks and prevention.

The educational activities are provided by the agency staff as well as peers who have received leadership and related health education training. The educational messages are presented via a variety of methods. Banners and posters with messages about pregnancy and STIs are the primary decorations. The youth participants visit a number of booths each focused on a different issue, such as, specific sexually transmitted infections (e.g., the HIV/AIDS booth, the chlamydia booth), contraception, adolescent pregnancy, and adolescent parenting. The booths provide packets to the youth with written materials on their issue and hygiene products (e.g., toothbrushes and toothpaste), personnel to discuss the issue and answer questions, and the opportunity to spin a Wheel of Fortune to win a prize if the participants are able to answer related questions correctly and further education if they answer incorrectly. (The distribution of condoms to minors is restricted in the city facilities, and, therefore, condoms could not be included in the packets.) A RAP contest has also been held in which various youth competed by composing and performing RAP songs related to pregnancy and STI prevention.

Every hour to hour and a half, the music is stopped and staff members go on stage and ask random questions regarding pregnancy and STI risks and prevention, with prizes provided to participants who offer correct answers. Prizes include music CD's and movie tickets. As further motivational devices, a number of "giveaways" are also provided to the youth who attend: key chains, less expensive music CD's, posters, etc. All youth who complete the posttest measure receive a free t-shirt and are eligible for raffle prizes (e.g., more expensive CD's, gift certificates to specific stores) including the grand prizes: sets of tickets to a local go-cart speedway.

METHODS

A repeated measures design was employed to determine the effectiveness of the intervention. That is, the adolescents completed pretests and posttests which determined the accuracy of their knowledge and the congruence of their attitudes with the program objectives. The data were collected from four separate GIG events held in academic year 2001-2002.

The Sample

The sample was comprised of self-selected adolescent participants who responded to local school and community advertisements regarding the events and/or friends and relatives from other communities invited by local youth. The local community is comprised of three small, incorporated cities in Los Angeles County with a combined population of 103,652 and which are 92.2% Latino (United Way of Greater Los Angeles; 1998-99).

Only those participants who completed pre and posttests that could be matched were included in the sample. Because the posttest was completed towards the end of the evening, this excluded those adolescents who left the event earlier for a variety of reasons. The only bias that might have resulted was in terms of age, since the majority of those who left early were young adolescents who were picked up by their parents. Thirteen (13) and 14 year olds accounted for two-thirds of the approximate 300 pretests for which there were no matching posttests. Moreover, using only those participants who remained through the entire event increased uniform exposure to the intervention. Because of the "one shot" nature of the intervention, maximum exposure was important.

A total of 609 Latino adolescents completed matched pre and posttest measures. Males constituted a slight (15%) majority, accounting for 57.0% (n = 347) of the respondents and females 42.5% (n = 259); three failed to indicate gender. The age range of the group was quite broad, from 10 to 22 years of age with the majority (n = 460; 75.5%) in the 15 (n = 147; 24.1%) to 17 (n = 132; 21.7%) age range and 16 (n = 181; 29.7%) the median and modal age. A very small number of individuals comprised the younger (10-12: n = 4; .9%) and older (19-22: n = 11; 1.8%) end of the continuum with larger numbers for ages 14 (n = 81; 13.3%) and 18 (n = 41; 6.7%), representing middle school students who will be transitioning to high school the next year and 18 year old high school seniors.

Corresponding to the age distribution, the majority of the respondents were in high school grades 9 through 11 (n = 443; 72.8%), with nearly equal numbers of 10th and 11th graders. Forty (6.6%) of those who completed the measures were middle school students, and 17 (2.8%) were in college, probably recent high school graduates. Although 42.7% (n = 260) of the students attended the local high school and 10.8% (n = 66) a second high school in close proximity, 55 other schools were represented by small numbers of students, from 1 to 25. This is in contrast to the composition the previous year, when the overwhelming majority of those attending the event were from local schools. It appears that the GIGs have developed a reputation as a desirable social event to attend.

The Measure

Given the setting, the creation of a pretest/posttest measure was challenging. It was determined that the measure would need to be brief, the response categories simple, in the students' vernacular, and in a casual format appropriate to the event. Photographs of four Latino adolescents from a popular teen magazine were placed across from the questions to meet the last criterion. The measure was pilot tested for feedback on content, format, and readability with the peer educators and a small number of students in one of the other program interventions and revised. Further revisions resulted from use in earlier GIG events that served to pilot test the intervention as well. For the sake of brevity, minimal demographic data are obtained: gender,age, grade, school, and zip code. Initially all participants were Latino and from the local area, so that no information regarding ethnicity was necessary. As the reputation of the event has increased, it appears that the population may become more diverse, so ethnicity will be included on the measure for the subsequent year.

The measure is comprised of 15 statements (see Figure 1) based on the objectives listed above (see PURPOSE). Five (5) statements refer to pregnancy and/or parenting issues and 11 to sexually transmitted infections. Three items overlap, referring to risk or prevention of both pregnancy and STIs. One of the remaining items deals with coercion and the last with substance use and safe sex. The statements are phrased primarily in the first person so that the youth will respond from his/her perspective. For each statement, the respondent circles "right" if he/she believes the statement is correct and "wrong" is he/she believes it is incorrect. The instructions clarify that right and wrong refer to correct and incorrect so that the respondent does not think that the terms refer to moral positions. A question mark is circled if the respondent is unsure whether the statement is correct or incorrect. This option was added to reduce the frequency of guessing on unknown items and to serve as another measure of change. That is, the youth were expected to answer "unsure" (?) less often after participating in the intervention. Total scores are calculated based on the number of items marked accurately with regard to factual information and consonant with the intervention goals in terms of attitudes. All question marks are treated as incorrect answers.

Data Collection Procedures

The youth were divided into two lines, males and females, for entrance into the event. For security purposes, all participants were searched and were required to show a school identification card. Upon completion of the pretest measure, they were given entry to the event, two tickets for raffles held throughout the event, an identification badge with a number for matching the pre and posttests, and their hands were stamped. To provide motivation for completion of the posttest towards the end of the event, major raffle prizes were awarded contingent upon its completion. That is, the music was stopped and all present were given posttests to fill out, which upon completion entitled them to tickets for larger raffle prizes. The identification number given to each student upon entry to the event was placed on both the pre and posttest

FIGURE 1. GIG Measure Items

1. I can tell if someone I'm going to have sex with has an std (sexually transmitted disease).
2. I believe it's mostly the woman's responsibility to keep herself from getting pregnant.
3. I don't want to get an std, so I have to use a condom *every* time I have sex.
4. A guy should ignore a woman when she says "stop" or "no" to sex, 'cuz she's just playin' with him.
5. If I have a baby now, it can keep me from finishing school and getting a good job in the future.
6. I could have sex with lots of people, but I don't because that would make it easier for me to get std's, including HIV/AIDS.
7. Pulling out before coming is a good way for me and my partner to prevent pregnancy and std's.
8. If I get herpes from my sex partner, I will have herpes for the rest of my life.
9. If I have HIV, but don't feel sick, I can't give it to people I have sex with.
10. Abstinence (not having sex) is the only way for me to be 100% safe from std's and pregnancy.
11. I can get hepatitis B from having sex and not know it until I get really sick later.
12. Using drugs and alcohol make it harder for me to have safe and responsible sex.
13. I'm safe from pregnancy or std's if I only have unprotected sex one time.
14. I need a blood test and a medical check-up to know whether I have an std or not.
15. If I get an std, including HIV/AIDS, the doctor can cure it with a shot or pills.

measures to allow for matching of the measures for the analysis while maintaining anonymity.

Data Analysis

Paired t-test analyses were conducted to determine if the differences between the pretest and posttest means reached statistical significance for the total score on the 15 item measure and for separate summated scores for items related to sexually transmitted infections and items related to pregnancy prevention. ANCOVA analyses were performed to determine if there were gender or grade differences on the posttest scores using the pretest scores as the covariate. Finally, frequencies, percentages, and gain scores were calculated for the individual items to examine changes in specific attitudes and areas of knowledge from pretest to posttest.

FINDINGS

The effectiveness of the GIG intervention was measured by comparing the total pretest and posttest scores on the 15 item GIG Measure. The total score was a simple calculation of the number of items marked correctly, that is, demonstrating specific knowledge and attitudes consonant with the messages offered in the instruction on STI and pregnancy risks and prevention during the event.

Total Scores were calculated and paired t-tests were conducted on the means for the matched measures (see Table 1).

As noted in Table 1, the increase in the total mean score from pretest to posttest was found to be statistically significant. These findings indicate that the GIG experience was effective in increasing the participants' accurate knowledge regarding STI and pregnancy risks and prevention and in changing their attitudes in the desired direction (consonant with intervention objectives). Although the means appear to indicate a modest increase, the change represents an increase in scores from 72% to 82% correct responses on the measure. A comparison of the distribution of the total scores demonstrates the considerable positive change in knowledge and attitude over this brief period of time. For example, at pretest, 47.2% ($n = 289$) of the adolescents scored 12 or above on the measure, whereas at posttest this had increased to 60.0% ($n = 366$). Moreover, while only 6.4% ($n = 39$) obtained a perfect score of 15 at pretest, at posttest 26.4% ($n = 161$) achieved this score. In summary, the majority of this group of adolescents appears to have met the intervention objectives.

As Table 2 indicates, the initial level of knowledge (pretest) varied by grade as would have been expected, with the scores increasing by grade. ANCOVA analyses indicated that when the posttest scores were adjusted with the pretest as the covariate, no statistically significant differences were found among the three grades at posttest [$F = 1.695$; $df = 2$; $p = ns$]. It is noteworthy that middle school knowledge levels became comparable to the others at posttest and that even the college students increased their scores at posttest.

Males scored lower on the pretest (10.663) than females (11.127), but both had comparable scores at posttest, 12.084 for males and 12.467 for females. The ANCOVA performed on the data with the pretest as the covariate determined that there were no differences between the posttest scores of males and females when adjusted by the pretest scores [$F = 1.810$; $df = 1$; $p = ns$].

TABLE 1. t-test: GIG Measure Total Score (N = 609)

	M	SD	df	t
Pretest	10.85	2.92		
			608	−10.552***
Posttest	12.24	2.53		

***p < .001

TABLE 2. Means: Total Score by Grade

	Pretest	Posttest
6-8	9.625	12.150
9-12	10.837	12.132
college	12.882	13.647

The items on the measure were then divided into those related to pregnancy and parenting and those related to sexually transmitted infections, with separate total scores calculated followed by paired t-test comparisons between pre and posttest means. The results appear in Table 3.

As demonstrated in Table 3, statistically significant increases were found on the total scores for the 5 items dealing with pregnancy and parenting issues and the 11 items regarding the transmission, diagnosis, and treatment of sexually transmitted infections. Improvements in knowledge and attitude indicate that the intervention objectives were met with regard to both pregnancy and STIs.

A clearer understanding of the specific knowledge gained can be gleaned from the item by item data display in Table 4. Note that, for the sake of brevity, the general content of the item is indicated rather than the wording of the specific item.

It is important to note the high percentage of adolescents whose responses demonstrated accurate knowledge and attitudes consonant with the program objectives. This percentage increased noticeably at posttest. For example, at pretest only 2 items were answered correctly by more than 80% (81.4-85.2%) of the participants while at posttest 8 items (more than half) were answered correctly by 80% or more participants, and one item by more than 90% of the youth. Moreover, at pretest, 6 items had correct responses in the 62-69% range; no items at posttest fell below 72%.

TABLE 3. t-test: Pregnancy and Parenting Total Scores (N = 609)

	M	SD	df	t
Pretest	3.675	1.29		
			608	−6.725***
Posttest	4.076	1.09		

***p < .001

t-test: Sexually Transmitted Infections Total Scores (N = 609)

	M	SD	df	t
Pretest	7.993	2.19		
			608	−11.424***
Posttest	9.081	1.89		

***p < .001

TABLE 4. GIG Measures: Correct Responses (N = 609)

	Pretest		Posttest		Gains
	f	%	f	%	
STI's					
1 can tell has std	454	74.5	529	86.9	+75
3 condom every time	519	85.2	555	91.1	+ 36
6 multiple sex partners	420	69.0	494	81.1	+74
8 herpes is life-long	448	73.6	525	86.2	+77
9 HIV transmission	378	62.1	495	81.3	+117
11 hepatitis B transmission	423	69.4	461	75.7	+38
14 std: medical diagnosis	451	74.1	507	83.3	+56
15 pills cure std/HIV/AIDS	423	69.5	484	79.5	+ 61
STI's and Pregnancy/Parenting					
7 withdrawal as prevention	385	63.2	514	84.4	+129
10 abstinence 100% safe	496	81.4	492	80.8	−4
13 unprotected sex 1 time	471	77.3	474	77.8	+3
Pregnancy and Parenting					
2 bc woman's responsibility	444	72.9	540	88.7	+96
5 baby affects future	442	72.6	462	75.9	+20
Coercion					
4 ignore when says "no"	438	71.9	477	78.3	+39
Substance Use					
12 substance use and safe sex	416	68.3	444	72.9	+ 28

(Item numbers correspond to measure items in Figure 1.)

The figures in Table 4 indicate that substantial numbers of the youth increased their knowledge in all but a few areas. With regard to effective methods of STI and pregnancy prevention, two important items saw noteworthy increases at posttest: (1) recognition of withdrawal as an ineffective method had a 20% (+129) increase; and (2) recognition of the need to use a condom every time they have sex reached the highest level of all of the items, over 90%. Moreover, there was a substantial attitude change as well, with an approximately 16% (+96) increase in those recognizing that birth control was the responsibility of both partners (to 88.7%). However, the correct response rate for two items related to protection are of concern: (1) recognizing the risks of having sex even once without protection, and (2) understanding abstinence to be the only 100% effective method. The former appears to have hit a ceiling level of 77%, and the latter experienced a decline, though still maintained an 80+% rate.

Important increases were noted in accurate knowledge regarding the transmission, diagnosis, and treatment of sexually transmitted infections. The largest increase (19.2%; +117) was the recognition that an asymptomatic HIV positive individual could transmit the infection. This is particularly noteworthy, because only 62.1% thought this was the case at pretest. Recognition that transmissible hepatitis B can also be asymptomatic lags somewhat behind, with an increase of 6.3%. Recognition of the incurability of herpes also had a large increase at posttest (12.6%; +77) to one of the highest percentages of correct responses (86.2%). Although a 10% increase was seen at posttest, fewer than 80% understood that HIV/AIDS is not curable at this time.

Few maintained the naive belief that one could "tell" if a sexual partner had a sexually transmitted infection. The item with the lowest posttest percentage correct dealt with the possibility that substance use might interfere with one's judgment regarding protection. Even with a small increase, fewer than 75% recognized this as a problematic situation.

The slight decrease in recognizing abstinence as the only 100% safe method is difficult to explain, except that perhaps the use of "100% safe" in the wording of the statement may have led them to consider the question wrong after listening to information on various methods of "safe sex."

Finally, a reduction in the number of "don't know" (?) responses from pretest to posttest further demonstrates the extent of learning that occurred at the GIG. The number reduced by almost half, from 110 at pretest to 60 at posttest. As would be expected, the frequency of the "don't know" responses was inversely related to age, so that the middle school students had the greatest number of "don't know" responses (both at pretest and posttest), the high school students a lower frequency, and the college students only one "don't know" response by posttest. No gender differences were noted in the number of "don't know" responses.

LIMITATIONS

While the findings are promising in terms of the ability of an intensive intervention to effect short-term changes in knowledge and attitudes regarding pregnancy and STI prevention, there is no way to determine if the gains are maintained, since follow-up is not feasible. Moreover, it is assumed that accurate knowledge and favorable attitudes are precursors to changes in risk-taking behavior. There is, however, no way to verify this hypothesis, because longitudinal data are not available, particularly with regard to behavior. Finally, the intervention needs replication in other communities to determine the generalizability, since the sample will always be self-selected.

DISCUSSION

Having examined the data from various perspectives leads one to conclude that the intervention was successful in reaching its objectives with respect to knowledge and attitude change with the great majority of the respondents. It is particularly noteworthy that these knowledge gains occurred in such a short space of time in comparison with most health education intervention programs. Even when the level of knowledge at pretest was high, the intervention effected additional change. Moreover, exposure to the intervention also served to reinforce accurate thinking and counter myths and misinformation.

It is important to note that a significant factor in the intervention's success may be its accommodation to the youth culture. That is, the design of the intervention carefully takes into account factors that will increase receptivity of the content by the youth and an atmosphere that will motivate youth to engage in the educational process. This creative intervention appears to have succeeded exceptionally well in this respect, attracting large numbers of youth from both the immediate community and diverse communities throughout the city. This exemplifies the type of community-based intervention recommended by Ross and Williams (2002): "Diffusion of intervention through existing social networks further extends the intervention into the community and acts to reinforce and maintain changes in peer norms towards safer sexual behavior" (p. 58). The first (and pilot) year the GIG's were conducted, the participants were nearly all students from the two major high schools in the area. Although this is still the case for the majority of the youth, the age range has broadened somewhat, and the participation from youth across the Los Angeles area has increased substantially, representing 55 other schools. The message and content of the interventions appears to be diffusing through a broader youth cohort.

An important contributor to this diffusion process is the use of peer educators who, in addition to providing accurate information, also serve as peer role models who help define peer norms and who, according to Ross and Williams (2002), are more likely to employ an approach that is culturally appropriate. Researchers have repeatedly identified the use of peer educators as one of the characteristics of successful pregnancy and STI prevention programs (Kirby, 2002; Ross & Williams, 2002; Siegel et al., 2001; Coyle et al., 1999).

The intervention also displayed a number of the components identified by Kirby (2002) as characteristic of effective prevention programs. First of all, the various educational activities and the physical environment (e.g., posters) presented "a clear message about sexual activity and condom or contraceptive use and continually reinforced that message" (p. 53). Second, the education at the various booths and the educational materials (e.g., pamphlets and packets) provided to the youth offered accurate information about risks involved in sexual activity and means of protection from both pregnancy and STI's. Third, the intervention employed a great variety of methods to instruct the participants. Most of these methods were interactive, engaging the youth on a one-to-one basis to "personalize the information" (p. 53) in addition to the group level intervention. Fourth, the instructional methods chosen were appropriate for the specific population being served. Fifth, sufficient time was provided for the educational activities to be completed as a 16 hour block of time was devoted to each GIG event. And sixth, peer educators were selected who held strong beliefs regarding the importance of the program and risk reduction in general, and were properly trained and given responsibilities during the event.

Overall, the GIG needs to be viewed as an educational process that continues to reinforce important knowledge and attitudes, rather than a single educational event that will bring about changes in risk-taking behavior. The aim is to help translate knowledge into behavior by reinforcing accurate information, breaking down myths and denial, and establishing a new milieu and youth culture that recognizes risks as undesirable and prevention as a preferable alternative. The analyses of the data clearly demonstrate that the GIG intervention is a very successful vehicle for educating youth regarding pregnancy and STI risks and prevention, capable of achieving the proposed objectives in a relatively short period of time with a very substantial number of youth. Similarly, Jermont et al. (1992) were able to achieve changes in knowledge, attitudes, intent, and risky behavior in a single 5 hour educational AIDS risk reduction intervention. Moreover, the youth were provided with several opportunities for re-education, as four GIGs were offered during the year, and for a segment of the participants, the GIG was just one component of a multi-component pregnancy and STI intervention program in which they participated. Research has identified a diverse, multi-component intervention as having greater likelihood of success (Kirby, 2002; Coyle et al., 1999).

It is important that significant improvement was noted on items dealing with high risk behaviors related to pregnancy (e.g., ineffectiveness of withdrawal) and STIs (multiple sex partners and asymptomatic transmission of HIV/AIDS). Moreover, the message regarding protection appears to have been communicated, as the need to use a condom for every sexual contact was acknowledged by the greatest number of participants. There is some contradiction in the data, however, as a considerably smaller percentage did not recognize the risks of having unprotected sex even one time. This may be the result of considering "the odds," that is, considering the relative risks of a pattern of lack of protection and a single failure. The tendency for adolescents to have a sense of personal invulnerability (described by Elkind, 1967, as "the personal fable") may contribute to this discrepancy.

There is some concern that despite the increases, an average 20 to 25% of the adolescents lack accurate knowledge in some of the areas covered by the measure. Since most items deal with substantial risk factors, this means that one-fifth to one-fourth of the youth are at risk for pregnancy and/or STIs. Additional methods for reinforcing the information need to be devised for inclusion in the intervention. Also of concern is the percentage of participants who do not recognize the added risks for pregnancy and STI posed by substance use, especially given empirical evidence of a positive association between the two (Millstein & Moscicki, 1995). At the same time, it is critical to remember that the intervention was a single educational experience that interspersed education with entertainment in a casual, non-didactic format. The very factors that increase the adolescents' receptivity to the information do not allow for the repeated reinforcement of the information that instruction over a period of time provides. However, even with these limitations, the data demonstrate that the intervention has been extremely successful in helping youth acquire more accurate knowledge regarding sexual behavior, pregnancy, and sexually transmitted infections.

IMPLICATIONS AND RECOMMENDATIONS

The findings demonstrate that a community-based intervention that combines a large scale educational component with individual one-on-one instruction in an intensive experience can effect changes in knowledge and attitudes in a relatively short period of time. Information saturation appears to be important in bringing about change. Because of this, loss of the younger participants earlier in the intervention poses some problems in terms of evaluation. Specifically, if they complete the posttest as they leave, they will have received less of the intervention than the remaining participants. This is particularly problematic since their pretest scores tend to be lower. One possible solution is having them complete the posttest as they leave and having staff indicate the time left on the measure so analyses by amount of exposure to the intervention can be conducted. Incentives would also be needed, such as small prizes upon completing the measure. With regard to the shortened intervention, a simple laminated card with the main messages regarding risks could be provided to assure that the basic content had been covered.

The GIG intervention is quite costly given the need for an appropriate venue, security, a disc jockey, and multiple prizes and incentives for the participants. Inasmuch as Ross and Williams (2002) identify partnering with other community stakeholders, such as local businesses, as factors that contribute to successful community-based interventions, such a partnering could assist with the financial burden of the intervention.

Because the intervention is aimed at ultimately changing peer norms, it is important that at least some of the peer educators be natural peer leaders and that the format of the event reflects the culture of the particular adolescent population.

Because the same youth are likely to attend more than one GIG, the pretest level may begin to climb and make it less likely that change can be achieved in the future. On the other hand, attending multiple GIGs may be the best way to continue to reinforce the content presented in the intervention. The effect of attending multiple GIGs can be easily examined by adding an item to the measure for the students to indicate the number of GIGs attended.

If funding permits, further reinforcement of the content could be achieved by having the students fill out address cards so that periodic mailings reiterating basic information learned at the GIG could be conducted. Surveys of knowledge, attitudes, and behavior could also be mailed as a long term follow-up with some form of concrete incentive for returning the completed measure. The GIG disc jockeys and local radio celebrities could be used to present public service messages regarding risk protection and link the content to both past and future GIG events.

The GIG intervention demonstrates a number of the elements of effective protocols which Kirby (2002) described as "brief, modest interventions" that were "quite encouraging" (p. 57) and in need of further study with rigorous evaluation. To this end, replication studies of this innovative intervention are needed in different communities with diverse adolescent populations to determine if the findings can be generalized beyond the self-selected participants in this community.

In sum, this innovative approach is reaching ever-increasing numbers of youth and provides an environment that appears to increase their receptivity to the educational content and facilitate changes in knowledge and attitude. It is important to note that this is one component in a multiple-intervention program that serves the important function of outreach to the larger adolescent population in the community.

Beyond the specific intervention, the findings have implications for social workers and public health professionals who work with at-risk youth, particularly in pregnancy and STI prevention. The findings suggest that for both school-based and individual (e.g., counseling) interventions, an intensive, single session community outreach component that draws large numbers of youth may serve a significant complementary function, diffusing information and influencing attitudes across a wide youth audience and, thereby, having a greater impact on youth norms. This diffusion effect is multiplied by repeating the intervention several times during the year. The school-based and individual interventions serve a core function, not only by reinforcing specific messages over time, but by providing skill development (e.g., negotiation, refusal, and communication skills) that is not possible in the larger scale venue. On the other hand, an intervention such as the GIG may allow for more generalization to social and interpersonal situations, because dealing with such issues has been normalized in a social milieu.

The research literature indicates that the ultimate aim of prevention programs is to foster the development of youth norms that view risk reduction and pregnancy and STI prevention as desirable and self-generated expectations. To increase the likelihood of achieving these outcomes, social workers and health care professionals need to include youth leaders in the design of interventions. Inasmuch as youth culture is very mercurial, the atmosphere of the event and the specific intervention activities need to be assessed regularly by the youth to assure their congruence with the culture of the present youth cohort. This is critical not only for attracting sufficient youth from the community to the event, but to engage them sufficiently in order to bring about change in a short period of time. If peer norms are to be affected, the youth need to feel that the experience speaks to their age and cultural cohort. This places a dual responsibility on the social worker or health care professional: (1) to find and train natural youth leaders to become an integrated part of the intervention, and (2) to learn to be open to feedback from these youth regarding the design and implementation of the intervention.

Finally, given the state of the present research literature, it is important that professionals who implement intervention programs include a methodologically sound evaluation component that is longitudinal or offers replication. This is crucial not only for their own accountability with regard to the outcomes of their intervention efforts, but to contribute to determining best practices and best practice models to guide the design of future intervention programs.

NOTE

1. GIG is a colloquialism meaning an event, usually involving live music. Musicians often refer to a job at such an event as a "gig."

REFERENCES

Aarons, S.J., Jenkins, R.R., Raine, T.A., El-Khorazaty, M.N., Woodward, K.M., Williams, R.L., Clark, M.C., and Wingrove, B.K. (2000). Postponing Sexual Intercourse Among Urban Junior High School Students–A randomized controlled evaluation. *Journal of Adolescent Health*, 27, pp. 236-247.

Alan Guttmacher Institute. (1999a). Teenage pregnancy overall trends and state-by-state information, pp. 1-10.

Alan Guttmacher Institute. (1999b). U.S. teenage pregnancy statistics: With comparative statistics for Women Aged 20-24, pp. 1-14.

Brindis, C. (2002). Office of Family Planning Audio Conference: Teenage Pregnancy Prevention Programs Evaluation Results and Next Steps, October 10, 2002.

Centers for Disease Control and Prevention. (2000). Adolescent Health Chartbook. *Health, United States, 2000.* DHHS publication No. (PHS) 2000-1232-1.

Centers for Disease Control and Prevention. (2002). HIV/AIDS among Hispanics in the United States, http://www.cdc.gov/hiv/pubs/facts/hispanic/htm, pp. 1-3.

Centers for Disease Control and Prevention. (2002). Young People at Risk: HIV/AIDS among America's Youth, http://www.cdc.gov/hiv/pub/facts/youth.htm, pp. 1-4.

Centers for Disease Control and Prevention. (2002). Trends in sexual risk behaviors among high school students–United States, 1991-2001. *MMWR Weekly*, 51(38), pp. 856-859.

Centers for Disease Control and Prevention. (2000). Youth Risk Behavior Surveillance–United States, 1999. *CDC Surveillance Summaries, June 9, 2000. MMWR 2000*, Vol. 49 (No. SS-5).

Coyle, K., Basen-Engquist, K., Kirby, D., Parcel, G., Banspach, S., Harrist, R., Baumler, E., and Weil, M. (1999). Short-term impact of Safer Choices: A multicomponent, school-based HIV, other STD, and pregnancy prevention program. *Journal of School Health*, 15, pp. 181-188.

Coyle, K., Basen-Engquist, K., Kirby, D., Banspach, S., Collins, J., Baumler, E., Carvajal, S., and Harrist, R. (2001). *Safer Choices: Reducing teen pregnancy, HIV and STD's*. Public Health Reports, 2001 Supplement, Vol. 114, pp. 82-93.

DiCenso, A., Guyatt, G., and Griffith, A.W.L. (2002). Interventions to reduce unintended pregnancies among adolescents: Systematic review of randomized controlled trials. *British Medical Journal*, 324:1426.

Driscoll, A.K., Biggs, M. A., Brindis, C.D., and Yankah, E. (2001). Adolescent Latino reproductive health: A review of the literature. *Hispanic Journal of the Behavioral Sciences*, 23(3), pp. 255-326.

Elkind, D. (1967). Egocentrism in Adolescence. *Child Development*, 38(4), pp. 1025-1034.

Hubbard, B.M., Giese, M.L., and Rainey, J. (1998). A replication of Reducing the Risk, a theory-based sexuality curriculum for adolescents. *Journal of School Health*, 68, pp. 243-247.

Howard, M. (1992). Delaying the start of intercourse among adolescents. In S.M. Coupey and L.V. Klerman (Eds.), *Adolescent Medicine: State of the art reviews.* Philadelphia: Hanley & Belfus, pp. 181-193.

Howard, M. and McCabe, J.B. (1990). Helping teenagers postpone sexual involvement. *Family Planning Perspectives*, 22, pp. 21-26.

Jermmott, J., Jermott, L.S., and Fong, G.T. (1992). Reductions in HIV risk-associated sexual behaviors among Black male adolescents: Effects of an AIDS prevention intervention. *American Journal of Public Health*, 82(3), pp. 372-377.

Kim, N., Stanton, B., Dickersin, K. and Galbraith, J. (1997). Effectiveness of the 40 adolescent AIDS-risk reduction interventions: A quantitative review. *Journal of Adolescent Health*, 20, pp. 204-215.

Kirby, D., Korpi, M. Barth, R., and Cagampang, H. (1995). Evaluation of education now and babies later (ENABL): Final Report. Berkeley, CA: University of California, School of Social Welfare, Family Welfare Research Group, 1995.

Kirby, D., (2002). Effective approaches to reducing adolescent unprotected sex, pregnancy, and childbearing. *Journal of Sex Research*, 39, pp. 51-57.

Levy, S., Perhats, C., Weeks, K., Handler, A. Zhu, C. and Flay, B.R. (1995). Impact of a school-based AIDS prevention program on risk and protective behavior for newly sexually active students. *Journal of School Health*, 65(4), pp. 145-151.

Millstein, S.G. and Moscicki, A-B. (1995). Sexually transmitted disease in female adolescents: Effects of psychosocial factors and high risk behaviors. *Journal of Adolescent Health*, 17, pp. 83-90.

O'Donnell, L., Stueve, A., Doval, A.S., Duran, R., Haber, D., Atnafou, R., Johnson, N., Grant, U., Murray, H., Juhn, G., and Piessens, P. (1999). The effectiveness of the Reach for Health community youth service learning program in reducing early and unprotected sex among urban middle school students. *American Journal of Public Health*, 89(2), pp. 176-181.

Ross, M.W. and Williams, M.L. (2002). Effective targeted and community HIV/STD prevention programs. *Journal of Sex Research*, 39, pp. 58-62.

Siegel, D.M., Aten, M. and Enaharo, M. (2001). Long-term Effects of a middle school- and high school-based human immunodeficiency virus sexual risk prevention intervention. *Journal of the American Medical Association*, 155(10), pp. 1117-1126.

Thomas, M.H. (2002). Abstinence-based programs for prevention of adolescent pregnancies: A review. *Journal of Adolescent Health*, 26, pp. 5-17.

United Way of Greater Los Angeles. (1998-1999). State of the County Report, 1998-1999.

U.S. Census Bureau, Census 2000, Table DP-1. Profile of General Demographics Characteristics of the United States: 2000.

Index

